Community Health Nursing

Community
Health
Nursing

Fourth Edition

Kathleen M. Leahy, M.S., R.N.
Late Professor Emeritus of Nursing
University of Washington, Seattle

M. Marguerite Cobb, M.N., R.N.
Associate Professor of Nursing
University of Washington, Seattle

Mary C. Jones, M.S., R.N.
Assistant Professor of Nursing
University of Washington, Seattle

McGraw-Hill Book Company

New York St. Louis San Francisco Auckland Bogotá Hamburg
Johannesburg London Madrid Mexico Montreal New Delhi
Panama Paris São Paulo Singapore Sydney Tokyo Toronto

This book was set in Times Roman by Jay's Publishers Services, Inc.
The editors were David P. Carroll, Mark W. Cowell, and David Dunham;
the production supervisor was Diane Renda.
The photo editor was Inge King.
New drawings were done by Jay's Publishers Services, Inc.
The cover was designed by Murray Fleminger.
R. R. Donnelley & Sons Company was printer and binder.

COMMUNITY HEALTH NURSING

1 2 3 4 5 6 7 8 9 0   DODO   8 9 8 7 6 5 4 3 2

ISBN 0-07-036834-1

Library of Congress Cataloging in Publication Data

Leahy, Kathleen M.
    Community health nursing.

    Includes bibliographies and index.
    1. Community health nursing.   I. Cobb,
M. Marguerite.   II. Jones, Mary C.   III. Title.
RT98.L4   1982   610.73'43   81-18636
ISBN 0-07-036834-1   AACR2

Chapter opening photo credits:

1 Visiting Nurse Service of New York
2 Ron Engh/Photo Researchers, Inc.
3 Erika Stone/Peter Arnold, Inc.
4 © Ellis Herwig, 1980/Stock, Boston, Inc.
5 Paul S. Conklin/Monkmeyer Press Photo Service
6 Visiting Nurse Service of New York
7 Ken Karp
8 © Guy Gillette/Photo Researchers, Inc.
9 Visiting Nurse Service of New York
10 Ken Karp
11 © Timothy Eagan/Woodfin Camp & Assoc.

In appreciation of past, present,
and future nursing students who,
by their questions, reactions,
critical appraisals, challenging
experiences, "stretch" the wisdom
of teachers beyond the mundane.

Contents

PART TWO

Preface

This is a consumer-oriented book. Its basic premise supports the inclusion of the client as a partner in managing his or her health care. To make full use of the client as a partner necessitates determining the client's learning ability; openly discussing differences in beliefs, values, attitudes; teaching essential health information which will facilitate informed decisions; supporting action beneficial for the client; and mutually rejoicing over outcomes attained. Nurses in partnership with clients are health care providers who share their expertise for the purpose of improved health status of clients. The satisfaction in working *with* clients, even when they are initially frustrating, is understood once it is experienced.

Senior nursing students are well prepared to enter the community and practice community health nursing. They have all the knowledge and skills required. All they have to do is to synthesize what they have learned in all fields of nursing, adjust and individualize this learning to fit the needs of each client situation, be willing to modify or change strategies or plans when progress is not evident, and objectively analyze factors contributing to growth and desired outcomes. The community is filled with interesting, unique people, each one a potential challenge. Herein lies the fascination of community health nursing! As mentioned in an earlier edition of this book, entering the field of community health nursing is not easy. It requires an assimilation of many ideas and activities which do not initially make sense to the beginning student. Looking at one's own behavior in addition to the client's and family's behavior can be extremely discomforting and sometimes traumatic at first. Coming into a community which we find familiar in some ways because we too grew up in a community, and which we find strange and complex in other ways because people live and interact so differently and incomprehensibly, requires adaptation and flexibility. Making the transition both physically and intellectually from an institutional setting to an amorphouslike community in which people appear, behave, talk, and act normally is distinctly startling and sometimes perplexing for the student starting out in the role of nurse. Learning to reach out, to initiate, to risk, to consent to new patterns of behavior takes courage, conviction, and determination. However, for those students who are willing to try, to experiment, to accept, the rewards are there—waiting to be discovered and treasured.

For teachers who elect to use this book as a text, it is not meant to be all-inclusive of the field of community health nursing. Many ideas are introduced that, dependent upon the discretion of the teacher, can be expanded upon in depth by lectures, audiovisual media, experiential assignments, library study, additional references, independent study, and current professional literature, not only in nursing and in public health sciences, but in supporting disciplines, such as sociology, psychology, cultural anthropology, and the humanities. The contents of the book are directed mainly to nursing students entering a community, opening their eyes to concepts and facets that exist, suggesting ways to ease entry, alerting them to phenomena for which to be watchful. The book is meant to be used as one of the tools of the teacher for preparing nursing students to perform community health nursing as it should be practiced.

We wish to express our appreciation to Kathleen Walsh Esper, Wayne State University, for her careful editing and suggested additions to Chapters 4, 5, and 6. Receiving validation that the content of the book is useful for nursing students in other parts of the United States is rewarding.

We are grateful for the chapter written by Carrie E. Hall. Her expertise and practical knowledge in the field of epidemiology contributed to the updating of Chapter 10; she added inestimably to the usefulness of the book.

Again, we are grateful for the written contributions of former nursing students, who, by sharing their feelings and experiences with their nurse instructors, added the extra dimension of humanistic appeal to the book.

M. Marguerite Cobb
Mary C. Jones

Part One

Chapter 1

Stepping into
the Community

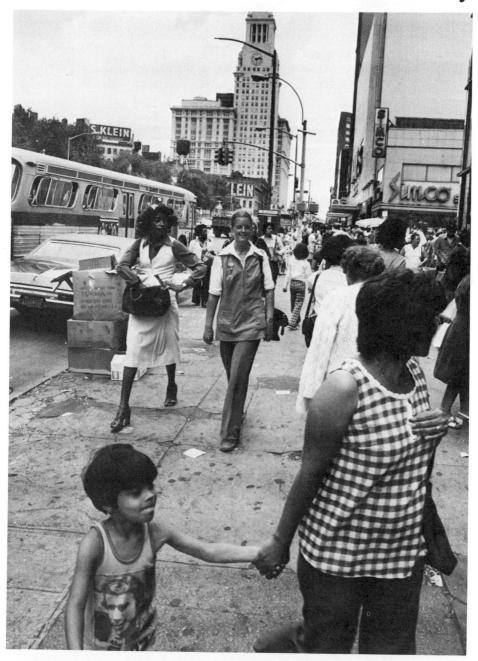

COMMUNITY HEALTH

The promotion and improvement of humankind's total health has a significant bearing on the social revolution now in progress throughout the world (see *The Family of Man*). New thinking and approaches to better health care become mandatory in solving such long-term problems as lack of compliance to primary prevention problems, sanitation, insufficient food and clothing, inadequate housing, and control of communicable diseases and such noncommunicable disease conditions as heart disease, accidents, or disaster. Emerging problems of family pathology, drug abuse and addiction, air and water pollution, polarization of the races, and overpopulation require new methods of solution. Increased scientific knowledge and more imaginative skills and techniques in teaching health care are in order for all community health work.

Community health or public health as a profession had its beginnings about a hundred years ago. Its early responsibility was the control of communicable disease, which was attempted by such measures as control of environment, better sanitation, and strict isolation procedures, particularly for typhoid fever and tuberculosis. As laboratory techniques were developed from increased knowledge of microbiology, earlier diagnoses became possible and medical care became more effective. Other control measures also were developed, such as immunization and the provision of safe water supplies and waste disposal.

Gradually the six basic functions of public health evolved—communicable disease control, environmental sanitation, laboratory services, vital statistics, maternal and child health care, and health education. Public health agencies began to base their programs on these six functions, the emphasis being on people. To carry out these functions effectively school and industrial health programs were developed, since large segments of the population could be reached in this way.

Community health programs built on the six basic functions, including school and industrial health programs, continue to be important, but nearly every nation is experiencing new health hazards that demand fresh approaches to their solutions. Problems stemming from the population explosion include environmental problems of overcrowding, air and water pollution, nuclear hazards, accidents, drug abuse, alcoholism, and child abuse. Current pollution of the environment affects not only human beings and domestic animals but also fish and wildlife in many parts of the world. This presents a pressing need for concerted community action as well as action on an international basis. Finally, there is the urgent need of many people for more care from the medical and paramedical professions—care that is better organized and equally available to all segments of society.

The significant social legislation passed by Congress during the 1960s and 1970s provided for increased health services and their funding. Examples of this legislation of interest to health workers include:

1   Heart Disease, Cancer, and Stroke Amendments of 1965 (P.L. 89-239)
2   Health Professions Education Assistance Amendment of 1965 (P.L. 89-290)
3   The Social Security Amendments Act of 1965 (P.L. 89-97)
4   The Housing and Urban Development Act of 1965 (P.L. 89-117)

5 The Comprehensive Health Planning and Public Health Services Amendments of 1966 (P.L. 89-749) and 1967 (P.L. 90-174)
6 The Health Planning and Resources Development Act of 1974 (P.L. 93-641)

Public health appears to be shifting its emphasis to both consumer and environment, accentuating the relationship of the total person to his or her total environment. Underlying this ecologic approach to public health is the vast amount of knowledge that has been accumulated within the past 50 years in the biologic, physical, and social sciences that must be adapted and utilized by the several professions, e.g., medicine, nursing, dentistry, and engineering, in the public health field. The field of public and community health becomes "the meeting ground of all areas of knowledge and professional activity relevant to the health of the public."[1]

COMMUNITY HEALTH NURSING

A description or definition of community health nursing should be based on an understanding and appreciation of the entire spectrum of nursing. Virginia Henderson considers the function of the present-day nurse to be unique. It is, she writes, "to assist the individual, sick or well, in the performance of those activities contributing to health or its recovery (or to peaceful death) that he would perform if he had the necessary strength, will or knowledge. And to do this in such a way as to help him gain independence as rapidly as possible."[2]

Primary prevention health teaching and counseling and the skilled care of the sick in their homes and other noninstitutionalized centers, by community health nurses from official or voluntary health agencies, is recognized as an essential service in the community's total health program. The nurse functions within the framework of both the nursing and the public health professions, utilizing knowledge of the content and methods of both professions in service to the individual, the client, the family, groups, and the community. There are many definitions of community health nursing, but the most comprehensive definition was established in 1973 by the American Nurses' Association:

Community Health Nursing is a synthesis of nursing practice and public health practice applied to promoting and preserving the health of populations. The nature of this practice is general and comprehensive. It is not limited to a particular age or diagnostic group. It is continuing, not episodic. The dominant responsibility is to the population as a whole. Therefore, nursing directed to individuals, families, or groups contributes to the health of the total population. Health promotion, health maintenance, health education, coordination and continuity of care are utilized in a holistic approach to the family, group, and community. The nurse's

[1] Hiliary G. Fry, in collaboration with William P. Shepard and Ray H. Elling, *Education for Manpower and Community Health,* The University of Pittsburgh Press, Pittsburgh, 1967, p. 8.
[2] Virginia Henderson, "The Nature of Nursing," *The American Journal of Nursing,* 64: 64–68, August 1964.

actions acknowledge the need for comprehensive health planning, recognize the influences of social and ecological issues, give attention to populations at risk and utilize the dynamic forces which influence change.[3]

Standards for community health nursing focus on the practice rather than the practitioner and are stated in a systematic approach to nursing practice in areas of assessment, planning, implementation, and evaluation. Based on the above definition, eight standards of community health nursing practice were stated to be:

    1 The collection of data about the health status of the consumer is systematic and continuous. The data are accessible, communicated, and recorded.

    2 Nursing diagnoses are derived from health status data.

    3 Plans for nursing service include goals derived from nursing diagnoses.

    4 Plans for nursing service include priorities and nursing approaches or measures to achieve the goals derived from nursing diagnoses.

    5 Nursing actions provide for consumer participation in health promotion, maintenance, and restoration.

    6 Nursing actions assist consumers to maximize health potential.

    7 The consumer's progress toward goal achievement is determined by the consumer and the nurse.

    8 Nursing actions involve ongoing reassessment, reordering of priorities, new goal setting, and revision of the nursing plan.[4]

Philosophy of Community Health Nursing

From the above definition, the philosophy of community health nursing, like that of all nursing, has always been based on the concept of the "worth and dignity of the individual." A hundred years ago, Octavia Hill, a social worker active in slum housing reform, expressed the same idea:

> It is essential to remember that each man has his own view of his life, and must be free to fulfill it; that in many ways he is a far better judge of it than we, as he has lived through and felt what we have only seen. Our work is rather to bring him to the point of considering, and to the spirit of judging rightly, than to consider or judge for him.[5]

Basic to the belief of all nurses is the acceptance that all persons have the capacity and the potential to develop better physical health and improve psychosocial well-being, dependent upon their desires, willingness to change, and adaptability to prescribed therapies. Nursing practice assists individuals and families in adjusting their health needs and wants, resolving health problems in the social, emotional, and physical environments, and facilitating coping abilities to achieve higher levels of wellness.

[3] Executive Committee and the Standards Committee of the Division on Community Health Nursing Practice. American Nurses Association, Kansas City, Mo., 1973.

[4] Ibid.

[5] Octavia Hill, "Through the Ages," *Family Welfare Association of America,* New York, n.d., p. 42.

Family health counseling and primary health care services appropriate to family and community health nursing practice assist individuals and groups to select, participate in, and evaluate health-related activities. Collaborative liaison actions and appropriate referral to other professionals to maximize client utilization of health care services for optimum health underlie all the community health process. As a social activist and consumer advocate, the nurse influences legislation and the legislative process to promote positive individual and collective health.

Each community health nurse develops a personal philosophy of nursing, tempered by background, preparation, experience, and personality. The nurse's philosophy will grow and deepen as experience in working with others is acquired—clients, families, communities, and coworkers—and as understanding is gained through continuous study, reading, and thinking. It has been said that "the community health nurse has lots to learn, to teach and to do."

The philosophy that community health nursing is based on "the worth and dignity of the individual" is identified closely with the age-old purpose of nursing, which Marion Sheehan so ably stated to be " . . .caring for, giving comfort and ease, helping persons with health problems to become healed in body and mind or helping them to live with their infirmities with grace."[6] The nurse who can successfully teach others to "live with their infirmities with grace" has that same ability and has achieved a philosophy in accord with that of community health nursing.

Roles and Functions

The community health nurse encounters problems and conditions never imagined by her or his predecessors. In addition to conditions previously mentioned, the nurse meets such situations as poverty amid affluence, urban sprawl and decay, social injustices, racial strife and tensions, and, in many areas, a decline in the quality and integrity of community life and efforts to improve it. Facing these situations requires marked objectivity on the part of the nursing and public health professions, coupled with the realization that specific knowledge and skills are essential in contributing to the solution.

The family is usually the unit of service for the nurse; therefore the major part of community health nursing is carried on in the home where health care is needed for clients of all ages. In many communities there is an increasing demand for skilled geriatric nursing, largely for the following reasons:

1 The increasing number of elderly people in the population, with many living alone rather than as part of a family group, as in former generations.

2 The growing incidence of chronic diseases usually found in older age groups, e.g., cancer and cardiovascular conditions.

3 The emphasis as placed today by the medical and nursing professions on commencing rehabilitation of the client at the onset of the disease or disabling condition or as early as possible.

[6]Marion W. Sheehan, "This I Believe about Nursing," *Nursing Outlook,* 11:641, September 1963.

In contact with the client and family, the nurse needs to develop opportunities and plans for teaching health concepts and practices to all members involved. Many parents need help in understanding and appreciating the growth and development—physical, mental, and emotional—of their children at differing age levels, including infancy, preschool, school age, adolescence, and early maturity. Parents sometimes need assistance in guiding their children not only to learn to accept the demands of living within their own group but also to learn to understand, respect, accept, live, and work with people of other races, cultures, mores, religions, and backgrounds.

When entering the home, the nurse is responsible for teaching the client, or the family member, or other person available for the client's daily care. This requires a sound knowledge of underlying principles of the physical, biologic, and social sciences, as well as the ability to teach, demonstrate, and use nursing skills, such as the application of sterile dressings to an open, draining wound to minimize the spread of infection and to teach the safe disposal of dressings that have been saturated with drainage. Although a comparatively simple procedure, it requires, if done safely, that the nurse have a knowledge of microbiology, anatomy and physiology, sanitation, and psychology, as well as a deft, sure nursing skill.

The nurse is concerned with the health of the entire family, including those in clinics, schools, industrial plants, and other places of work, as well as those in the home being visited. The nurse must be aware of extraneous community health hazards, such as poor housing conditions, insufficient and unsafe water supply and waste-disposal facilities, faulty fire protection, and traffic safety. The nurse must be cognizant of possible sources of disease in the community and the routes of spread and methods of their control.

A dimension added to community health nursing is the mental and emotional health services and their integration into the other services the nurse can offer in the home, the school, and places of employment. This integration has been triggered by a wider knowledge and awareness of behavioral sciences, and developing recognition by communities of their responsibilities toward their emotionally disturbed citizens, and a growing understanding of the value of the nurse-client and nurse-family relationships. Possibly, by the end of the twentieth century these and other services will have made an impact on the health aspects of people and communities similar to those results brought about by the control of diphtheria, smallpox, poliomyelitis, and insect-borne diseases in the past century. These changing social and health patterns have been the impetus for new and experimental programs and activities in community health services, including nursing.

The need is growing for more nursing services that will provide care and health supervision to clients of all ages and social and economic backgrounds. Nurses are expanding their skills in areas of physical assessment in order that a more complete and definitive nursing diagnosis can be made. There is some increase in nursing services through the provisions for nursing care and supervision in the various health insurance plans, both private and governmental, and programs for continuity of medical and nursing care between hospital and home in urban and rural areas. This increase in service to clients and families widens opportunities for teaching principles and practice of positive health as well as for nursing care of the ill. Group teaching is increasing wherever the nurse can bring like-interest groups together for such classes as prenatal care, child care, nutrition, health or wellness, and home nursing. The nurse should be on the alert for opportunities to develop such classes in housing projects, health centers, or clinics.

Primary Care

Many definitions of primary care are noted in the literature. An encompassing definition is the first or initial contact that the individual or family have with a health provider. It is continuous over time to the client in various states of health and illness. The health care provider may be a community health nurse, physician, nurse practitioner, or other type of health personnel that the client seeks for initial help. Actually the underlying concepts are not new to community health nurses as the community setting provided the basis for the model of primary care.

The community health nurse as a primary care provider assesses the situation and gives appropriate intervention, whether bedside, health promotion, or health maintenance. In the event the problem or concern indicates additional resources, the nurse determines the most appropriate available provider and makes a referral to that person or agency. Because of the long-term personal relationship with individual or family, the nurse is able to relate the full scope of health problems to the provider. The nurse follows up on the referral, coordinating the care of planning, establishing priorities, intervention and evaluation with the client, resuming responsibility for primary care.

Expanded Role

The concept of the *expanded role* for nursing had its beginning in 1964 when Dr. Loretta C. Ford (R.N.) and Dr. Henry K. Silver (M.D.) had a demonstration project for community health nurses. Since that time, there has been a proliferation of training and educational programs for family nurse practitioners and for the specialty areas of pediatric nurse practitioners, school nurse practitioners, gerontology, family planning, and diagnostic-disease specialties, to name a few.

The extended or expanded role was based on the premise that more care could be given at a lower cost and that more consumers could be served, especially in the crowded inner cities and rural communities. The Early Periodic Screening Development Test (EPSDT) for ages birth to 21 years required more labor to carry out the legislated program, as did the women, infant, children (WIC) program. This necessitated the nurse to acquire skills of physical assessment. Preparation of the nurses took place in a variety of ways from an apprenticeship with a physician, short-term courses, and continuing education to formal academic programs.

The utilization of the nurse in the expanded role as a major provider of health care and primary health care is gaining sanction. Nurses practicing in the expanded role are found in institutional and noninstitutional settings, i.e., ambulatory care, clinics, health departments, and individual practice in urban and rural settings.

Because nurse practitioners are able to function with relative independence in clinical settings under the general direction of physicians or a board of health, they are of particular value to health departments. The increasing trend for health departments to become more active in direct health care continues, utilizing the skills of nurses in giving direct health service to people. The expanded functions include some medical diagnosis and treatment which needs more study. The most important fact is that the role remain with nursing for role identity, as too many nurses look at their self-image aligned with medicine rather than with nursing. The reliability of the expanded role is dependent upon the availability of qualified personnel and physician and consumer acceptance. Nursing practice acts have been revised in some states to give special licensure for those nurses meeting the stated qualifications.

Family Nurse Practitioner

The family nurse practitioner, sometimes known as a family nurse clinician or family community nurse practitioner, is given to those community nurses who have had additional educational preparation. The majority of schools preparing nurse practitioners vary in length from 1 to 2 years and usually award a master's degree. The curriculum provides expanded knowledge, assessment skills, and therapeutic nursing intervention in providing primary, acute, and chronic or long-term care in ambulatory-care settings. In addition, health 'promotion, prevention, health counseling, and maintenance of health care are integral components of the curriculum. Systems analysis to maximize social action, capacities within leadership roles, and research are usually identified. Upon completion of an educational program, the nurse is considered a specialist-generalist as in-depth study is given to normal and abnormal findings in the life cycle. The family nurse practitioner has competencies in the ability to:

    1 Assess the past and present physical and psychosocial health status of children and adults
    2 Provide health promotion and education, care and referral for acute uncomplicated illness or management of stable conditions with medical collaboration for clients
    3 Provide family health counseling for health maintenance, family planning, child rearing, well-child development, and family relations
    4 Serve in leadership roles in community health services or education settings
    5 Conduct and use research to extend nursing theory and practice to improve the quality of health care and nursing services[7]

    The family nurse practitioner manages the care of upper respiratory infections, urinary tract infections, gastric upsets, gynecological problems, hypertension, diabetes, chronic congestive heart failure, obesity, osteoarthritis, and anxiety or crisis situations in the home.
    Family nurse practitioners are found in diverse settings in urban and rural communities. Practice may be in ambulatory clinics in or out of hospitals sponsored by public or private sectors; practice may be with a physician, or independent in an isolated area through collaboration with a physician. The family nurse practitioner is aware of the limits of practice and works closely and interdependently with all health professionals in order to provide the best possible health care to the people served. Acceptance by

---

[7]*Family Community Health Nurse Practitioner Program,* University of Washington, Seattle, 1975.

consumers, community, physicians, and other nurses is growing. Some hospitals where nurses and physicians collaborate are granting hospital privileges to family nurse practitioners.

Research has increased in the past few years giving evidence of positive results in utilizing nurse practitioners to improve the delivery of health care services in primary, acute, and chronic or long-term care. Studies in the areas of role, function, setting, preparation, strategies for care, and client outcome need to continue to further delineate the knowledge base for clinical practice. Like nurses in the expanded role, special licensure is given by state boards of professional licensure to those family nurse practitioners who meet the requirements imposed by the state in which the nurse practices.

The American Nurses Association provides a voluntary certification for Family Nurse Practitioners, as well as other specialties. Upon successfully completing the certification process, a certificate is awarded demonstrating excellence in the specific area of practice. Currently, the certificate is valid for 5 years. For continued certification after 5 years as a nurse practitioner, the nurse reapplies to the American Nurses Association to fulfill the process.

Pediatric Nurse Practitioner

The pediatric nurse practitioners working in community health serve infants, preschool, school, and adolescent populations. They function in clinics, mobile health units, schools, and home to provide assessment of normal growth and development and follow-through care for clients who are at high risk. Often the pediatric nurse practitioner participates in screening programs and conducts routine examinations for school, camp, and athletics. They provide formal and informal health education to individuals, family, and groups in the areas of growth and development, nutrition, child management, and usual childhood illnesses.

Preparation for role of pediatric nurse practitioner requires education beyond basic preparation. Schools of nursing in colleges and universities provide course of study through continuing education or masters degree programs. These programs vary in length generally from 6 months to 1 year. Certification for pediatric nurse practitioner is similar to the family nurse practitioner through the American Nurses Association or through the National Association of Pediatric Nurse Associates and Practitioners.

School Nursing

The scope of the nurse's activities in the school setting is changing. In 1902, Lillian Wald, the founder of the Henry Street Visiting Nursing Service in New York City, and at that time its director, convinced the city health department of the value of health services for the school child to give first aid and to implement the control of communicable diseases, especially such diseases as scabies, impetigo, scarlet fever, and diphtheria. The immediate success of the program was evident, and schools in other communities soon adopted it. Specialized school nursing continues to function in urban areas, but in some urban and most rural areas, it has become part of the program of county health departments.

The school nurse is a member of the professional educational team employed to aid children in developing their full potential in health and education. Objectives for the school health program are formulated within the philosophy of the school. The nurse organizes and carries out activities according to the standards, policies, and procedures of the specific school. Responsibilities include assessment of the health status of the pupils and school personnel, including health appraisals and screening tests. An important component of the role is the counseling of students, staff, and parents concerning identified needs and being an advocate and liaison between school personnel, medicine, and other disciplines concerned with health care and providing information to or referring the family to appropriate community resources. The nurse provides guidance and health instruction in informal and formal settings, such as in the nurse's office and in the classroom. As a member of the school staff, the nurse is cognizant of and participates in the maintenance of a healthful environment.

An important function is the implementation of emergency care for conditions occurring in the school. Some of the high-risk areas where injuries take place are physical education, industrial arts, and home economics. The nurse identifies students and personnel who are known to have high potential of the need for emergency care in such conditions as diabetes, convulsive disorders, drug or beesting allergies, bleeders, etc.

Record keeping, like in every area of nursing, from kindergarten through grade twelve, is essential. The health history, screening tests, immunizations, illnesses (physical and emotional), referrals to and from health personnel or agencies, conferences, treatments, and home visits should be recorded. The health record generally becomes a part of the student's academic record. Confidentiality must be adhered to at all times.

Home visits are made according to the school policies. Evaluation of the school health program demonstrates the effectiveness of the program and the performance of the nurse. The nurse conducts and/or participates in research of school nursing activities, methods, procedures, and accomplishments for the purpose of changing or upgrading standards.

Certification of school nurses by the state board of education is required by some states and seems to be a growing trend. Since school health programs differ in the 50 states, readers should explore programs and requirements in their own states. There is a potentially high rate of utilization for nurses in the expanded role or nurse practitioners in schools for health education, health screening, and basic diagnosis and treatment.

Occupational Health Nursing

This specialization as a field of community health nursing began in 1895 with the employment of the first occupational nurse by the Vermont Marble Works for the care of its employees. The expansion of the field of occupational health nursing services has since spread to many occupational settings including department stores, post offices, factories, industrial plants, hospitals, etc.

With the passage of the Occupational Safety and Health Act of 1970 by the United States Congress, interest in the health and welfare of working women and men was accelerated. The purpose of the act was "to assure so far as possible every working man and women in the nation safe and healthful working conditions and to preserve our human resources." Early provisions of the act included concern for

1 Control of worksite health hazards in the working environment
2 A mandatory reporting system
3 Enforcement of safety procedures
4 Standards for medical services, research, and training in the prevention and treatment of occupational diseases and injuries

The National Institute for Occupational Safety and Health (NIOSH) which is part of the Department of Health and Human Services was the federal agency designated to:

1 Investigate causes of workplace illness and accidents and determine if a substance, practice, or condition is a present or potential hazard. This includes on-the-spot evaluations as well as long-term follow-up.
2 Perform research and develop criteria documents that recommend exposure limits to hazardous chemicals, physical agents, and processes.
3 Test and certify personal protective equipment.
4 Provide for education of personnel responsible for occupational health and safety.
5 Develop sampling and measurement methods to evaluate workplace hazards.[8]

The Occupational Safety and Health Administration (OSHA) which is part of the Department of Labor was established as a regulatory agency to:

1 Inspect workplaces for violations of existing health and safety standards. Enforce standards by assessing fines or by other legal means.
2 Review criteria documents, hold hearings, and set new or revised standards for control of specific substances, conditions, or use of equipment.
3 Set and enforce requirements for use of personal protective devices.
4 Provide for consultative services for management and employer and employee training and education.

Working Adults The physical, social, and economic environments in which people live, grow up, and work also affect their health, susceptibility to illness, and the chances of responding to an insufferable milieu by pursuing unwholesome patterns of behavior.[9] Occupational health nurses in business and industrial settings and employee health nurses in hospitals broaden their general basic preparation in nursing with courses in industrial hygiene and safety, toxicology, industrial processes, and similar courses. These nurses learn how to assess quality of working conditions such as temperature, light, space, noise, toxicity of substances used, pollution, and confinement of work spaces. By knowing how to identify potentially risky work areas, they are able to

---

[8] "A Worker's Guide to NIOSH," U.S. Department of Health, Education, and Welfare, NIOSH Publication No. 78-171.
[9] Evelyn E. Meyer and Peter Sainsbury, *Promoting Health in the Human Environment,* World Health Organization, Geneva, 1975, p. 23.

contribute their expertise as members of industrial hygiene and safety teams toward creating safer and healthier work environments. The average adult worker accepts risks and hazards in the work environment and/or believes that work environments have been made safe. Rarely do workers assume their rights as outlined by the Occupational Safety and Health Act as follows:

1 The right to request information from employers on safety and health hazards in their work area

2 The right to ask for an inspection of the workplace by NIOSH or OSHA to see if safety or health hazards exist

3 The right to remain anonymous in this request

4 The right to protection from being fired or punished in any way for exercising these rights under the act

5 The right to have an employee representative accompany inspectors on plant safety and health inspections

6 The right to know the results of an inspection report

7 The right to appeal certain OSHA findings or orders

8 The right to become part of certain legal proceedings in which an employer appeals OSHA findings or orders

9 The right to obtain a copy of OSHA standards and other rules, regulations, and requirements

10 The right to a safe and healthful workplace[10]

Increasing publicity and attention has been focused on occupational safety and health factors considered beneficial and/or detrimental to the good of the working adult and American citizen. Recurring crises of diverse natures have been publicized nationally and received reactions of increasing consumer concern, i.e., chemical wastes dumped into waterways, nuclear accidents, fire hazards, etc. Knowing that the free enterprise system exists on profits causes an individual to wonder if social or economic "benefits" outweigh production risks that imperil workers or the community.[11] The goal of preventing or eliminating risks in occupational health in today's society is a complex problem involving many facets of the economic, social, behavioral, political, and cultural environment. The actual complexity of the problem combined with the urgency for instituting essential changes in the working environment constitutes an exciting basis for becoming involved in the field of occupational health nursing.

The Nursing Role in Occupational Health Every occupational health nurse accepts responsibility for functioning professionally as defined by the professional nursing organizations, i.e., American Association of Occupational Health Nurses, and the American Nurses Association. These responsibilities include implementation of

---

[10] "A Worker's Guide to NIOSH," op. cit.

[11] Erik P. Eckholm, *The Picture of Health*, W. W. Norton & Company, Inc., New York, 1977, p. 218.

nursing practice based on professionally based standards, utilization of the nursing process in the care of employees, maintenance of record systems in compliance with existing legal, medical, and governmental regulations. To be more specific, occupational health nurses must demonstrate expertise in taking occupational histories, doing physical assessments of essentially normal adults, giving emergent care and referring on to appropriate specialized medical services, doing special techniques such as audiometry and spirometry, promoting and teaching health practices and lifestyles of greatest benefit to employees, and maintaining records which clearly reveal data of importance in maintenance and improvement of health.

The occupational setting in which the nurse practices influences considerably the diversity of the practice, the priorities exercised, and the specialized functions carried out. For nursing students to be cognizant of the variabilities inherent within the occupational health nursing role, observation visits to the following settings can be enlightening.

1 Visits to the medical department of a large company and/or corporation
2 Visits to companies employing 500 or less workers and employing 1 nurse
3 Visits to industrial clinics within urban environments
4 Visits to employee health services of large hospitals
5 Visits to local, state, or federal government agencies employing occupational health nurses

In each occupational setting the nurse is first and foremost, a nurse, but she or he also functions (dependent on the work setting) in the capacity of a manager, consultant, teacher, counselor, data gatherer, record keeper, emergency expert, safety and health protection educator, coordinator of community services, evaluator of health services. In each work environment the nurse plays a critical role in shaping how health services are perceived and valued. In a highly rated health services department, nursing practice is top-notch and professional; nurses are favorably viewed by employees and management. The occupational health nurses have a thorough knowledge of the company, hospital, or agency for whom they work. This includes knowledge of company products or services provided. Nurses know about health care costs expended by the company, and the diseases and injuries for which employees are at risk. They are persuasive in promoting the use of protective equipment and clothing in situations that are hazardous. They are familiar with plant operations and processes, do plant surveys for the purpose of monitoring for potential health hazards and promoting health maintenance techniques for employees. To be comfortable with walk-through surveys, nurses are encouraged to take courses in industrial hygiene and safety, industrial processes, and toxicology. These courses (and related ones) give an overview of environmental hazards (physical, biological, chemical, and psychosocial), occupational diseases, carcinogenic agents, routes of entry, control of environmental hazards, and sampling techniques. These courses also affect the view of nurses regarding the valued services of industrial hygienists and safety personnel. Working as a team in an occupational setting, the nurse, industrial hygienist, and safety person perform invaluable services when influence for needed changes are necessary in the health care system of a company. By collaborating, occupational hazards can be measured, sampled, evaluated, monitored; data collection of recurring complaints and/or symptoms of employees can be synthesized with potential hazards or stresses in the work environment; engineering controls can be recommended; all for the ultimate goal of improved health care practices in the company.

Dependent upon the interests of the employing company and the cost-effectiveness of the action, nurses must be ready to engage in health and safety education and self-care programs for employee groups, promote physical fitness programs particularly for sedentary employees, and conduct small, well-designed pilot studies for the purpose of improving health practices. When clearly presented data are shown to management and to employees, the possibility for effecting needed changes in motivation and in policy is enhanced. As suggested by Collings, the occupational health field abounds with opportunities for the resourceful health professional willing to look for better ways to run a business. "Management in virtually all companies could use help in the health areas."[12]

Educator and Teacher

The community health nurse as educator and teacher of health imparts special knowledge to the family or group. Health education or health teaching is a process in which the client and nurse participate to increase their abilities to make informed decisions affecting their well-being. The process requires motivation of people to want to change to more healthful practices and lifestyles. Principles of learning are fundamental in the teaching process. Chap. 3 discusses health education, teaching, and promotion in detail.

Counselor

Another dimension of the nurse's role is counseling. Counseling is a helping process between the nurse and the client or family. This requires a relationship of friendliness, honesty, openness, and respect between the client or group and the nurse. It is a method for assisting others to identify feelings and to clarify beliefs and values about a concern in order to make appropriate decisions. Health counseling is a valuable way of assisting the client or group in improving health practices and self-care.

Facilitator

Removing barriers to care can be accomplished by the nurse as a facilitator. Facilitation is a process of listening, explaining, verifying, and describing a situation with the result that the client or group is involved in the decision-making process.

The nurse's knowledge of human behavior and learning allows the client or group to make decisions regarding better health outcomes. This may be in the areas of disci-

---

[12]G. H. Collings, Jr., "Management's View of the Nurse," *Occupational Health Nursing,* **27**:9–12, February 1979.

pline, parent-child groups, substance abuse, teenage pregnancy or self-care discussions. Chap. 7 describes the fundamentals of political participation by nurses. According to Aydelotte, the professional association provides the best vehicle through which nurses can work toward common goals and interests in an effort to resolve pressing issues.[13] Examples are changes in the nurse practice acts, third-party pay, and salary and fringe benefit increases in the work situation.

If nurses are to participate in putting political pressure on all levels of government, they must become a militant force in public policy-making. The more visible nurses become, the greater their strength will increase. By becoming active, assertive members on committees, boards, and organizations, changes in policies and legislation will be made. Nurses giving testimony at city or county councils or at the state legislature influence decisions to be made. Examples of the political process are found in Chap. 7.

HEALTH SETTINGS

Many members of different social and economic groups in society have a growing awareness of the intrinsic value of health to each individual. There is an increasing recognition that health is no longer a privilege of the few who can pay for it but a right to which every citizen is entitled. There is a definite trend on the part of many communities to accept this belief and to regard adequate health services as one of the responsibilities of government. Communities are realizing, more and more, that not only is a healthful environment essential but also that health services and health supervision are basic to the maintenance of the health of the entire community. This has led to an increase in the number of agencies organized to provide nursing service in homes, health centers, schools, and places of employment.

Community health nursing is practiced in a variety of settings including the official health departments, voluntary agencies, proprietary agencies, ambulatory clinics, schools, industry, free clinics, or special clinics to meet specific ethnic or population needs, such as senior citizen centers and low-cost housing centers. Whatever the setting, the nurse works within the framework set up to carry out certain health-related functions.

The official agencies are those that are tax-supported through federal, state, and local revenue. Examples of the official agencies are the United States Public Health Service, state health departments, and county, district, or city health departments and are generally referred to as *public health agencies.* Voluntary (nonofficial) agencies are private in nature, receiving various sources of support such as gifts, client fees, United Fund or United Crusade funds, and contracts with insurance companies and with medicare and medicaid. Examples of voluntary agencies are visiting nurse associations, the American Heart Association and its components, home health services, and community hospitals. These are generally referred to as *community health agencies.* Proprietary agencies are those in business to make a profit. Examples of this category are many nursing homes and some hospitals.

---

[13]Myrtle K. Aydelotte, "Unity for New Direction," *Washington State Journal of Nursing,* **50**: 13-17, Summer–Fall 1978.

Local Health Departments

Many counties in the 50 states have county, bicounty, or tricounty health departments or health districts. The idea of a county health department was organized in 1911. The first such departments were in Yakima County, Washington, and Guilford County, North Carolina, and they were set up almost simultaneously. In Yakima County, an organization was needed to control a typhoid fever epidemic, and in Guilford County, health promotion of school children was the immediate objective. All large cities and many smaller ones have municipal health departments, some having functioned since the beginning of the nineteenth century, when their main interest was the control of communicable diseases.

The legal basis for the authority of municipal, county, or district health departments lies in the laws of the several states and in the rules and regulations that define the mandatory activities of local government units relating to health matters. Local ordinances may define additional activities.

Historically, local health departments have come to be charged with responsibilities for (1) developing programs based on the health needs of the community, (2) providing necessary facilities and qualified staff to carry out these programs, and (3) making surveys of community needs and evaluating existing programs as necessary to ensure that these responsibilities are being met. Most local health departments developed their programs around the basic six functions, placing emphasis on the most pressing current problems; for instance, at one time tuberculosis, with its high incidence of death rates, was the most pressing problem in many communities. Health departments in those communities devoted much medical and nursing time to the prevention and control of this disease.

The nucleus of any local health department staff continues to be the health officer (usually a physician), the nurse, the environmental specialist, and the secretary, who is responsible for keeping records and vital statistics. Local programs were and still are instituted and maintained depending on community interest, health needs, budgets, the vision and leadership of the professional staff, and staff availability. As communities come to recognize their health needs and to demand additional professional services, they are more willing to support increased budgets for programs and staff.

With the shift of emphasis from concern for environment to greater concern for consumer, health departments are changing their roles. This results in part from laws recently enacted in the 1960s and 1970s by the United States Congress in relation to social security. Some states followed the federal government and passed similar legislation to meet emerging health problems in their jurisdiction.

This period of transition from the old, accepted "prevention" programs to the wider, more comprehensive, and direct approach to the solutions of health problems with emphasis on the individual and his or her family, raises questions regarding the adequacy of health departments as now organized and administered to meet current problems. Many shifts of practice and emphasis in the health organizations and their administration will become necessary in the near future. There is need also for a careful appraisal of the spending of available financial resources so that the greatest benefit for all people in the community may be obtained, for air pollution and other environmental hazards that directly or indirectly affect the health of people in every part of a community.

This changing concept of community health needs should be implemented by constant study and evaluation of health problems of the individual—such as physical and mental diseases, physical defects, and maternal and child health needs—and of environmental dangers—such as traffic accidents, poor housing, and unsafe dairies and other sources of foods. Following such studies, programs for community protection and safety can be established. The social and economic components of illness must be considered in any assessment and program planning.

Within the metropolitan areas, population shifts have modified the needs for certain health programs and services, and intensified the needs for others. For example, the child population tends to be centered in the suburbs today, thus increasing the needs there for more maternal and child health services; an older age group tends to become centered in cities, necessitating such programs as nursing homes and long-term home nursing services. Furthermore, it is becoming obvious that the child population remaining in the metropolitan areas is to be found, for the most part, in the dependent and low-income groups, who have many health needs.

Many urban, suburban, and rural communities in the past two decades have been experimenting with methods of merging local health departments. The weight of their experiences has shown that essential health services can be maintained with greater efficiency and economy and more effective use of staffs by a combined agency of some type. Various patterns of merged health agencies have been developed by communities, depending on local needs, resources, customs, government, and the interest and participation of the citizens.

Mergers range from a permanent consolidation of two or more agencies into a "combined health district" to the "contract-for-services" type, which allows for an annual contract between two or more health agencies or health departments, stating the specific services to be rendered by one agency to another and the financial obligations and administrative responsibilities involved.

The experiences of agencies that serve wide geographic areas show that communities can be served more efficiently if there is a decentralization to several health districts but with all of them functioning under the same health department policies and practices. Community planning for health programs will continue, but in order to meet new needs and to provide better and more efficient health services, other approaches to health agency reorganization must be developed and tested. The implementation of the Health Planning and Resources Development Act of 1974 (P.L. 93-641) through the designated health services area should improve the health of the residents without increased cost and unnecessary duplication of health resources.

Combination Public Health Nursing Agencies

This type of nursing service has been defined as an agency that is "administered jointly by a voluntary and an official agency, and supported by tax funds, community chests and united funds, earnings and contributions, in which the combined field of service offered by the participating agency is rendered by a single staff of nurses."[14]

During and immediately following World War II, many communities began searching for more effective utilization of the services of the public health nurse. Professional and lay leaders recognized that the duplication of travel and services of both staffs was costly in time and money. Studies relating to the situation revealed that staff nurses from both official and voluntary agencies were visiting the same families, often on the same day.

Combined public health nursing agencies function in approximately 100 communities in the United States, as a part of both health departments and visiting nurse organizations and in some instances as a part of the schools. The degree to which a combination or merging of nursing services takes place varies with the community. Experimentation with this form of nursing service continues, and new patterns in organization will emerge with study, research, and experience.

State Health Departments

Massachusetts established the first state board of health in 1869. Today, all 50 states have health departments functioning as a recognized part of state government. These departments are charged with the responsibility for assisting local health departments— city, county, district—to promote health in all its phases and provide the safest possible environment for all members of the community.

State health departments are administered in most states by qualified health officers assisted by staff drawn from the many public health disciplines mentioned previously. Other specialists are added depending on the types of industries, health problems, and hazards peculiar to any one state. Each state develops individual programs according to its own needs and resources. Health programs appropriate to Alaska might not meet the needs or be feasible in Kansas or Connecticut.

In the early part of this century, programs were developed to meet pressing community health needs. These programs were built on the six basic functions mentioned before. Programs were developed around these functions, with nursing participating to some degree in all of them. While it is still important to carry out *these* functions, other functions and programs have become necessary if current community problems are to be attacked. In addition to those previously mentioned, these problems include an increase in recognized mental illness, the need to provide and extend medical care, the toll of accidents with resultant deaths or severe disabling injuries, the increase in drug addiction, alcoholism, and venereal diseases, and the need for family planning and abortion counseling.

Some state health departments provide direct services, including community health nursing services, to local communities. This may be done for demonstration purposes or, especially in remote areas, from necessity because of a lack of local facilities or scarcity of nursing personnel.

A trend apparent in some states is combination of state departments of welfare

---

[14] *Nurses in Public Health*, U.S. Department of Health, Education, and Welfare Publication 785, 1964, p. 52.

and health into one organization. There is insufficient experience at present to determine the feasibility of this move. Students should watch for developments of this and similar trends in their own states.

The Public Health Service

The agency now known as the Public Health Service of the Department of Health and Human Services was established in 1798. Its main work then was to protect the young nation from disease from without by providing hospitals for ill and injured American and foreign seamen, and to protect the country as a whole from diseases that might spread from one state to another.

Although these original functions are still important, other functions have developed to meet increasing health needs. These include: (1) to carry on research and training in medical and related sciences and community health administration; (2) to aid communities in their planning and development of hospitals, health centers, and related facilities; and (3) to assist states and possessions with finances and trained personnel to apply new knowledge in prevention and control of diseases, maintenance of healthful environments, and development of appropriate community health services.

Medicine, nursing, dentistry, epidemiology, engineering, veterinary science, health education, nutrition, and biostatistics are among the disciplines making specific contributions to the carrying out of these functions. Effective use also is being made of the social sciences. Anthropology, psychology, sociology, political science, and public administration have enabled health workers to gain increased knowledge and understanding of people, aiding them in their work with clients, families, neighborhoods, and the wider community.

Home Health Service

Home health services had their beginning in the early 1880s with the beginning of the Visiting Nurse Association. With the advent of medicare in the 1960s, other agencies were established to give skilled nursing care in the home or place of residence, such as a home health agency of a special area or a community home care service of a city or county health department assuming more responsibility for extended care.

Home health services are health services provided on an intermittent basis to individuals of all ages. These services are provided to aging, disabled, sick or convalescent individuals who require care on either a short- or long-term basis. Home health services may be specialized or comprehensive depending upon the needs of the client requiring treatment and the level of care provided. The levels of care generally available in home health care include: intensive-acute, intermediate-restorative, maintenance-preventive, and hospice.

Home health services are provided according to specific needs of the client as determined by a single professional or a multidisciplinary team. Services generally offered are nursing, physical therapy, social work, speech, occupational therapy, nutrition, and home health aide services.

Most major hospitals today have a home health or home care coordinator program that becomes involved with planning and coordinating care in the home prior to discharge of the client. The nurse makes referrals to agencies as appropriate, for example, home health services or meals on wheels. Some hospitals and especially health maintenance organizations (HMO) employ community health nurses to provide extended care in the home.

PRECEPTS PRACTICED IN COMMUNITY HEALTH NURSING

As community health nursing developed in large cities and rural areas, changing socioeconomic conditions pinpointed precepts that should be observed to enable the nurse to practice with safety and meet the needs of client, family, and community. These changing conditions include new findings and practices relating to health, economic, social, and industrial changes, and changes in attitudes of clients, families, and neighborhoods toward health values.

Precept 1 Community health nursing is an established activity, based on recognized needs and functioning within the total health program.

As an activity to meet recognized community health needs, nursing provides supervision and counseling for health promotion, health appraisal, rehabilitation, and prevention of disease and provides care for the sick, toward cure or a peaceful death, in their homes. In addition to the home, nursing services may be carried out in the health center, clinics, schools, and places of employment. Community health nursing is an integral part of the total public health program, coordinating its plans and activities with those of other social and health agencies, and does not function or stand alone in the community.

Nursing services are supported by public and private funds to the degree that the community understands and appreciates its own health needs. The community has the obligation to study and evaluate continuously the nursing services it receives to determine trends of changing family and community needs, to develop new programs as necessary, and to discontinue those no longer pertinent. The decrease in communicable disease incidence resulting from education, immunization, and other control programs, and the increasing need to provide nursing service and rehabilitation for persons in their homes are examples.

Precept 2 Community health nursing agencies have clearly defined objectives and purposes for their services.

The multiplicity of social and health agencies in any given community demands that each agency have clearly defined and stated objectives and purposes in order to prevent duplication of certain community services and omission of others. Objectives and purposes vary with the type of agency and the community but should be related to the goals of the agency for nursing service, so that every citizen may be helped to achieve and maintain optimal health.

The philosophy, now in evidence, of the consumer of nursing service having a voice in the development of the objectives and purposes of community nursing is important to implementation of this precept. Such constructive participation by the consumer can result in a more effective nursing service.

The community health nurse works within the administrative framework of the agency, being fully aware of its objectives, purposes, and policies and adhering to them carefully. For the most part, the nurse works alone in the district and frequently is faced with decisions that relate to the work with families and coworkers, such as social workers, school, and industrial personnel. The nurse's complete knowledge and understanding of the agency's objectives, purposes, and policies will help prevent errors that might involve the agency and even community health nursing itself.

Precept 3 An active, organized citizens' group, representative of the community, is an integral part of the community health nursing program.

Community health nursing agencies, public and private, need to share their problems with and seek advice from representative community groups. Nearly every community includes, among its citizens, men and women who have been a part of its past and who will continue to be a part of its future. Their knowledge and experience, shared with the professional workers, can be of inestimable value to the community as a whole and can provide the professional workers with an understanding and awareness of the elements of the complex backgrounds of the community's life, development, and experiences.

An active, organized citizens' group, representing the public, should be invited to participate in the planning and development of health programs that will meet community needs and interests. Such a group can provide continuity for the planning and service of the agency and contribute to the interpretation of community health nursing. It can serve also as a valuable liaison between the agency and the community.

The composition of this group varies according to whether the community is urban, suburban, or rural. Since consideration of community needs is an important function of the group, members should be selected for the contribution they are able to make. Their period of service should be limited, e.g., to 3 or 6 years, depending on the needs of the community and its resources. Members may be drawn from such organizations as parent-teacher associations, men's civic and service clubs, women's organizations, church councils, professional groups such as lawyers or physicians, schools, labor and management, and industrial and agricultural groups. Representatives of diverse religious and ethnic groups will aid in the general understanding of community problems, e.g., housing and unemployment.

A citizens' group functions in various ways. Its members may make selected home calls with the nurse so that they can interpret the nurse's work with more understanding to other community groups. They can point out to the agency needs for nursing services as they see them in their neighborhoods, districts, or parishes. They can discuss and offer solutions to problem cases presented by the agency. They can assist in the extension and development of nursing services, either geographically or in depth. They can keep the agency informed of trends relating to the economic and social conditions in the community; this is especially valuable when a trend is just beginning. The interest and assistance of this group can also be of great value at budget planning time.

The precept that a citizens' group should be an integral part of the community health nursing program points up that just as the public health nurse should work *with* client and family, rather than *for* them, community health nursing should plan health programs *with* community members, rather than *for* them.

An advisory committee should meet at regular intervals to be kept informed of the agency's program and to contribute from their personal and community experiences to the solution of problems. They are entitled to share in the successes of the program as well as the failures. Recognition and implementation of this precept is important, as many citizens spend practically their entire life in the community and have much invested in it, and the valuable contributions they can make to the work and success of the public health agency should not be lost.

On occasion, nurses will find small, informal groups of residents in their districts who can be of great help to them in their work. These groups can interpret the local needs, cultures, and mores of their neighborhood. Many of these men and women have a potential for leadership and might be considered for membership on communitywide health committees, where their experience and understanding of such neighborhood problems as lack of health centers, child-care centers, and hospital facilities can contribute to the entire community. Recognition and utilization of this resource can add stability and continuity to the agency's program.

Precept 4 Community health nursing services are available to the entire community regardless of origin, culture, or social and economic resources.

Community health nursing is a field of specialization within the broad spectrum of organized public health practice. Its services should be available to all persons according to their health needs, physical and emotional, and regardless of ethnic origin, cultural background, or social and economic resources. Deviation from health of any one member of a family or of the community may affect the health of the entire family or community. The background of the individual or family should not interfere with their receiving the needed services the nurse can provide, e.g., skilled nursing care and health teaching relating to maternal and child care, nutrition, immunizations, and mental and emotional problems. Although community health nursing had its inception in the work of the early church, it is not necessarily a charity and has adapted itself to changes in the social order.

Nonofficial agencies, such as visiting nurse associations, charge for nursing care if the family can arrange to pay. Fees should be within the range of the family's financial resources and should reflect the value placed on the service by the community, the family, and the agency. Fees for visits are charged on a full- or part-pay basis, depending on the ability of the family or client to pay, especially when the client is the family's breadwinner. The nurse needs to estimate the period of time care will be needed, as it will be a factor in establishing the fee. Many families who might be able to pay full fees for the nurse's visits for a short-term illness might be unable to do so if faced with a long-term illness, such as cancer. When the family can arrange to pay at least part of the fee, they should be encouraged to do so. Necessary nursing care should not be discontinued because of an inability to pay for it. Part of the nurse's plan is to assist the client and family in their rehabilitation to attain optimal health so that they may function independently and assume, as soon as possible, their responsibilities for their own health problems. But when for economic reasons a client has to forego essential nursing care, the goals of the nurse and agency are lost. In some agencies after the nurse has assessed the situation, arrangements for fee collection are made by the clerical help.

Current policies in most official nursing agencies do not provide bedside nursing care except on a demonstration basis. In some areas this practice is changing; the present trend is for local health department staffs to provide bedside nursing when the community lacks other home nursing facilities. Some states have passed legislation that makes it possible for local official agencies to charge for these nursing visits when feasible.

The precept that community health nursing services are available to everyone is broad in its concept. It permeates all nurse-client and nurse-family relationships. It contributes to the goals of the overall community health nursing program.

Precept 5 In community health nursing the *family,* rather than the *individual client,* is recognized as the unit of service.

The community health nurse's work is family-centered, rather than client-centered, with the home being the usual setting. This is a different approach from that of client-centered care in the hospital environment. It recognizes the client or family as the hostess and the nurse as the guest in the situation. The effect of health or illness (physical or emotional) of any one member on the lives of other family members is more obvious in the home than in the hospital, and the nurse is able to observe more closely in the home than in the hospital the effect of suffering, fear, and death on members of the family.

In studying and trying to understand the home situation, the nurse draws widely on knowledge and background of the social and behavioral sciences. On the basis of knowledge of the family composition, its history, resources, and current problems, the nurse employs the epidemiologic approach in meeting family needs. The nurse makes frequent appraisals of the health progress of the family and client. The nurse recognizes that the family is a segment of the community and of society and utilizes the available community resources in the planning. Frequently the nurse functions as a liaison person with other community agencies in securing health and social resources for the family.

The nurse's ultimate goal is to make the entire family independent and knowledgeable regarding health principles and practices. Achieving this goal is facilitated when the nurse plans *with* them rather than *for* them. Emphasis is primarily on health promotion for all the family through health counseling, emotional support and understanding, teaching, demonstrating, and nursing care; at the same time the nurse provides for the client's needs.

Precept 6 Health teaching, health promotion, and counseling for client, family, and community are integral parts of community health nursing.

Teaching health concepts and practices to the community, family, and client is interwoven throughout the work of the community health nurse. On a community level the nurse participates with other members of the health team in planning and carrying out community health education concerning immunization programs, safety programs, dependable food and water supplies, reliable waste disposal, or development of mental health programs. Media used to provide community health education include news stories, films, posters, radio and television programs, and talks to individuals and groups. County and state fairs offer excellent opportunities for educating the general public about heart disease, diabetes, and other diseases, and for programs on vision conservation, better nutrition, and accident prevention, among other topics.

In the home the nurse works closely with client and family in health counseling, focusing on individual needs. The nurse plans with them to meet their goals in health promotion, rehabilitation, and independence in health matters. Teaching the family the importance of immunization and environmental sanitation and teaching prospective parents the care of mothers and babies are examples. As far as possible, the nurse should coordinate the teaching in the home with that of the family physician.

In the schools, the nurse cooperates with principals and teachers in health matters. The nurse acts as a resource for health education, and is available for conferences on health matters with children, parents, teachers, and administrative personnel. In industrial plants, the nurse assists supervisory personnel and others in instituting health and safety programs and coordinates her or his work with other health education activities in the plant and in the community.

The general public is interested in many health matters and fairly well informed regarding them. However, since much of the lay person's information is received from current lay periodicals, the nurse needs to be aware of this source of "health" literature, as it sometimes contains half-truths and needs interpretation. On the other hand, the nurse also needs to keep well informed regarding knowledge currently presented in the literature of the medical, nursing, and allied fields.

The nurse's goal in all health teaching and health counseling is to help the individual, the family, and the community to be so well informed regarding sound health principles and practices that they achieve and maintain optimal health by means of their own knowledge and efforts.

Precept 7 Individuals and families participate fully in all decision making relating to goals for the attainment of health.

The community health nurse recognizes and respects the right of client and family to participate in all decision making relating to their health goals. The nurse's function is to help the client and/or family to recognize the existence of a health need, to assess all aspects of the situation, to consider appropriate activities that will improve the situation, and to arrive at the decision which is deemed most suitable by the client and family. Implicit in the decision-making process is that the client and family comprehend fully the meaning of the decision and accept the responsibility for consequential events. An example is the parents' decision to have a rubella immunization for their child after weighing the pros and cons of immunization versus voluntary exposure to a "childhood disease," rubella.

A more involved situation would be the decision a client and family would have to make regarding open-heart surgery. Although this surgical technique has reached a fairly high degree of safety, there are certain elements of danger in individual cases. The nurse needs to be objective in teaching, helping the client and family to make their own decision, and at the same time help them to make a free and responsible choice on their own and to gain independence for future decision making through the experience.

The nurse also observes this precept when working with community groups. The aim is to involve community members in the planning and provision of health care to the highest possible degree and to help create independent thinking and action on the part of consumers, as well as the ability to live with their decisions. If a community fails to pass a bond issue for necessary money to ensure safe water supplies or a well-equipped fire department, they may have to accept the results of a water-borne epidemic or a heavy loss of life and property following a disastrous fire, but the decision should lie with the community.

Precept 8 Periodic and continuing appraisal and evaluation of the health situation of the community, family, and client are basic to community health nursing.

Although this precept has been recognized for a long time, its importance has been accentuated in recent years by the rapidly changing patterns in community and family life and by the new discoveries in medicine that shorten recovery and convalescent periods. In some situations, changes in the circumstances of the community, family, or client may be so subtle that they pass unnoticed unless the nurse and the agency maintain continuous appraisal and are fully aware of their implications. The term *periodic* is a fluid one, and its meaning depends on many factors. In a family, community, or neighborhood experiencing rapid changes, it may mean every month or oftener; in other situations a review or appraisal might not be necessary more than once every 6 months.

The family health appraisal is a tool for the nurse in helping the family to achieve health independence. Family situations can be dynamic, a birth or death may cause a complete family reorganization, and a severe illness or change in the health status of any one member may have repercussions for every member. Also a change of residence or a change of occupation with resultant change in income may have marked effects on the physical and emotional health situation. At intervals, these changes need to be assessed by family and nurse in the interests of planning for the family health program. By consultation with family and client and by careful observation and case recording, the nurse can evaluate the family health progress, determine the priorities, and adjust the nursing plans.

An awareness of the progress that is being made and of the degree of independence that the family seems to be achieving helps the nurse to establish priorities in planning for daily work in the district and the home calls to be made.

Communities, too, are dynamic and changing constantly for better or worse, some at a quicker rate than others. Periodic study of the neighborhoods in her or his district enables the nurse to be informed of changes that will affect the lives of the families there. What changes are taking place in relation to population shifts, age groups, business areas, recreational facilities, and housing? Changing transportation facilities, such as an increase or decrease in bus routes, parking lots, arterials, and highways, affect a neighborhood. The need for additional buildings for schools and hospitals, or their abandonment, points up community changes involving growth or decay.

From these periodic appraisals of client, family, and community, the nurse gains a basis for evaluating the effectiveness of the work and of her or his own growth and development.

Precept 9 The nurse is prepared professionally to function as a health worker in the community.

A hundred years of experience with community health nursing has proved to society that the nurse must be prepared professionally to serve as health worker in the community and that this preparation should be based on a firm foundation of nursing knowledge and skills, including theory and practice in community health procedures. The nurse needs special competence in adapting learned nursing procedures to the home care and rehabilitation of the client. Since community health nursing is a family-centered activity rather than a client-centered one as in the hospital, the nurse also needs a broad background in such social and behavioral sciences as anthropology, sociology, and psychology to meet effectively problems that involve interpersonal relationships, community organization, and social pathology.

The community health nurse brings not only broad preparation and technical skills to the work, but also must continue to grow and to improve performance skills in interviewing, teaching, problem solving, group work, and leadership. The nurse needs to keep up with recent knowledge in nutrition, social work, epidemiology, and behavioral sciences as well as in nursing and medical care.

This precept that the nurse be prepared professionally for work is the cornerstone in the foundation of community nursing, for without previous professional preparation and an awareness of current knowledge in nursing and medical care, as well as in the allied fields, the nurse's work could not measure up to the community's needs.

Precept 10 The community health nurse functions as a member of the health team in serving community, family, and client.

All successful teamwork is based on a common interest of the team members and there should be no division of concern among them. The community health nurse often functions on various teams at one time or another. One such team would include members from the agency or nursing division such as other staff nurses, paranursing personnel, students, the district supervisor, the nursing director, clerks, volunteers, and other nonprofessional personnel, all of whom work together to provide the best possible community nursing service.

The nurse also participates on a community team composed of workers from the allied health fields and interested community members. Although the ultimate goals of this team are the same as those of the nursing team, the emphases may vary. This interdisciplinary team usually includes, besides the nurse, a health officer, family physician, social worker, nutritionist, and environmental specialist. Members of other health disciplines can be added as needed, as well as such interested community members as school personnel, clergymen, volunteer community workers, and in most situations, the client or the client's family.

The nurse has several roles on the interdisciplinary team. The nurse acts as an interpreter of nursing in the team's assessment of the client's physical, mental, and social needs and in planning means to meet these needs, and in turn keeps the nursing team aware of the thinking and action of the community team. The nurse also participates in the team action regarding improvement of environmental resources. The nurse also functions as a leader by influencing the quality of health and nursing care that can be provided to the community by helping it to become aware of the need for health programs.

With the recognition of the value of continuity of nursing care, it is possible that a third team is emerging composed of hospital personnel as the head nurse, staff nurse, resident, intern and/or family physician, and the community health nurse, all of whom would know the client. This team can coordinate plans for continuity of nursing care, thus providing for fewer interruptions in the care of the client during the transition from home to hospital to home. The client and family frequently participate on this team and assist with the making of plans and their implementation.

In making the team effective, each member must recognize the contribution of all other team members in achieving the planned goals and objectives, which are the health, safety, and comfort of client and community.

Precept 11   The community health nurse provides nursing care for the individual client as ordered by the client's physician.

The provision of nursing care for the individual client as ordered by the client's physician is basic to all nursing. Every nurse caring for the sick works under the direction of the physician in charge of the client. Violation of this precept jeopardizes the entire community health nursing program. The nurse receives orders for care from the physician responsible for the medical care and supervision of the client. In most instances this is the family physician, but it might be a physician from a hospital clinic, a school system, or an industrial plant.

When a family or client refuses medical care, although it appears necessary to the nurse, there is no recourse but to withdraw from the situation. This has occurred on occasion. It is a difficult step for the nurse to take, especially if the client is an infant or a child, but this precept must be held inviolate. Before taking such a radical step, however, the nurse should report the situation to the nursing supervisor or health officer. Except in great emergency, a nurse does not care for a sick client without medical orders.

Most community health nursing agencies have a policy, approved by the local medical society, that the nurse may make, without medical supervision, two nursing visits to a family with illness for the purpose of providing nursing care. If during the first visit, the nurse believes that the client should be under medical supervision—and he or she is not—the nurse must advise the family that a physician should be called. Depending on judgment, the nurse may give nursing care during the visit according to the agency's standing orders, which have been approved by the medical advisory committee of the agency, the county medical society, or the local health officer. At this time also the nurse may counsel the family on health matters such as general nutrition, rest, comfort, and safety of the client. The next day, the nurse may visit the family to see whether a physician was called and to ascertain the physician's orders for nursing care. If the family has not called a physician and does not plan to do so, the nurse should determine their reasons. If it is a matter of finances, the nurse can explain the community resources for free medical care. If the family does not wish to have medical care for other reasons, the nurse cannot continue to provide nursing care.

As in the hospital, the nurse in the public health field reports regularly to the physician in charge, regarding the client's condition, and secures additional orders as necessary. When visiting the home for health teaching and counseling, the nurse keeps the family physician informed, in writing or by telephone, so that they may work together in assisting the family to achieve independence and self-sufficiency in health matters.

Precept 12 The community health nurse makes full use of family and other service records.

The maintenance of accurate records and their use are important to both family and agency. The family record is indispensable to the nurse's daily work and is an important element in making continuity of nursing care possible. Good recording covers all nurse-family, as well as nurse-client, contacts and interaction. The nurse uses client and family records in planning for home visits and for other means of serving the client. The nurse's visit plans will be based on the accomplishments of previous visits that she or he and other nurses, if any, have made to the family or client and on the current situation of the client or family. Records are invaluable to the nurse assuming care of the client for the first time. A review of the records prior to the first visit will save both the nurse's time and that of the family. The nurse's knowledge and understanding of situations will reduce family stress at the time of a first visit by a new nurse.

The quality of the agency's services to the community is reflected in its records. A periodic critical study of them helps the agency to evaluate its program in relation to its current objectives, and assists in determining its long-term objectives. The records are a source of statistical information and are valuable in determining costs, in ascertaining needs for additional staff members, and in planning budgets. They provide a guide in making staff assignments to the different nursing districts.

Community health nursing agencies have legal authorization to operate, their records are legal documents and as such are subject to subpoena by the courts, but in all other situations they are strictly confidential. Within the policies of the agency, a report of the contents of the record is shared with the family physician or with a professional staff member of another agency, such as a social worker, when requested.

The staff nurse is responsible for maintaining records so that they are current, accurate, complete, and legible. The information should be recorded objectively, the nurse being aware at all times of the many uses the agency will make of the record.

Precept 13 The community health nurse does not provide material relief but directs the client or family to appropriate community resources for necessary financial and social assistance.

The community health nurse does not provide material relief, since there are community agencies organized for this purpose. The nurse's concern is for the client's immediate health needs and for the promotion of health, physical and emotional, and prevention of disease. By providing material relief, even transportation to the clinic or health center, except on the request and approval of the cooperating agency, the nurse might be jeopardizing the long-range planning of other community workers. The nurse is responsible for knowing the programs and functions available from social agencies and for cooperating with them, utilizing their services, and referring clients and families to them.

The timing for the referral and the family's readiness to accept it needs careful consideration. The family should participate in the planning for the referral, which should never be made against their will but only with their understanding and acceptance.

It is basic to this precept that when providing material relief, no matter how little, the nurse tends to nullify her or his teaching. Unconsciously, the nurse is buying client and family cooperation in health matters, for instead of incorporating the teaching into their thinking and making it their own practice and action, they are waiting to be paid for it.

Precept 14 Nursing supervision of the staff nurse is provided by qualified nursing personnel.

Supervision is an educational and advisory relationship between supervisor and staff nurse. Its aim is to develop the abilities and skills of the nurse so that she or he can meet professional responsibilities with an increasing productivity and effectiveness.

Supervision in community health agencies by qualified nurses is essential for continuous improvement of the nursing service to client and family, for the overall planning of the staff nurses' work, and for coordination of their activities within the agency. It is also a stimulus and guide for the staff nurse in health teaching, family counseling, and nursing service, and for her or his own growth and development.

Methods of supervision vary with agencies, but the methods most frequently employed include planned and continuing staff orientation, joint study and review of family case records by supervisor and nurse, supervised home calls or clinic experiences, and individual and group conferences relating to the nurse's work and to the continuing development of the agency's program. Staff members need to be aware at all times of the agency's planning and work if a balanced development is to be maintained. An adequate and satisfactory program of supervision will assist not only in the growth and development of each staff member but also in the continued improvement of the quality of nursing service that the agency provides the community.

Precept 15 Community health nursing agencies provide continuing staff education programs.

Such a staff education program is essential to maintain sound nursing practice in hospitals and community health agencies. Planning for in-service education takes into account the professional needs and interests of the staff nurses. Consideration is given also to the special skills and knowledge required by the agency. The staff must be kept informed of new situations and conditions arising in the community, such as a sudden increase in the incidence of a communicable disease, a change in the health and welfare resources in the community, e.g., the formation of a local council for alcoholism, and new federal, state, and local regulations relating to health matters.

Periodic, planned staff meetings for sharing experiences and information with other members of the health team in the community also provide an opportunity for widening professional knowledge and skills, not only in nursing but also in other phases of the community health program. Many agencies send one or more staff members to conferences, institutes, summer schools, or professional meetings in other parts of the state or country on the premise that the entire staff will share in the reports of these educational experiences.

A sound in-service program is based on the dynamics of medical and nursing care and an appreciation of the ever-increasing body of knowledge with which the nurse must be familiar and the additional skills needed in the daily practice with clients and families and in contacts with coworkers.

Precept 16   The nurse assumes responsibility for her or his own continuing professional development.

The responsibility of the nurse for continuing professional development is a precept basic to all nursing; it is the other side of the coin of the precept just stated relating to the agency's recognized responsibility and obligation for providing in-service and staff development programs. The staff nurse is equally responsible for continuing professional growth and education. It has been said that the ultimate goal of an education program is to shift to the student the burden of pursuing her or his own education. Continuing education is considered by many leaders in all fields to be the greatest single challenge to professional personnel.

Each nurse needs to establish immediate and long-term goals in order to continue building and developing her or his education, both professional and general. This can be done by various methods, such as reading professional journals and periodicals on nursing and allied subjects, attending and participating in the meetings of professional organizations, and not neglecting books, journals, and lectures in the humanities and the arts. For the most part, the nurse will find libraries, art galleries, concert and lecture series available in either her or his own community or an adjacent one. As a professional person, the nurse should plan to invest some time and money in growth and development through attendance at summer sessions in colleges and universities, and by working toward higher degrees whenever possible.

SUMMARY

The precepts of community health nursing relate to the *organization* of community health nursing, to the *work* of the individual nurse, and to the *nurse* herself or himself. They are guidelines only and are to be followed in any situation with sound judgment and common sense. The majority of these precepts pertain to nursing in general, not to community health nursing alone. Their implications for all nursing will tend to increase as the philosophy and practice of continuous care of the client from home to hospital to home becomes accepted by client, family, and community, as well as by the nursing, medical, and allied professions. Students of nursing have become aware of many of these precepts from their experience in clinical situations in the hospitals. They are stated here, however, within the framework of community nursing.

The responsibilities of today's community health nurses are succinctly summarized by Cline and Howell as "to help individuals, families and communities to develop and utilize their potential for healthful living through cultivation and use of their own and external resources, and to provide nursing care for the sick and disabled in their homes."[15]

The means by which the nurse carries out these responsibilities include visits to client and family; work with neighborhood groups, such as parents' classes and prenatal classes; health supervision in places of employment; and assistance to teachers of children of all age groups. Community health nursing must be based on an understanding and appreciation of the needs, social relationships, and cultural mores of the client, family, or group.

SUGGESTED READINGS

American Nurses Association, Division of Community Health Nursing, *A Conceptual Model of Community Health Nursing,* American Nurses Association, Kansas City, Mo., 1980.

Archer, Sarah Ellen, and Ruth Fleshman: "Community Health Nursing: A Typology of Practice," *Nursing Outlook,* **23**:358–364, June 1975.

Archer, Sarah Ellen, and Ruth Fleshman: *Community Health Nursing Patterns and Practice,* 2d ed., Duxbury Press, North Scituate, Mass., 1979.

Bergeson, Paul, and Nancy Melvin: "Granting Hospital Privileges to Nurse Practitioners," *Journal of the American Hospital Association,* **49**:99–101, August 6, 1975.

Blum, Henrik L.: *Health Planning,* Human Sciences Press, New York, 1974.

Brown, Mary Louise: *Occupational Health Nursing: Principles and Practices,* Springer Publishing Company, New York, 1981.

Bryan, Doris: *School Health in Transition,* The C. V. Mosby Company, St. Louis, 1973.

Department of Health, Education, and Welfare, Public Health Service, *Healthy People: The Surgeon General's Report on Health Promotion and Disease Prevention,* Government Printing Office, Washington, D.C., 1979.

Draye, Mary Ann, and Lorrie Anderson Stetson: "The Nurse Practitioner as an Economic Reality," *The Nurse Practitioner,* **1**:60–63, November–December 1975.

Dunn, H. L.: *High Level Wellness,* R. W. Beatty Co., Arlington, Va., 1961.

Farrand, Linda L., and Marguerite Cobb: "Perceptions of Activities Performed in Ambulatory Care Settings," *The Nurse Practitioner,* **1**:69–72, November–December 1975.

Green, Lawrence W.: "Educational Strategies to Improve Compliance with Therapeutic and Preventive Regimens: The Recent Evidence" in Brian Haynes, D. Wayne Taylor, and David L. Sackett (eds.), *Compliance in Health Care,* The Johns Hopkins University Press, Baltimore, Md., 1979.

Guidelines for the School Nurses in School Health Program, American School Health Association, Kent, Wash., 1974.

Hanlon, John Jr.: *Public Health Administration and Practice,* 6th ed., The C. V. Mosby Company, St. Louis, 1974.

[15] Nora Cline and Roger W. Howell, "Public Health Nursing and Mental Health," in Stephen E. Goldston (ed.), *Mental Health Considerations in Public Health,* U.S. Department of Health, Education, and Welfare, Public Health Services and Mental Health Administration, National Institute of Mental Health, Chevy Chase, Md., 1969, p. 146.

Igoe, Judith Bellaire: "The School Nurse Practitioner," *Nursing Outlook,* **23**:381–384, June 1975.

Institute of Medicine Division of Health Manpower and Resource Development, *A Manpower Policy for Primary Care,* National Academy of Sciences, May 1978.

"An Interview with Dr. Loretta Ford," *The Nurse Practitioner,* **1**:9–12, September–October 1975 (editorial).

Milio, Nancy: *9226 Kercheval: The Store Front That Did Not Burn,* The University of Michigan Press, Ann Arbor, 1971.

McNeil, Jo, M. N. Bergner, and Lawrence Bergner: "Use of Mobile Units to Provide Health Care for Preschoolers in Rural King County, Washington," *Public Health Reports,* **90**:344–348, July–August 1975.

Oda, Dorothy S.: "Increasing Role Effectiveness of School Nurses," *American Journal of Public Health,* **64**:591–595, June 1974.

Skrovan, Clarence, Elizabeth T. Andrews, and Janet Gottschalk: "Community Nurse Practitioner," *American Journal of Public Health,* **64**:847–852, September 1974.

Splane, Verna Huffman: "Community Health Nursing in Canada," *The Nursing Clinics of North America,* December 1975, **10**:687–778.

Tinkham, Catherine V., and Eleanor F. Voorheis: *Community Health Nursing and Process,* Appleton-Century-Crofts, New York, 1974.

U.S. Department of Health, Education, and Welfare, Secretary's Committee to Study Extended Roles for Nurses: "Extending the Scope of Nursing Practice," *American Journal of Nursing,* **71**:2346–2351, December 1971.

Williams, Carolyn A.: "Nurse Practitioners Research: Some Neglected Issues," *Nursing Outlook,* **23**:172–177, March 1975.

Williams, Carolyn A.: "Community Health Nursing—What Is It?" *Nursing Outlook,* **25**:250–254, April 1977.

Conceptualizing a Model for Community Health Nursing

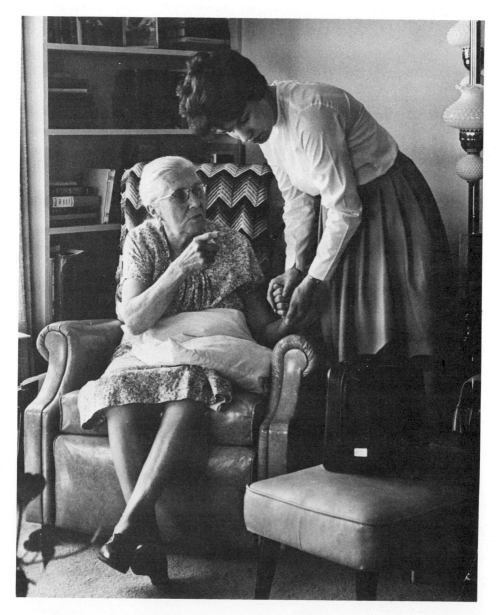

To practice community health nursing successfully, the nurse must (1) perceive the nursing role with clarity, (2) recognize clients with health needs as having participatory decision-making skills, and (3) interact in language and actions that are understandable and that communicate warmth and consideration to clients. Developing a framework for the practice of community health nursing therefore requires an understanding of interrelationships of descriptive terms or concepts, the utilization of selected theories, and objective evaluation of outcomes.

PRACTICAL PURPOSE FOR USING THEORIES

The range of theory usage is broad. For the practitioner, the level of theory usage differs markedly from that of a researcher seeking to create new knowledge. The practitioner is seeking practical directions that will lead to potentially successful outcomes. Practice in the real world is tangible and can be either ineptly or skillfully accomplished. Most nursing students have the innate desire to demonstrate nursing practice in an illustrious manner. For practice to be assured and competent, the usage of selected practice theories is recommended.

Miller argues for the practical art of using theory by diagramming a progression of practices which lead to outcomes predictably determined successful or unsuccessful. The progression is shown as follows:

Practices $\longrightarrow$ practices
This is a monkey see, monkey do operation. The nurse sees another nurse doing an action and imitates it.

Practices $\longrightarrow$ hunch $\longrightarrow$ practices
This indicates that various actions are considered, and a hunch is followed in selecting the action that will best suit the situation.

Practices $\longrightarrow$ hunches $\longrightarrow$ principles $\longrightarrow$ practices
Past experiences and hunches are reviewed to establish guidelines or rules to use in the selection of the most appropriate action to take. This step is at a higher level than trial and error.

Practices $\longrightarrow$ hunches $\longrightarrow$ theory $\longrightarrow$ principles $\longrightarrow$ practices
Theory provides a rational and systematic view of the situation and serves as a guide in the selection of appropriate principles for action. The results of practice either support or question the theory. Modification of theory usage can provide a basis for new action.[1]

When a group of students discusses problems that have occurred in the field and then theorizes (speculates) regarding elements of the problem, usage of the theory, and possible outcomes, they develop a means for coping with new problems when they

---

[1] Van Miller, "The Practical Art of Using Theory," *The School Executive,* 77:60–63, 1958.

occur. This kind of discussion represents thoughtful mental consideration of problems and theory usage as practiced in the field. Such a discussion tends to be unifying for the group because experiences are shared from the standpoint of learning and generalizing from experiences rather than critiquing what actually happened in specific situations. Discussion of theory usage in the field is most satisfying and educational when it helps students understand and improve their own practice as community health nurses.

THEORY USAGE IN COMMUNITY HEALTH NURSING

Assumptions regarding the practice of community health nursing are stated as precepts in Chap. 1. In recognition of the precepts as stated, a set of descriptive terms or concepts is required of the community health nurse to incorporate into a framework for practice. These concepts provide building blocks to theory usage. Utilization of selected theories yield rules of conduct (principles) designed for desired outcomes. For the community health nurse initiating the use of a specific theory in the field of practice for the first time, tolerance for ambiguity is essential. As explained by Stevens, nursing theory regarding the nature of nursing is in an early stage of development; by accepting conflict and diversity among theories, nursing as a discipline is progressing.[2]

Practice theories are intellectual tools and form the basis for applying concepts and direction to nurses who seek knowledge, understanding, and prescriptions for effective actions. Practice theories provide guidelines for successful actions. By applying a conscious use of a selected theory while studying an individual, family, or community, the community health nursing student is enabled to synthesize classroom theory with actual practice. In so doing, the student learns that theory has practical value; that new and useful data are elicited because of the requirements of the theory; that individuals, family members, and community clients learn and understand new ways of behaving when the theory is completely explained; and that they become aware of positive results as a consequence of their experimental change of behavior.

OPTIMAL HEALTH OR WELLNESS AS A GOAL

Historically, it has been said that the goal of community health nurses was to "help patients help themselves." Today this goal implies "self-care." Upon meeting a client for the first time, the community health nurse mentally visualizes or imagines that individual at a more optimal state of health or wellness than observed at the moment of introduction. The nurse begins immediately to utilize the nursing process and guides the client toward desiring a better state of health. Recognition, conscious or subliminal, has always been given to the fact that clients play an important role in facilitating or sabotaging nursing guidance or actions. For purposes of most committed community health nurses, the goal toward which practice is aimed is optimal client health or wellness based on each client's needs, wants, and desires. Optimal health is viewed as a total life process and is attained differentially by each individual. For progress toward

[2]Barbara J. Stevens, *Nursing Theory: Analysis, Application, Evaluation,* Little, Brown and Company, Boston, 1979, pp. xi–xiii.

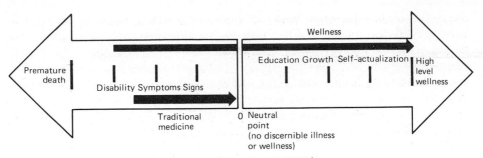

Figure 2-1   The wellness-illness continuum. (*After Travis, 1977.*)

a higher level of health to be demonstrated, each client must be responsible for exercising some modicum of self-care according to personal limits of motivation.

The following definitions of health and wellness have some common dimensions.
Health is viewed as a total life process and/or a dynamic state in the life cycle of an
individual. This implies continuous adaptation to stresses in the internal and external
environment through optimum use of one's resources to achieve maximum potential
for daily living.[3] In other words, life is a continuous growth process during which situations, events, or developments must be seen as opportunities for increasing wellness if
optimal health is the goal of the individual. Health encompasses the whole person and
is related to the way in which the individual deals with the stresses of growth and development while functioning within the cultural milieu.[4]

Wellness is an integrated method of functioning that is oriented to maximizing the
individual's and family's potential within their environment.[5] Both definitions recognize environmental influences and emphasize the individualization of resources and/or
coping skills for the client's achievement of greatest potential. Greatest potential infers
a positive direction toward wellness or optimal health.

Travis has depicted a wellness-illness continuum[6] as shown in Fig. 2-1. The center
of the scale at zero shows the absence of illness. Moving from the center toward the
left indicates the presence of illness as manifested by signs, symptoms, and obvious
disabilities. When an individual becomes aware of a pain, general discomfort, or dysfunction of a body part, a physician or health care provider is sought out. Recognition
of illness or any manifestation of a change from an accustomed functional state is easily identified by individuals no longer at the neutral point of the scale.

Moving from the center toward the right indicates an increasingly positive state of
health. Clients for the most part are unfamiliar with the idea of positive states of health
on a graduated basis. They nonchalantly tend to accept health and ability to do activities of daily living. For the average individual, states of wellness and illness fluctuate
back and forth on the scale as temporary negative and positive feelings (such as stom-

[3] Imogene M. King, *Toward a Theory for Nursing,* John Wiley and Sons, Inc., New York,
1971, p. 72.
[4] Ibid., p. 67.
[5] Halbert L. Dunn, *High Level Wellness,* R. W. Beatty Co., Arlington, Va., 1961, pp. 4–5.
[6] John W. Travis, *Wellness Workbook for Health Professionals,* Wellness Associates, Inc., 42
Miller Avenue, Mill Valley, Calif., 94941. Copyright 1977 John W. Travis, M.D. Reprinted with
permission.

achaches and/or momentary peaks of exuberance) are experienced. When clients become aware of a *persistent* headache or uncomfortable symptom, however, the movement toward the left end of the scale sends a different message. Realization that the symptom may have serious consequences and permanence produces various reactions. Clients are generally well acquainted with resources dealing with illness and disease. On the other hand, moving toward the right on the scale is unfamiliar territory for many clients. These people must be taught that better states of health can be attained through education and practice of selected health habits or activities. A greater feeling of wellness can be achieved and sustained for those clients willing to extend the effort. Chap. 8 expands on health teaching measures intended to improve existing states of health.

A FRAMEWORK FOR COMMUNITY HEALTH NURSING PRACTICE

A suggested paradigm for community health nursing which recognizes the participation and decision-making ability of the client is shown in Fig. 2-2. Discussion of the paradigm will start with a description of nursing. The community health nursing process is described completely in Chap. 6.

Nursing

Nursing has been defined repeatedly, with each new definition attempting to focus more precisely on its basic nature. Henderson's definition continues to be widely accepted. "Nursing is to assist the individual, sick or well, in the performance of those activities contributing to health or its recovery (or to peaceful death) that he would perform if he had the necessary strength, will or knowledge. And to do this in such a way as to help him gain independence as rapidly as possible."[7] Kinlein, a nurse who has set up an independent practice, characterizes the professional nurse as an extension of the client, and as being known by the care given to the client. She defines nursing as "assisting the person in his self-care practices in regard to his state of health."[8] Within this definition the knowledge and practice of the nurse is directed toward teaching, ministering, referring, and evaluating as needed and desired by the client. Orem's view

[7] Virginia Henderson, "The Nature of Nursing," *The American Journal of Nursing,* **64**:64–68, August 1964.

[8] M. Lucille Kinlein, *Independent Nursing Practice with Clients,* J. B. Lippincott Company, Philadelphia, 1977, p. 23.

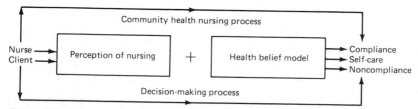

Figure 2-2   A suggested paradigm for community health nursing.

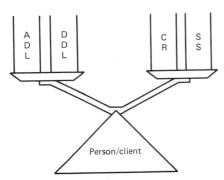

Figure 2-3 The Carnevali and Patrick definition of nursing suggests that the nurse's concern is with balancing the activities of daily living (ADL) and demands of daily living (DDL) on the one hand and coping resources (CR) and support systems (SS) on the other hand. (*From Carnevali and Patrick, 1979.*)

regarding nursing is concern for "man's need for self-care action and the provision and management of it on a continuous basis in order to sustain life and health, recover from disease or injury, and cope with their effects."[9] The nurse's special interest is providing continuing therapeutic care which the client requires.[10] From Orem's perspective, the nursing focus takes into account both the medical point of view and the client's point of view. Kinlein moves away from the medical model which considers the nurse as an extension of medicine, and structures the nurse in direct primary contact with the client when the client feels the need for a nurse. Following the establishment of a nurse-client relationship, the nurse helps the client recognize and express needs regarding health status and goals, then the nurse and client together determine how the needs can be managed best. The context of Kinlein's approach is feasible for community health nurses particularly when they work with clients utilizing preventive and/or health promotion measures in community and home settings.

Another perspective of nursing has been developed by Carnevali and Patrick which states, "Nursing's primary focus to be that of helping the individual and his family to manage the activities and demands of daily living as these affect and are affected by health and illness, at the same time taking into account the individual's lifestyle." This definition of nursing suggests that the nurse's concern is with balancing the activities and demands of daily living on the one hand and coping resources and support systems on the other, since each of these aspects is influenced by health, illness, and associated experiences.[11] The visualization of this perspective is shown in Fig. 2-3.

The following terms are central to Carnevali and Patrick's definition of nursing (see Fig. 2-3).

Activities of daily living (ADL) are the usual events and behaviors engaged in by the individual during the course of the 24-hour day.

Demands of daily living (DDL) are personal expectations derived from the self or others and which determine personal priorities, choices, routines, and pace. They may suggest areas of discomfort if disruption occurs, the explicit or implicit personal

[9]Dorothea E. Orem, *Nursing: Concepts of Practice,* 2d ed., McGraw-Hill Book Company, New York, 1980, pp. 1–2.

[10]Ibid., p. 49.

[11]Doris L. Carnevali and Maxine Patrick, *Nursing Management for the Elderly,* J. B. Lippincott Company, Philadelphia, 1979, p. 7.

"shoulds." This includes expectations of compliance with prescribed medical or health care regimens.

Coping resources (CR) are personal capabilities (i.e., strength, endurance, knowledge, desire, sensory capability, courage, creativity, problem-solving ability, and past coping patterns). These are the intrapersonal resources that enable the individual to manage to some degree the challenges to the individual's lifestyle.

Support systems (SS) are external environmental and personal forces that sustain and maintain the individual in a preferred or required lifestyle, such as family and important others, equipment, architecture, supplies, housing, neighborhood, stores, finances, transportation, ecologic environment, and laws.

Lifestyle (LS) is the totality of an individual's approach to living, often evidenced by preferences, pattern, and pace in daily living and use of resources or support systems. It incorporates such characteristics as preferences for independence vs. dependence, high vs. low stress levels, spontaneity and change vs. structure and regularity, extroversion vs. introversion, rapid vs. slow pace, and high vs. low physical activity. These preferences are translated into observable behaviors in approaching routine as well as unusual events.[12]

The model as shown in Fig. 2-3 presumes the person or client to be "in balance." Generally, most persons are out of balance to some degree and the scale is tipped due to multiple possible variables such as an unhealthy habit, acute stress for a given day, feelings of wellness or illness, etc. For the community health nurse, this perspective is useful for assessing and gathering the nursing database inclusive of subjective and objective data and identifying client problems in terms of the balance between activities and demands of daily living and available coping resources and support systems. An example of a housewife with four children is shown in Fig. 2-4. The ADL and DDL are such things as the demands of her husband for a smoothly operating and clean house and the demands of the children for transportation and money. This woman feels stressed and therefore complains, drinks large quantities of coffee, and smokes. She indicates no support from her husband and children and feels depressed as a consequence. The nursing judgment regarding the client's needs and problems specifies the nature of the coping deficits, the cause of the deficits, and the areas of impact on immediate or long-term patterns of living. In this case, the diagnosis can be stated as stress based on minimal support from family and/or stress based on current health hab-

[12] Ibid., p. 7.

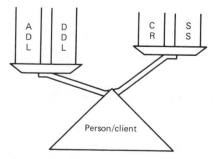

Figure 2-4 The Carnevali and Patrick model as it appears out of balance for a housewife with four children. The imbalance occurs between the activities of daily living (ADL) and the demands of daily living (DDL) on the one hand and coping resources (CR) and support systems (SS) on the other. (*From Carnevali and Patrick, 1979.*)

its. The nursing plan and implementation would involve making adjustments in any or all four of the areas based on the client's willingness to act. In the example given, the focus of the plan might be initiated by (1) building the client's internal coping resources (e.g., by assisting the client with time management techniques, or developing the client's perceptions of her own innate strengths and capabilities); or (2) exploring the status of external resources or support systems (e.g., scheduling a family conference with husband and children, or referring the client to specific professional services such as a stop-smoking clinic). The initial concern of the nurse would be directed toward getting the client into a better balance which would involve shifting and adjusting the weight more equitably from ADL and DDL to CR and SS. As changes would occur, even though minute, evaluation of the changes would lead to new plans which could be instituted as feasible with the client. For the community health nurse using this model, the idea of a better-balanced scale and the factors contributing toward keeping it in relative balance are helpful in utilizing the nursing process for the management of client concerns.

A succinct definition of nursing was endorsed by the American Nurses Association (ANA) in December 1980. It says, "Nursing is the diagnosis and treatment of human responses to actual or potential health problems." The human responses that nurses treat are "often multiple, episodic or continuous, fluid and varying, and are less discrete or circumscribed than medical diagnostic categories."[13] The scope-of-practice policy statement delineates four characteristics of nursing: phenomena, theory application, nursing action, and evaluation of effects of action. These terms closely correspond to the steps of the nursing process (data collection and/or assessing, planning, treatment and/or implementing, and evaluation). As explained in the policy statement, the core of nursing practice is the basis for nursing care—the "phenomena" of human response to actual or potential health problems. Through observation and diagnosis, nurses identify and treat such responses as "self-care limitations . . . pain and discomfort . . . impaired functioning in areas as sleep, rest, activity, circulation, nutrition, etc." (See Nursing Diagnosis, Chap. 6). Nursing practice is described as having boundaries that expand in response to changing needs, dimensions which encompass settings for practice and other distinguishing characteristics such as a humanistic philosophy, a high regard for self-determination, accountability, etc., intersections with other health professions that are not hard and fast lines, and a core (the phenomena of human response). Study of the scope-of-practice policy statement is encouraged since it represents an official and national endorsement of nursing as it is recommended to be practiced universally. Copies of the text, *Nursing: A Social Policy Statement,* can be ordered from the ANA, Kansas City, Missouri.

Perception of Nursing Whichever definition of nursing is internalized by the nurse, this is conveyed to a client by the nurse's words, actions, and manner. It is important for the nurse to have and be able to articulate a conscious conviction about nursing. It is equally important to elicit the client's perception of nursing. If the two

---

[13] American Nurses' Association, "Scope of Nursing Policy Statement Issued by ANA," 81(2): 263–300, February 1981.

viewpoints are divergent, communication is apt to be dysfunctional or nonproductive. The client who sees the nurse primarily as an extension of the medical model will have a different perception of her or his own health concerns and situations than the nurse with the professional attitude of an independent agent dealing with health concerns. Both client and nurse will have individual perceptions of reality and each will act accordingly. For example, if the nurse presumes to offer suggestions regarding a health concern which is not necessarily in accordance with the client's physician's views, the client may respond negatively. The nurse will react with distress and/or bewilderment when it becomes apparent that the suggestions were unacceptable. Eliciting the client's perceptions of nursing will facilitate sharing of ideas and raising the client's consciousness regarding the position of nursing as a helping profession. As the nurse's and client's perceptions of nursing come closer to congruency, there will be a supportive basis for future action.

A Practice Theory: The Health Belief Model

A variety of practice theories can be utilized effectively by community health nurses as they interact with clients in community and home settings. A description of the health belief model (HBM) (see Fig. 2-5), which is a partially developed theory, is included in the paradigm for community health nurses because of its great potential for equipping nurses with improved strategies for change and efficacious health guidance.

The HBM evolved from a psychological theory of decision making attributed to Lewin. Lewin and his associates hypothesized that behavior depends mainly on two

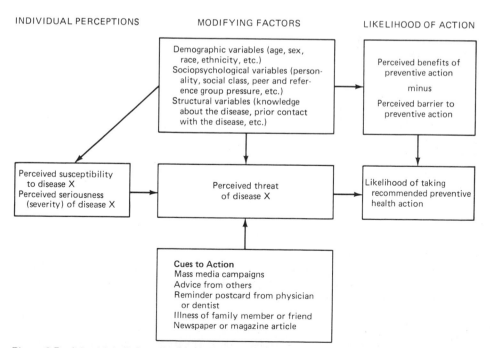

Figure 2-5 A health belief model. (*From Becker, 1974.*)

variables: (1) the value placed by an individual on a particular outcome, and (2) the individual's estimate of the likelihood that a given action will result in that outcome.[14] Hochbaum, Leventhal, Kegeles, and Rosenstock formulated the HBM to assist in the explanation of preventive health behavior. The HBM "analyzes an individual's motivation to act as a function of the expectancy of goal attainment in the area of health behavior."[15] The model assumes that "motivation is a necessary condition for action and that motives selectively determine an individual's perceptions of the environment."[16]

Considerable research has been done regarding the utilization of the HBM to explain health behavior, illness behavior, and sick-role behavior. *Health behavior*[17] as defined by Kasl and Cobb is "any activity undertaken by a person who believes himself to be healthy for the purpose of preventing disease or detecting disease in an asymptomatic stage." *Illness behavior* is "any activity undertaken by a person who feels ill, for the purpose of defining the state of his health and of discovering suitable remedy." *Sick-role behavior* is "the activity undertaken by those who consider themselves ill, for the purpose of getting well." The HBM gives a useful perspective with all behaviors but as yet needs much more study and refinement. The model has great educational potential for community health nurses as they deal with the wide range of health issues existing in community settings. Application of the model when dealing with health behavior, illness behavior, or sick-role behavior assists the nurse in gaining useful data and determining creative, individual, and germane strategies for change.

Variables of the HBM The original conception underlying the HBM was of an "individual existing in a life space composed of regions some of which were positively valued (positive valence), others of which were negatively valued (negative valence), and still others of which were relatively neutral."[18] One's daily activities were seen as a process of being pulled by positive forces and repelled by negative forces. For example, the person who has a deep fear of contracting lung cancer will be repelled by forces (such as cigarette smoking) that are believed to contribute to contracting that disease, and will respond to positive forces such as sitting in no-smoking areas at public places, requesting smokers to put out their cigarettes, etc. All persons have negative, positive, and neutral valences in their life space and live their lives responding to these valences in individually characteristic ways.

The HBM was developed on the idea that to avoid a disease an individual would need to believe three things.

1 A personal *susceptibility* to the disease is present.
2 The occurrence of the disease would have at least moderate *severity* on some component of the individual's life.

[14]Lois A. Maiman and Marshall H. Becker, "The Health Belief Model: Origins and Correlates in Psychological Theory," in Marshall H. Becker (ed.), *The Health Belief Model and Personal Health Behavior*, Charles B. Slack, Inc., Thorofare, N.J., 1974, p. 9.
[15]Ibid., p. 21.
[16]Ibid., p. 22.
[17]Stanislav V. Kasl and Sidney Cobb, "Health Behavior, Illness Behavior, and Sick-Role Behavior," *Archives of Environmental Health*, 12:246, February 1966.
[18]Irwin M. Rosenstock, "Historical Origins of the Health Belief Model," in Marshall H. Becker (ed.), *The Health Belief Model and Personal Health Behavior*, Charles B. Slack, Inc., Thorofare, N.J., 1974, pp. 2–3.

3 Taking a particular action would in fact be *beneficial* by reducing susceptibility to the condition. If the disease were present, the benefit could occur by the reduction of the disease's severity. In either case, the particular beneficial action should not entail overcoming important psychological *barriers* such as cost, convenience, pain, and embarrassment.[19]

Perceived Susceptibility Susceptibility refers to the subjective risks of contracting a condition. The response of the individual to a perceived risk can be denial, admittance of a statistical possibility, or a sense of real danger.

Perceived Seriousness Perceived severity of a health condition is often linked to an individual's knowledge about the condition and its possible consequences. Implications of severity range from an emotional response to concern regarding possible restrictions affecting self, employment, family life, and social relations.

Perceived Benefits of Taking Action A person's behavior is thought to depend on how the various beneficial alternatives are believed to be feasible, acceptable, and/or desirable. "The person's beliefs about the availability and effectiveness of various courses of action, and *not* the objective facts about the effectiveness of action, determine what course he will take."[20] In addition, the norms and pressures of social groups influence individual behavior.

Perceived Barriers to Taking Action Barriers to action can be attitudes, unpleasant alternatives, or negative forces that produce conflict within the individual and thereby influence actions. For example, an individual may perceive cigarette smoking as an action that will increase the threat of disease, i.e., lung cancer or emphysema, but believe the action of giving up smoking to be too inconvenient, unpleasant, painful, or upsetting. Negative aspects of a health action serve as barriers to action and affect readiness to act. Expense of a given action is an additional and realistic barrier for many clients, and interventions seeking to remedy costs can be effective strategies for eliminating this barrier.

Cues to Action Factors that serve as cues or triggers toward appropriate action are usually necessary before clients are motivated to act overtly. Instigating events or cues can be internal (e.g., imagining a body part as disfigured), or external (e.g., visiting a terminally ill family member). The intensity and timing of appropriate cues with specific clients are variables that need further testing.

Other Variables[21] Demographic variables (age, sex, race, ethnicity), psychosocial variables (social class, personality, social group pressures), and structural variables (knowledge about health conditions, previous contacts with individuals having a disease), are variables of importance to the community health nurse. Consideration of these variables is useful when ascertaining risk factors, determining individual perceptions and perceived benefits of particular actions, and eliciting data pertinent to specified health concerns.

The HBM as a theoretical model has particular relevance for community health nurses as they interact with sick or well clients. The HBM is helpful when utilizing the nursing process to gain information about client perceptions of health providers, health services, existing health concerns, and outcomes believed achievable. As data are gath-

[19] Ibid., p. 3.
[20] Ibid., p. 4.
[21] Ibid., p. 7. (See model of HBM.)

ered based on the variables of the HBM, nurses are equipped to help clients make decisions that are appropriate and feasible for each situation under study and lead to outcomes considered satisfactory. In influencing behavior, nurses must recognize the limits of each client's cognition, motivation, and possible action.[22] This entails eliciting the client's beliefs, opinions, and factual knowledge in relation to health needs, health goals, and overall values. To create a positive motivational structure within the client, a proposed action must be seen as a feasible means for reaching the particular goal. To create the action structure, specific actions must be defined which demand definite decisions before the situation can be altered or modified.

Decision-Making Process

The decision-making process is similar to steps used in problem solving. A judgment is made regarding an existing state of affairs or health concern. The judgment influences the action that results from the decision. Action is implicit in a decision. The decision-making process is made up of the following steps:

1 Recognition, definition, and limitation of a problem
2 Analysis and evaluation of the problem leading to potential courses of action and possible outcomes or consequences
3 Establishment of criteria or rules by which a solution will be evaluated or judged as acceptable and adequate
4 Formulation and selection of the preferred solution
5 Implementation of the preferred solution
6 Evaluation of the results in terms of achievement of satisfactory or unsatisfactory outcomes.[23]

In assisting clients with the decision-making process the nurse must (1) be sensitive to the client's perceptions, values and beliefs, and demographic, psychosocial, and structural variables; (2) be creative and flexible in exploring and discussing all possible alternatives for action or health guidance; (3) accept and facilitate the client's decisions even if the choices do not appear to be the wisest; and (4) evaluate outcomes fairly and objectively with the client. In Chap. 3 a pencil and paper tool called the decision tree is described which nurses can use as a visual aid. Choices, risks, objectives, monetary gain, and information, can be outlined and clarified for clients as they ponder all aspects involved in making complex decisions.

Compliance

As it is commonly used by health professionals, the word *compliance* means the extent to which a client's behavior coincides with a therapeutic plan.[24] It is the wish of all health providers that clients will comply 100 percent with treatment plans designed to improve their health status. For compliance to be actuated, the client must understand

---

[22] Dorwin Cartwright, "Some Principles of Mass Persuasion," *Human Relations,* 2:253, 1949.
[23] Daniel E. Griffiths, *Administrative Theory,* Prentice-Hall, Inc., Englewood Cliffs, N.J., 1959, p. 95.
[24] David Sackett and R. Brian Haynes, *Compliance with Therapeutic Regimens,* Johns Hopkins University Press, Baltimore, Md., 1976.

the purpose of the therapeutic plan, believe in the efficacy of the plan, be aware of consequences or side effects that may occur when the plan is carried out properly or when it is not followed faithfully, and have the abilities required for adhering to the plan. All too often, when compliance is not complete, one of the above factors has been omitted or not properly interpreted for the client. However, client compliance is much more complex than just gaining acceptable adherence to a therapeutic plan. Weintraub[25] uses the term *capricious compliance* to describe a common problem during which clients as a matter of convenience follow a therapeutic plan based on their varying daily activities and individual schedules. A client might forget, be unable to follow a complicated regimen due to other social pressures of the day, or substitute "reasonable" alternative methods for the treatment plan. Clients are not customarily disobedient, they just like to assume a degree of autonomy in matters relating to themselves and their health. If nurses accept the belief that clients can assume responsibility for promoting certain aspects of their health status, they are less likely to urge complete obedience to therapeutic regimes. It's not therapeutic to command, "Do as I say and don't ask questions!" The nurse should realize that education is a significant correlate of good health and should thereby teach clients the necessary information required for optimizing health practices. Every capable person has the right and responsibility for self-care or to exercise a choice in the maintenance of life and health.

Self-Care

Self-care as defined by Levin is a "process whereby a layperson functions on his/her own behalf in health promotion and prevention and in disease detection and treatment at the level of the primary health resource in the health care system."[26] Self-care connotes that it is a voluntary, self-limited, nonorganized, universal activity. Self-care can be viewed "as a decision-making process which involves self-observation, symptom perception and labeling, judgment of severity, and choice and assessment of treatment options."[27] As described by Powers and Ford,[28] most clients are capable of recognizing when they need help to remain healthy, or identifying symptoms indicative of illness before independently seeking professional services. Before taking action, clients often will discuss their concerns with a variety of resources (friends, spouse, others) before making an appointment with a health provider. They maintain control of their life and affairs and are self-directive until they reach the health provider's office and submit to an examination of their body. At that point the health provider assumes control, and the client becomes participant-observer of the assessment, diagnostic, and treatment processes.

Survival in today's society provides a motivational basis for purposeful self-care. The growing holistic health care movement, which advocates optimal health and well-

[25]Michael Weintraub, "Intelligent Noncompliance and Capricious Compliance," in Louis Lasagna (ed.), *Patient Compliance,* Futura Publishing Co., New York, 1976, p. 44.

[26]Lowell S. Levin, Alfred H. Katz, and Erik Holst, *Self-Care: Lay Initiatives in Health,* Prodist, New York, 1976, p. 11.

[27]Ibid., p. 11.

[28]Marjorie J. Powers and Loretta C. Ford, "The Best Kept Secret: Consumer Power and Nursing's Potential," in Louis Lasagna (ed.), *Patient Compliance,* Futura Publishing Co., New York, 1976, pp. 53–54.

ness for all individuals, is based on the following premises:

1 That every client who comes for care is understood and treated as a whole person within her or his total environment. This includes tailoring of treatment to meet the genetic, biological, psychosocial, cultural, and familial needs of each individual.

2 That every client is an active partner in achieving an improved health status and is responsible for her or his own health.[29]

By responding positively to the self-care movement, nurses have a unique educational opportunity to assist clients in attaining higher levels of health. They can engage in self-care education. Its goals are derived from the learner's perceived needs and preferences, the desired outcomes based on the learner's decision as to which risks to avoid, and the content that is determined and evaluated in terms of the learner's own criteria.[30] Self-care encourages autonomy in matters relating to the client's health. Attributes which must be considered by the nurse to determine each client's ability to engage in self-care during the time of need include state of growth and development, age, self-image, social roles, capacity for engaging in self-care, and capability for learning.[31] After assessing the requirements of a given situation, the nurse must often synthesize or unify a variety of care elements into a process of self-care for the client. As pointed out by Orem, positively therapeutic self-care "helps to sustain life processes, maintains integrated functioning, promotes normal growth and development, and prevents or controls disease and disability and their effects."[32] The nursing focus is directed toward assisting clients to achieve health results they have defined and decided to be worth attaining. Community health nursing is one field of nursing that is particularly qualified to promote self-care as a desirable requirement for every responsible person.

Noncompliance

Noncompliance occurs when a client refuses to accept a therapeutic plan. The refusal may be based on lack of knowledge or understanding, conflict with cultural beliefs and values, negative and overruling personal forces, inconvenience, expense, deep-seated fears, and a variety of other reasons. The client may indicate no intention of compliance or may seemingly accept the treatment plan in words and behavior, but does not subsequently engage in self-care or therapeutic treatment practices as advised. When noncompliance occurs, the nurse must attempt to elicit data that may explain the noncompliant behavior. Reasons for noncompliance are often valid and reasonable ones. If reasons are not valid or reasonable after the client has been made as knowledgeable as possible regarding the situation, the client still retains the right to make decisions regarding the state of health.

---

[29] James S. Gordon, "Holistic Medicine: Introduction and Overview," *Holistic Medicine*, Institute of Noetic Sciences, San Francisco, 1979.

[30] Lowell S. Levin, "Patient Education and Self-Care: How Do They Differ?" *Nursing Outlook*, 26:170–175, March 1978.

[31] The Nursing Development Conference Group, *Concept Formalization in Nursing: Process and Product*, Little, Brown and Company, Boston, 1973, p. 166.

[32] Orem, op. cit., p. 41.

CASE STUDY

Laura is a nursing student assigned to work with a family for 2 months. Initial information about the family after one visit is as follows. Betty is a 22-year-old single parent of two daughters. She is overweight and talkative, and her only income is through welfare. Her 2-year-old daughter Joy is in the process of being toilet trained. Betty's 5-month-old daughter Pam has cradle cap, diaper rash, and symptoms of circulatory problems.

Regarding the home environment, Laura said, "It was difficult to be nonjudgmental in the face of such filthy living conditions. It really hit home that I value cleanliness as being next to healthiness. I wanted to jump right in and say, 'Clean up your act and your kids and you might be healthier for it!'"

Needs and/or problems as assessed by Laura:

Poor hygiene practiced in the home.
Follow up on potential circulatory problems of Pam.
Reinforcement of toilet training techniques for Joy.
Growth and Development education.
Betty has a tendency to procrastinate in all behaviors.

Needs and/or problems as stated by mother, Betty:

Need for transportation to well child clinic.
Need for job—would like to be a salesperson.

Weekly visits were made during which Laura listened nonjudgmentally to Betty, gave special attention to Joy and Pam, and consciously praised any behavior or suggested potential behaviors that she saw as contributing toward better health practices. In the course of the visits, she learned that the children were immunized and visited the well child clinic regularly. Laura screened both, using the Denver Developmental Screening Tool and found them to be within the normal developmental profiles for their ages. The nurse learned that Betty was an intelligent woman, was not a high school graduate, had married an alcoholic husband, had her tubes tied after Pam's birth, and had a boyfriend. Inasmuch as possible, the nurse was supportive of Betty's expressed ideas, provided they were based on sound health principles. Since Betty expressed a need for transportation, the nurse made a contract with her to call a local voluntary resource whenever she had a need for transportation.

On every visit the nurse held Pam, inspected her feet and hands, which were always cold, wrapped her up more warmly, and expressed concern regarding a possible circulatory problem. Betty stated that this condition was common in her family history. As the nurse-client relationship progressed, small changes began to become apparent. Pam's cradle cap and diaper rash gradually disappeared and Joy's toilet training progressed more smoothly.

Laura found the home to be smelly and offensive, and after careful thought said to Betty, "Does it ever bother you to have to walk around animal feces on the floor?" On subsequent visits, the cat was found to be litter trained and the housekeeping had improved perceptibly.

At long last, Betty was induced to take Pam to a local physician who made the diagnosis of acrocyanosis. No treatment was instituted but encouragement was given to watch the circulatory condition closely.

Before the nurse terminated her visits, Betty had been persuaded to take graduate equivalency tests in lieu of completing high school. Betty had excellent potential to pursue a goal of finding a job.

QUESTIONS

1 How was the nurse perceived by the mother, Betty?
2 In what ways did the nurse communicate the essence of nursing to Betty?
3 Did Betty perceive Pam's possible circulatory problems to be serious?
4 Did the nurse perceive Pam's possible circulatory problems to be serious?
5 What were the perceived benefits for Pam if a visit to a physician were arranged?
6 What were the barriers preventing a visit to a physician?
7 In your opinion, what motivated the mother to take Pam to the physician?
8 Were any other practice theories used by the nurse while visiting this family?
9 Would you judge this mother to be compliant, noncompliant, or utilizing self-care options?

SUMMARY

A model for community health nursing practice is developed in this chapter based on the client and nurse sharing their perceptions of the role of nursing preparatory to the initiation of nursing actions. The use of theories is recommended to provide a rational and systematic view of each client situation and to serve as a guide for determining appropriate and feasible nursing actions. The health belief model is suggested as a theory having great potential for equipping nurses with effective strategies for change. The decision-making process experienced by clients determine whether they will comply, not comply, or modify treatment options based on their capability for self-care. This model exists in every transaction between nurse and client whether it is explicit or implicit. A case study providing exploration of the model is described.

SUGGESTED READING

Aguilera, Donna C., and Janice M. Messick: *Crisis Intervention, Theory and Methodology,* 3rd ed., The C. V. Mosby Company, St. Louis, 1978.

Bakker, Cornelis B., and Marianne K. Bakker-Rabdau: *No Trespassing!,* Chandler & Sharp Publishers, Inc., San Francisco, 1973.

Becker, Marshall H. (ed): *The Health Belief Model and Personal Health Behavior,* Charles B. Slack, Inc., Thorofare, New Jersey, 1974.

Bevis, Em Olivia: *Curriculum Building in Nursing,* The C. V. Mosby Company, St. Louis, 1973.

Carnevali, Doris L., and Maxine Patrick, *Nursing Management for the Elderly,* J. B. Lippincott Company, Philadelphia, 1979.

Dunn, Halbert L., *High Level Wellness,* R. W. Beatty Co., Arlington, Virginia, 1961.

Duvall, Evelyn Millis: *Family Development,* J. B. Lippincott Company, Philadelphia, 1962.

Erikson, Erik H.: *Childhood and Society,* W. W. Norton & Company, Inc., New York, 1950.

Festinger, Leon: "Cognitive Dissonance," *Scientific American,* October 1962.

Glasser, William: *Reality Therapy,* Harper & Row, Publishers Inc., New York, 1965.
Gordon, Thomas: *Parent Effectiveness Training,* Peter H. Wyden, Inc., Publisher, New York, 1970.
Hardy, Margaret E., and Mary E. Conway: *Role Theory, Perspectives For Health Professionals,* Appleton-Century-Crofts, New York, 1978.
Harris, Thomas A.: *I'm OK–You're OK,* Harper & Row, Publishers, Inc., New York, 1969.
Holmes, Thomas H.: "The Social Readjustment Rating Scale," *Journal of Psychosomatic Research,* **11**:213–218, 1967.
Jourard, Sidney M.: *The Transparent Self,* D. Van Nostrand Company, Inc., Princeton, N.J., 1971.
King, Imogene M.: *Toward a Theory for Nursing,* John Wiley & Sons, Inc., New York, 1971.
Kinlein, M. Lucille: *Independent Nursing Practice with Clients,* J. B. Lippincott Company, Philadelphia, 1977.
Kubler-Ross, Elisabeth: *On Death and Dying,* The Macmillan Company, New York, 1969.
Levin, Lowell S., Alfred H. Katz, and Erik Holst: *Self-Care: Lay Initiatives in Health,* Prodist, New York, 1976.
Maslow, Abraham H.: *Motivation and Personality,* Harper & Brothers, New York, 1954.
Orem, Dorothea E.: *Nursing: Concepts of Practice,* 2d ed., McGraw-Hill Book Company, New York, 1980.
Otto, Herbert A.: *Guide to Developing Your Potential,* Charles Scribner's Sons, New York, 1967.
Patterson, Gerald R., and M. Elizabeth Gullion: *Living with Children,* Research Press, Champaign, Ill., 1968.
Rogers, Carl R.: *On Becoming a Person,* Houghton Mifflin Company, Boston, 1961.
Satir, Virginia: *Conjoint Family Therapy,* Science and Behavior Books, Inc., Palo Alto, Calif., 1967.
Satir, Virginia: *Peoplemaking,* Science & Behavior Books, Inc., Palo Alto, Calif., 1972.
Stevens, Barbara J.: *Nursing Theory: Analysis, Application, Evaluation,* Little, Brown and Company, Boston, 1979.
Travis, John W.: *Wellness Workbook for Health Professionals,* Wellness Associates, Inc., Mill Valley, Calif., 1977.
Werner, Joanne R.: "Effective Community Health Nursing: A Framework for Actualizing Standards of Practice," *Nursing Forum,* **15**(3):265–276, 1976.
Williams, Carolyn A.: "Community Health Nursing–What Is It?" *Nursing Outlook,* **25**(4):250–254, April 1977.
Zimbardo, Philip, and Ebbe B. Ebbesen: *Influencing Attitudes and Changing Behavior,* Addison-Wesley Publishing Company, Inc., Reading, Mass., 1969.

Chapter 3

Starting Where the Consumer Is

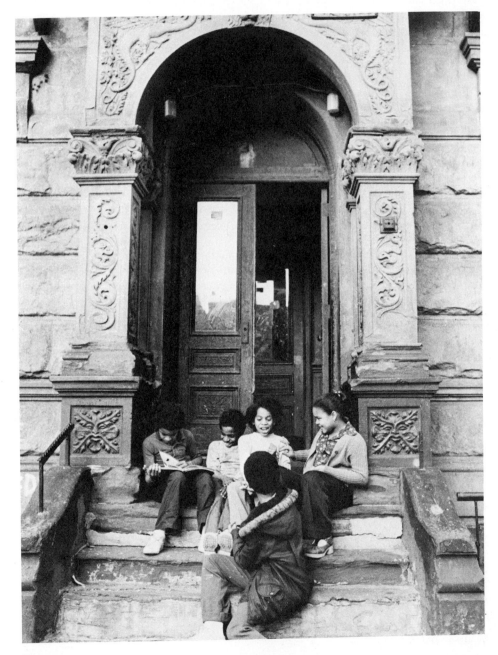

For the nurse beginning to practice community health nursing, the necessity for relating effectively and productively with others is known to be a crucial determinant for subsequent practice. Because of inner awareness of this knowledge, many nurses often approach the first families with high anxiety and attempt to practice the role of the community health nurse according to accurate or inaccurate preconceived ideas, past experiences with community health nurses, and expectations of proper professional nurse behavior. What happens thereafter is dependent upon the innate skills of the nurse and the behavior of the family receiving the visit.

The nurse must know *why* contact is being made with the family, and must be able to convey the purpose for the visit in words that the family can understand and accept and with behavior that is congruent with the explanation. Openness, honesty, and genuineness are essential. With an approach like this, the family is inclined to reciprocate with similar behavior. Because it is important to work *with* families, understand reciprocal verbal and nonverbal communications, and work toward goals which are agreed upon together, it is vital that the nurse initiate the relationship process in a way that the family member can accept and support.

SELF-IMAGE OF NURSING STUDENTS

Not all nursing students exhibit a self-image that strengthens, sustains, or promotes confidence. This may be attributed to an internal sense of inadequacy, based in part on distortions and misinterpretations of statements made to them regarding competence during the early phases of their nursing learning experiences. Consequently, many students behave more compliantly than is prudent for the role of professional nurse.

According to Douglas, Field, and Tarpey there are five types of images that an individual can have of self. They are

1 The real self
2 The ideal self
3 The self-image
4 The apparent self
5 The reference-group image[1]

When applying these images to the role of professional nurses, explanations of each image are described as follows: (1) The real self is the nursing student as an objective entity. This self is more nearly what that person is fundamentally, and the real self is never completely understood or observed. Contained within the real self are a person's basic physical and emotional requirements and characteristics. (2) The ideal self is what the nursing student would like to be. This self concerns the person's aspirations, strivings, and desire to do and be better. The ideal self is never fully achieved. A person always finds something new to strive for. (3) The self-image is how the nursing student sees self. It is a combination of the real self and ideal self, and it contains the person's understanding of self and one's aspirations. The self-image guides much of the nursing

[1]Douglas, John, Field, George A., and Tarpey, Lawrence X., *Human Behavior in Marketing*, Charles E. Merrill Publishing Company, Columbus, Ohio, 1967, pp. 64–67.

student's behavior. (4) The apparent self is how others see the nursing student. Mainly, what others see is some combination of the ideal self, the real self, and the self-image. The impressions that others hold of the nursing student have a direct bearing on social interactions. (5) The reference-group image is how the nursing student thinks others with whom she or he associates or identifies perceives the student. It is not the image others necessarily have, but the reference-group image is an important motivator, for we tend to behave as we think others want us to behave. Thus, the way we think others see us (namely, nursing instructors, or nursing mentors, or nursing friends) is important to our behavior.

In recognition of the motivational power of the reference-group image and ideal self-image, it is essential for reference-group members (namely peers and instructors) to encourage nursing students to acknowledge existing strengths and to demonstrate the potential latent strengths that each one possesses. As self-confidence increases, nursing students are better able to risk experimental behavior changes, perform as positive influences in their interaction with consumers, and behave as autonomous, self-assured, creative, professional nurses.

Talking and Listening

The spontaneously talkative nurse must be aware of the effect of verbosity on the client. If the constant output of words is repelling or elicits few responses from the client, the purpose of the encounter may be nullified. The gabby nurse needs to be able to control the talkativeness, be sensitive to dominating the dialogue, and maintain a discipline of self-articulation. On the other hand, the quiet nurse who finds it difficult to verbalize extensively is often a good listener and is therefore generally able to elicit responses from patients fairly easily. Difficulty arises when the client is another quiet person and the conversation is filled with frequent uncomfortable silences. The quiet nurse needs to be prepared with specific information to which the consumer may be responsive during a home visit and must particularly be able to talk when the conversation takes a lull and needs direction. Role playing or rehearsal of information giving before making the home visit may make the nurse feel more at ease during the actual visit. Learning to talk effectively is facilitated when the nurse is accepting of self, honest, spontaneously open to experiences, and does not hide behind the mask of being a quiet person.

Intelligent and effective listening takes conscious effort and is the key on which a successful interview is based. Listening to a client takes skill, which is best accomplished in a competent, professional, and friendly way. It denotes a voluntary effort to comprehend meanings and can be used in several ways. It can mean that (1) the nurse acts as a sounding board against which the client can ventilate and recognize feelings; (2) the nurse elaborates and expands the words the client has used and gives a sense of prestige and importance in exerting greater effort to clarify or crystallize meanings; (3) the nurse provides psychological support by listening to the client's feelings in relation to the problem, and the burden is lessened because the problem is shared; (4) the nurse creates an environment in which the client is comfortable in expressing thoughts; and (5) the nurse is willing to expend energy toward gaining greater understanding and empathy with the client.

A client's willingness to verbalize is highly dependent upon the nurse's response to what is said, and by sensitive listening the nurse plays a major role in facilitating recognition of the client's expressed needs. Wilson stated that it is desirable for nurses to do reflective listening and described it as a process that involves the listener's conscious or unconscious assessment and selection of clues from the auditory influx of data, the listener's interweaving and interconnecting of this data with her or his own existing psychic organization, and the resultant behavioral responses.[2] Reflective listening implies an integral *relation* between verbalization, listening, and response and promotes a creative, progressive relationship between nurse and client that is dependent on their mutual listening abilities. When both nurse and client experience feelings of satisfaction about their interactions, this implies cooperation and responsibility regarding the purpose of their exchange and provides impetus to strive toward accomplishment of their mutually set goals.

Friendliness and Professionalism

Many nurses feel a deep concern about their manifestation of professionalism. They wish to be open, honest, and genuine, but these attributes seem to conflict with their concept of professionalism. Nursing students report that they receive ambivalent messages from experienced nurses about the characteristics of professionalism. Can a professional nurse be a friendly nurse? Can the nurse reveal self as a personable being?

Not many years ago the professional nurse image purported to be organized, orderly, clean, courteous, and knowledgeable with a manner of crisp efficiency. The nurse never revealed any personal characteristics that would betray human weaknesses. This image tends to persist even though behavioral scientists currently encourage more openness, genuineness, and warmth.

To be involved in a helping relationship, Carl Rogers has set some penetrating questions upon which to reflect. They are:

1   Can I *be* in some way which will be perceived by the other person as trustworthy, as dependable or consistent in some deep sense?

2   Can I be expressive enough as a person that what I am will be communicated unambiguously?

3   Can I let myself experience positive attitudes toward this other person—attitudes of warmth, caring, liking, interest, respect?

4   Can I be strong enough as a person to be separate from the other?

5   Am I secure enough within myself to permit him his separateness?

6   Can I let myself enter fully into the world of his feelings and personal meanings and see these as he does?

7   Can I receive him as he is? Or can I only receive him conditionally, acceptant of some aspects of his feelings and silently or openly disapproving of other aspects?

8   Can I act with sufficient sensitivity in the relationship that my behavior will not be perceived as a threat?

---

[2] Lucille M. Wilson, "Listening," in Carolyn E. Carlson (ed.), *Behavioral Concepts and Nursing Intervention,* J. B. Lippincott Company, Philadelphia, 1970, pp. 153-168.

9 Can I free him from the threat of external evaluation?

10 Can I meet this other individual as a person who is in process of *becoming,* or will I be bound by his past and by my past?[3]

By internalizing these questions and using them as a guide for behavior with the client, the nurse is less apt to hide behind a mask of "professional" helpfulness and is more inclined to be genuine and honest with the client. The nurse should be comfortable about revealing significant personal thoughts and feelings and sharing past experiences when a disclosure seems purposeful and has potential meaning for the client.

In a nutshell, the friendly nurse also can be the professional nurse. The friendly nurse is preferred by most consumers. The difference between a purely friendly and a professional relationship is that the professional is purposeful and goal-directed in behavior with the client, whereas the friend responds to interactions spontaneously and with no particular intent to change behavior.

Well and Sick Clients

Since most nurses are perceived as persons who work mainly with sick clients, an initial difficulty for some beginning community health nurses is to relate with well persons as the focus of their attention. They may be accustomed to working with clients who are sick enough to be bedridden or who are in the process of being rehabilitated to activities of daily living. Such clients have the advantage of a diagnosis and a prognosis, and the nurse feels comfortable in the role of care giver. However, many of the consumers of health services in community nursing are well persons who are coping in their own way with the conditions of their world. The community health nurse is an intervener who becomes acquainted and offers services in an effort to improve their health status. They may recognize a need for improved health but are not always cognizant of the role that a community health nurse can play in assisting them. This fact requires the nurse to interpret and communicate to the consumer a special ability to relate, to give services purposefully and in a nonthreatening manner, and in so doing, to imply that the coping measures of the consumer will be greatly enhanced by the nurse's intervention and will be more effectively adaptable to ever-changing daily tasks.

To elaborate, all human beings experience some degree of tension daily and have individual ways of coping with stress, which they regard as perfectly normal or as their own idiosyncrasies. In an effort to maintain balance or order in their lives, they make use of coping measures which have been satisfying to them in the past, such as chewing gum, cursing, taking a long walk, and other common activities which help to release excess energy. However, when equilibrium is not achieved at a particular time and tensions seem to mount, as evidenced by exaggerated or irritated reactions to minor daily events, coping devices inevitably become more pronounced and are less effective in alleviating stress, and a state of emergency or crisis ensues. It is at this strategic time that the nurse intervener can most effectively initiate a helping relationship. Jones cited the case history of a woman who was pregnant, had marital problems, an alcoholic husband, and little money. The client was coping with her problems by feeling

---

[3]Carl R. Rogers, *On Becoming a Person,* Houghton Mifflin Company, Boston, 1961, pp. 50–55.

discouraged, eating quantities of bread and jam, and constantly criticizing her husband. The nurse on early acquaintance was responsive to the client's concerns, listened to the description of her worries with sensitivity, and by means of discussion, encouraged ideas or activities that the client could try that she had not considered or attempted previously. As a result of the progressively supportive nature of the relationship between the client and nurse, changes occurred within the family because the client voluntarily started to try new methods of coping, such as dieting and attempting to praise her husband instead of nagging him. As the client noticed subtle, perceptible improvements within her household, her self-confidence gradually returned and her eagerness to try more and more measures to alleviate trying conditions within the home was accentuated. She reported her accomplishments to the nurse with satisfaction and pleasure.[4]

Positive Presentation of Self

In community health nursing the nurse sometimes recognizes that she or he may be mistakenly received as a salesperson at the door. To counteract such an impression the nurse launches into a personal introduction, provides the name of the agency represented, and gives a purpose for visiting. At the same time, if the visit is the first one to the family, the nurse presents the most favorable and convincing appearance possible in order to gain entrance into the home. Because of the initial need to "sell" self and services, the nurse must be conscious of personality style, approach, strengths, and limitations. The nurse must also be aware of behavior on an initial visit if anxious and uncomfortable, so that accurate evaluations of nurse-client interactions later can be studied alone or with the help of a consultant or supervisor. The nurse can increase awareness of personal style by attempting to objectively view the self as a third party by writing process recordings of interactions with clients, by listening to self and client on a tape recorder, or by use of videotapes if they are available. Preceding a home visit an anticipated situation can be role-played with other nurses or with the supervisor, or following a home visit, a description of an actual situation can be reenacted with the nurse playing either the role of self or of the client. New insights are often gained through role playing or psychodrama because the enactment of a role not only causes words to be spoken but actual physical sensations to be felt that are autonomous to the situation. Another effective method of increasing self-understanding is to role-play yourself in a given situation with another person, followed by a reversal of roles. Observing another person playing your role according to their perception of your behavior can be illuminating and clarifying.

In a study of community health nurses interacting with patients, Mayers found that each nurse had a basic, generally unchanging, interactional style. In other words, if the nurse was inclined to be a nondirective listener, that style was used in every client situation. If the nurse was directive, that style was also consistent. Of importance about this finding is the fact that each nurse has an individualistic consistent style.[5]

[4]Mary C. Jones, "An Analysis of a Family Folder," *Nursing Outlook,* 16:48–51, December 1968.

[5]Marlene Mayers, "Home Visit–Ritual or Therapy?" *Nursing Outlook,* 21:328–331, May 1973.

However, how many nurses have an accurate perception of their own interaction style? Many tend to avoid conscious appraisal of themselves as an act of humbleness or avoidance of knowing. Many intellectually explain how they come across to others, based on their *intended* messages. However, most individuals dislike hearing their own voice on a tape recorder when they first listen or seeing their body language by means of videotape. Consequently, their interactional style can be quite different from what they believe it to be. Learning about your own interactional style *accurately* and *objectively* is sometimes jolting and difficult; however, it must be done, and as a nurse you must learn to accept your voice, your appearance, and your behavior. Accurate feedback is gained from tape recordings, videotapes, and honest feedback from others.

Another important finding from Mayers's study was the high correlation of client-focused interactions with positive client response. In other words, nurses who were client-focused communicated a sense of concern and caring, followed up on client cues, and consequently had more successful interactions—regardless of their individualistic style. Nurses who were nurse-focused were more inclined to react to client's cues from their own perspective, act upon their own idea of solutions without consulting the client, and seemed less involved with the client's situation.[6]

It is possible for all nurses to be client-focused and learn to interact therapeutically, even though individual styles vary. To be client-focused requires the desire to be so, the ability to listen and observe sensitively and accurately, and the initiative to follow up on verbal and nonverbal cues coming from the client.

THERAPEUTIC RELATIONSHIP SKILLS

When the nurse meets a family for the first time, a relationship is initiated which has the possibility for moving in any number of directions. A nurse who is offering skills to help the family with a health problem wants the relationship to be a therapeutic one. Initially, as two people interact, they work out together what type of communicative behavior will take place in their relationship. From all the possible messages given to each other, they select which messages are acceptable or unacceptable. The cues for acceptability or unacceptability are given verbally or by nonverbal behavior. In this way they reach a mutual definition of the relationship. For example, on making a home visit and meeting a mother with a young baby for the first time, the nurse may enter the living room of the home and say, "That is a beautiful flower arrangement. Did you do it?" The mother may respond with pleasure and the conversation will focus on flowers temporarily. Later in the interview, the family cat may choose to jump on the nurse's lap, whereupon the nurse reacts with horror and pushes the cat away. The look of displeasure on the mother's face will be a cue to the nurse that the behavior with the cat was unacceptable. By being observant of all cues and initiating different subjects for discussion, the nurse and client consciously and indirectly agree on limits within which the relationship can be developed.

In order for any relationship to be successful, Truax and Carkhuff state that three characteristics are essential for the therapist to possess. These are accurate empathy,

---

[6] Ibid., p. 331.

nonpossessive warmth, and genuineness.[7] To be facilitative toward another human being requires that the therapist be deeply sensitive to the other's moment-to-moment experience, grasping both the core meaning and significance and the content of experiences and feelings. To understand empathically means that the therapist must have some warmth and respect for the other person. This is best expressed by being "real" or truly genuine with the other person. To be *genuine* means to be honest and open, to meet the other person without defensiveness or without playing a role that is "phony." Nonpossessive warmth is of central importance to any trusting relationship. The warm person has a sense of liking people and practices a friendly interest and acceptance of the other, regardless of differences or appearances. The quality of being nonjudgmental is of vital importance and has to be constantly exercised before it becomes a natural aptitude. To have a truly empathic understanding of another person, warmth, respect, trust, and even love for that person must be mutually communicated.[8] It is caring deeply about what is happening and what might happen to that person. It is at this point that a therapeutic relationship is established and the growth of the client begins to take place. The development of a therapeutic relationship takes time and several contacts; it does not happen immediately.

Rapport and Therapeutic Relationship

Rapport can happen immediately between two persons, but not necessarily between all persons. Rapport is a process, a happening, an experience undergone simultaneously by the nurse and client. It is composed of a cluster of interrelated thoughts and feelings which are transmitted and communicated to each other. The nurse and client remain separate and distinct human beings who share a series of mutually significant experiences.[9] Both are involved. They perceive each other and relate as human being to human being, instead of as nurse to client. For example, when two people's eyes meet and something "clicks," it often means a good rapport in which meanings of words are understood, enthusiasm is transmitted, and a mutual warmth of liking for each other occurs. Humor is shared and all behavior is accepted at face value. However, if two people meet, are courteous to each other, listen attentively and politely to all words spoken, but nothing is communicated when the eyes meet, this represents a pleasant acceptance but not necessarily a rapport. Because there are individuals in the community who have had little opportunity to experience moments of relatedness, it is particularly vital for the community health nurse, if possible, to facilitate the vivid awakening of a meaningful human-to-human encounter with specified clients. Rapport is a dynamic process and is developed with consecutive contacts and interactions, which lead eventually to a therapeutic relationship.

The therapeutic relationship may be developed slowly or rapidly, depending on the circumstances of the nurse-client situation. The nurse facilitates the development

---

[7]Charles B. Truax and Robert R. Carkhuff, *Toward Effective Counseling and Psychotherapy,* Aldine Publishing Company, 1967, p. 25.

[8]Ibid., p. 32.

[9]Joyce Travelbee, *Interpersonal Aspects of Nursing,* F. A. Davis Company, Philadelphia, 1966, pp. 155–156.

of trust by being warm, open, honest, genuine, and flexible, and by creating an atmosphere in which the client feels free to express feelings, whether positive or negative. The nurse actively tries to understand why the client feels as he or she does and assists in developing personal understanding. Listening must be done keenly, sensitively, and with complete attention. The nurse communicates a genuinely caring attitude. The client responds to the relationship by feeling secure and comfortable. Any initial anxiety is reduced and a reassuring sense of worthiness and respect develops. The client feels that perhaps help can be obtained and becomes ready to change any views or behavior if it seems expedient. All interactions are directed purposefully toward a mutually agreed goal of health. During the early stages of the relationship, there are periods of progression and regression. It is the nurse's task to be sensitive to the moments of regression and identify possible reasons for the client's behavior. Assistance from special consultants may be needed to define the weakened link in the process and to be able to intervene subsequently in a helpful manner with the client.

In conclusion, the therapeutic relationship is a connection or bond between nurse and client that connotes mutual trust, respect, caring, sharing, and understanding. By its nature, it facilitates the growth of the client toward a goal of health which the client desires and is made possible through the purposeful intervention of the assisting nurse.

UNDERSTANDING CONSUMER BEHAVIOR

When community health nurses talk about individuals for whom they are giving services, they commonly identify them as clients and/or consumers. Consumers are persons who use services to satisfy their needs. Each term is acceptable for describing recipients of the varied services of community health nurses.

Great emphasis is being directed by the government toward the responsibility of health care consumers to represent their own kind and participate increasingly on decision-making bodies concerned with health care planning, legislation, policies, and services. The trend toward consumerism has escalated since President Kennedy's speech in 1962 during which he stated that consumers have four rights:

1 The right to safety
2 The right to be informed
3 The right to choose
4 The right to be heard[10]

Health care providers and health care consumers are often dichotomized. All too often, health care providers tend to regard consumers as objects, dependents, recipients, unsophisticated regarding the technology of the professional health care system and services. It is the premise of this text that health care consumers must be perceived more on a parallel basis, that there can be an exchange between provider and consumer

[10]Warren G. Magnuson, "Consumerism and the Emerging Goals of a New Society," in R. M. Gaedeke and W. W. Etcheson (eds.), *Consumerism,* Canfield Press, San Francisco, 1975, p. 4.

that is mutually beneficial. As a consequence, more attention must be directed toward the study of consumer behavior.

Consumer behavior is human behavior. So a look at human behavior motivation is worth reviewing. As outlined by Craig and Craig, it includes:

1   *Basic survival*   To do what is necessary to survive.

2   *Competence*   To be spontaneously active and to exercise all of one's capacities.

3   *Exploring and mapping*   To explore and develop a comprehensible and orderly map of one's social and physical world. As experiences evolve in one's life, they are stored in memory and mental maps serve as quick reference records whenever needed.

4   *Self-determination*   To exercise personal control over what happens to one's self.

5   *Social interchange*   To openly express feelings, to honestly exchange information, and to cooperatively share companionship and love.

6   *Self-esteem*   To feel good about oneself.[11]

Remembering these six tendencies while interacting with consumers serves as a foundation for helping nurses to exercise greater flexibility in implementing health services and solutions satisfying to consumers.

The Decision-Process Approach and the Multimediation Model

The "study of consumer behavior, if it is to be realistic, must be based upon an understanding of social, individual, and institutional variables as they influence and constrain consumer decisions."[12] Engel, Kollat, and Blackwell use an analytical framework to describe the decision process undergone by consumers when faced with a problem needing some type of decision. The advantage of the decision-process approach is the view of behavior as a process rather than as a discrete act, and the study of how a decision is reached.[13]

The Engel, Kollat, and Blackwell model is presented in this text for the purpose of broadening the perspective of community health nurses regarding the complex nature of decision making, the multiple variables influencing actual or potential decisions of consumers, and the need for constructing innovative strategies which will induce consumers to desire improved health practices. An understanding of consumer behavior will enable nurses to determine most variables impinging on a consumer decision, and thereby predict probability of consumer response to a health need or problem and proposed solution. When nursing actions are based on accurate assessments of consumer behavior, successful outcomes are more likely to occur.

Engel, Kollat, and Blackwell describe the model as a *multimediation model* of consumer behavior. *Multimediation* refers to the "fact that many processes intervene or mediate between exposure to a stimulus and the final outcomes of behavior."[14]

---

[11] James H. Craig and Marge Craig, *Synergic Power beyond Domination and Permissiveness,* Proactive Press, Berkeley, Calif., 1974, pp. 13–14.

[12] James F. Engel, David T. Kollat, and Roger D. Blackwell, *Consumer Behavior,* 2d ed., Holt, Rinehart and Winston, Inc., New York, 1973, p. 7.

[13] Ibid., p. 47.

[14] Ibid., p. 49.

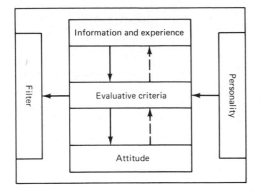

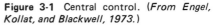

Figure 3-1 Central control. (*From Engel, Kollat, and Blackwell, 1973.*)

Two of these processes are identified as information processing and the decision process. They are processes always in a state of interaction at various levels. For an understanding of the fundamentals of the model, the psychological makeup of an individual is pictured as the central control unit in Fig. 3-1.

Central Control Unit of Consumer Behavior The *central control unit* includes both memory and the basic facilities for thinking and directing behavior. The important components for understanding consumer behavior are information and experience, evaluative criteria, and attitudes. Each of these variables is affected by personality, and they interact to form a filter through which incoming stimuli are processed.[15]

Information and Experience The consumer learns from experience and retains this information in either conscious or unconscious memory. Thus the individual learns to respond to stimuli of all types in consistent and predictable ways.[16]

Evaluative Criteria Evaluative criteria refer to specifications used by consumers to compare and evaluate available choices. These criteria are concrete manifestations of the consumer's personality (traits and motives), stored information, and various social influences. They vary with each consumer in terms of strength or conviction, number of criteria used to make a decision, and relative importance of the criterion. For example, one consumer with a health problem will decide to attend a neighborhood clinic because it is inexpensive. The criterion of greatest importance is price. Another consumer will choose to visit a private physician because of the desire for an accurate diagnosis. The criterion of importance for this decision is quality, based on a perception of the probable performance of a qualified, experienced physician. The purpose of evaluative criteria is to serve as a standard or guideline against which alternatives are compared and evaluated.[17]

Attitude An attitude is a mental state of readiness to respond which is organized through experience and exerts a directive and/or dynamic influence on behavior.[18]

[15] Ibid., p. 50.

[16] Ibid., p. 50.

[17] Ibid., pp. 50–51.

[18] Gordon Allport, "Attitudes," in C. Murchison (ed.), *Handbook of Social Psychology*, Clark University Press, Worcester, Mass., 1935, pp. 798–884.

Attitudes toward alternatives reflect an evaluation of health services utilizing evaluative criteria stored in the central control unit. Alternatives receiving the highest rating summed across the evaluative criteria have the greatest probability of being accepted. The solid arrows in the model show a direct relationship of the variables, attitude, stored information and experience, and evaluative criteria. The dashed line connecting the variables indicates the feedback relationship between variables. When an attitude is crystallized, there tends to be a restriction on changes in evaluative criteria and stored information as a protective mechanism from contradictory elements being filtered.[19]

Personality Each individual has a particular way of thinking, behaving, and responding that makes everyone unique. The sum total of these factors is personality. As shown in the model, personality exerts a direct influence on evaluative criteria. Environmental influences affecting personality include income, culture, family, social class, physical and other factors.[20]

Filter "All the variables in the central control unit interact to form a filter through which incoming stimuli are processed."[21] Stimuli are discarded, attenuated, or admitted. When admitted, evaluation is based on the pertinence or importance of the stimulus to the consumer for processing and storing in memory. For the nurse working with a consumer, the assessment phase of the nursing process is a critical one because the collection of data about the client, observation of cues, and elicitation of necessary information in the health history leads to a nursing judgment or diagnostic statement. The effectiveness of any nursing intervention depends on the accuracy of the nursing diagnosis. Before reaching a nursing judgment, the following factors must be weighed: what the client knows about a given health condition; information about past experiences that are pertinent; criteria important to the client; cultural, social, economic, familial, environmental, and other influences impinging on the client.

Information Processing

Information processing as depicted in the multimediation model (see Fig. 3-2) is described for the purpose of imagining the actual or potential influence the nurse exerts when interacting with a consumer regarding a health problem or need and proposed intervention.[22] The health care services as characterized by the presence of the nurse represent incoming stimuli that the consumer must process through the central control unit.

Incoming stimuli pass through the filter within the central control unit and are processed in four distinct phases: (1) exposure, (2) attention, (3) comprehension, and (4) retention. The information processing is illustrated in Fig. 3-2. Each phase is a distinct entity but does not necessarily relate sequentially. In other words, a stimulus is not necessarily comprehended even though it captures attention. The solid arrows and dashed arrows show what happens at each phase of the process by entering the filter and providing feedback.

[19] Engel, Kollat, and Blackwell, op. cit., p. 51.
[20] Ibid., p. 51.
[21] Ibid., p. 52.
[22] Ibid., p. 52.

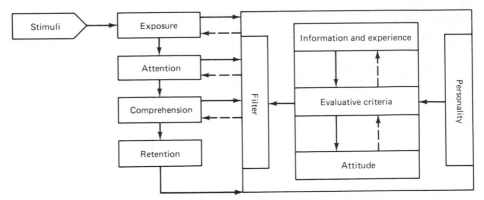

Figure 3-2 Information processing. (*From Engel, Kollat, and Blackwell, 1973.*)

Exposure Every individual is continually bombarded with stimuli of all types. The multiplicity and complexity of stimuli can be characterized as originating from many factors such as physical and sensory sensations, demands of family members, expected patterns of behavior in social settings (norms), behavior of friends, environmental factors such as weather, traffic congestion, etc.[23]

Attention Attention is the selection by the mind, in clear and vivid form, of one of several simultaneously possible trains of thought. Attention is highly selective. An individual who is aroused by a state of bodily need will be highly selective in what is seen, heard, touched, felt, and smelled. The aroused need activates an "on-off" switch to attention.[24]

To attain selective attention of a consumer stimuli must be developed to maximize the probability of being processed. Some mechanisms that can be considered for attracting the consumer's attention are novelty and surprise approaches, intensity of a message, use of color, readjusting the consumer's perception of the environment, etc.

Comprehension Even though attention is secured, it does not ensure comprehension. The central control unit filter has the capacity to attenuate and distort stimulus input in such a manner that certain attributes are amplified and others are diminished or ignored. Consumers can miss the point of a persuasive communication, or they can attribute a meaning that never was intended. This distortion occurs to make the stimulus more consonant with the consumer's beliefs and preferences.[25] The consumer has full capacity to screen out any message which contradicts strongly held beliefs. For this reason it is vitally important to elicit consumers' perceptions regarding their health needs, assess their health status, and employ action strategies congruent with their beliefs and values and reinforcing of tendencies leading toward desired outcomes.

Retention Information processing is selective in the way it is stored in conscious memory. Not every comprehended message enters into working memory. Retention is

[23] Ibid., pp. 52–53.
[24] Ibid., p. 53.
[25] Ibid., p. 53.

tested by asking for verbal or written feedback from the consumer following exposure. Obviously, during the information processing phase of assessment, the initial task of the nurse is to secure the attention of the consumer. This can be accomplished by experimenting with innovative ways of interacting with consumers. Before the client can be expected to comprehend any persuasive message, the nurse must have knowledge of the client's (1) beliefs, attitudes, and values regarding a health need or problem; (2) image of the present situation and its anticipated extension in the future if no action is taken; (3) image of various alternatives that might be achieved and that seem applicable to the situation; and (4) expectations of satisfactions and dissatisfactions that would flow from selected alternatives. It helps to remember that people are often out of touch with their basic desires and urges and are unable to identify or imagine experiences that would satisfy them. Instead, they tend to strive for things or conditions that their culture or advertisements promote as important and satisfying. For example, social drinking, smoking, or traveling to distant countries is advertised as highly satisfying. However, not all people who sample these behaviors find them satisfying. Exploring alternatives or experiences uniquely suited to each consumer is the challenge with which every community health nurse is confronted. Determining the client's retention of critical information requires that the nurse request verbal or written feedback at the end of each interaction or conference to ensure that the exchange between nurse and client has congruent meaning.

The Decision Process

The decision process begins with problem recognition and is inclusive of search and evaluation of alternatives, decision, and outcomes.[26]

Problem Recognition Problem recognition occurs when the consumer perceives a difference between a desirable and an actual state. It can occur through several means, one of which is need activation. Need activation causes the individual to become alert, responsive, and vigilant because of the resulting feelings of discomfort or dissatisfaction. It can be activated through a process of imaging or visualization. For example, the nurse can talk about a desirable solution to a problem in such persuasive language that the consumer feels aroused to act. Not all perceived discrepancies between desirable and actual states will lead to action in terms of perceived problems because of external influences which may intervene; for example, the withdrawal of necessary family support. When an external influence becomes a constraint, a *hold* is introduced in the decision-making process; the recognized problem remains but action is postponed until the constraints are removed. Some factors which can facilitate or constrain a decision include income, cultural values, family desires, social class, physical, and other factors.[27]

Alternatives Search and Evaluation When a problem is recognized and no constraints intervene to halt the decision process, the consumer automatically assesses alternatives for action. The initial step is a search of stored information and experience

[26] Ibid., p. 54.
[27] Ibid., p. 55.

to determine if alternatives are known and have been satisfactorily evaluated.[28] It is important for the nurse to elicit alternatives known and familiar to clients. Oftentimes, these alternatives are much more pertinent and satisfactory than ones formulated by the nurse. If feedback shows that attitudes toward alternatives are formed and fully operative, a satisfactory decision can be made. However, if known alternatives are not suitable or preferred, further information must be secured regarding external resources which are applicable to the problem. The community health nurse is an expert in the exploration and search of external resources. Discussion regarding the pros and cons of all possible alternatives and the facilitating or constraining factors can clarify all aspects contained in the decision process for the consumer. Oftentimes, the consumer needs a lot of information and assistance to visualize what can and must be done to achieve the desired goal.

Decision and Outcomes   Once a decision is made, the consumer may be satisfied and confident about outcomes. However, when the consumer has doubts about a decision, a reconsideration of evaluative criteria and facilitating and constraining factors can assist in weighing all factors much more carefully.

The complete multimediation model of consumer behavior is shown in Figure 3–3. It is essential for the consumer to perceive a health problem or need before the nurse can activate any of the consumer's thinking leading to the decision-process approach. Factors that facilitate or constrain must be considered when examining possible

[28] Ibid., p. 56.

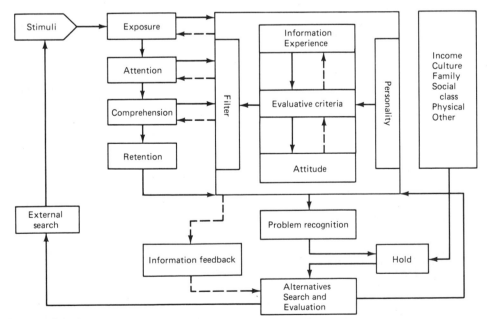

Figure 3-3 Multimediation model of consumer behavior. (*From Engel, Kollat, and Blackwell, 1973.*)

alternatives. Suggested tools that nurses can utilize while working with clients as consumers are described under Educating Consumers below.

EDUCATING CONSUMERS

Consumer education is not a luxury but a necessity if clients are to receive maximum benefit from today's knowledge of treatment, prevention, and control of disease.[29] Winslow lists the following factors cited by nurses as interfering with health teaching:

1 Lack of time, heavy work load, and inadequate staffing.
2 Lack of knowledge.
3 Inadequate preparation to teach.
4 Lack of nursing service support.
5 Poor communication between members of the health team.
6 Belief that sharing knowledge with the client decreases the nurse's power.
7 The client does not request information.
8 The doctor will not "let" the nurse teach the client.[30]

All of the above factors can be legitimately challenged provided the nurse believes in the client's "right to be informed."

A key function for community health nurses to activate is skill in health teaching of clients and client groups. Health teaching and/or health education is defined in many ways in the literature. Green defines *health education* as any combination of learning opportunities designed to facilitate voluntary adaptations of behavior conducive to health.[31] Green's definition is particularly appropriate for nurses seeking individualized and feasible teaching strategies for use with clients in particular situations.

Somers identifies consumer health education as subsuming a set of activities which:

1 Inform people about health, illness, disability, and ways in which they can improve and protect their own health, including more efficient use of the delivery system
2 Motivate people to want to change to more healthful practices
3 Help them learn the necessary skills to adopt and maintain healthful practices and lifestyles
4 Help other health professionals to acquire these teaching skills
5 Advocate changes in the environment that facilitate health conditions and healthful behavior
6 Add to knowledge via behavioral research and objective evaluation concerning the most effective ways of achieving the above objectives

---

[29] Elizabeth Hahn Winslow, "The Role of the Nurse in Patient Education," Elizabeth Hahn Winslow (ed.), *The Nursing Clinics of North America,* W. B. Saunders Company, Philadelphia, June 1976, p. 220.

[30] Ibid., p. 217-218.

[31] Lawrence W. Green, "Educational Strategies to Improve Compliance with Therapeutic and Preventive Regimens: The Recent Evidence," in R. Brian Haynes, D. Wayne Taylor, and David L. Sackett (eds.), *Compliance in Health Care,* The Johns Hopkins University Press, Baltimore, Md., 1979, p. 160.

In brief, consumer health education is a process that informs, motivates, and helps people to adopt and maintain health practices and lifestyles, advocates environmental changes as needed to facilitate attainment of this goal, and conducts professional training and research to this end.[32] Somer's definition is comprehensive and descriptive of the parameters included in the field of health education. It is of interest that the term "health education" is sometimes misunderstood and misinterpreted by clients as cited by Newman.[33] For that reason, henceforth in this text the words *health teaching* and *health promotion* will be used as a substitute for the term "health education."

A classification of levels of health promotion was developed by a health systems agency committee in the northwestern United States. The classification differentiates components of health promotion at five levels and suggests settings congruent with behaviors to be promoted. The classification is shown in Table 3-1.[34] The classification levels make distinctions that assist nurses in developing discrete teaching plans based on the needs of clients for health promotion. The variety of settings in which health teaching can be focused suggests a widening base for nurses to make known their skills as health promoters.

Teaching Adults

It is important to remember that education is the key to "nurse power." When educating adults, nurses must utilize teaching strategies that are different from those with which they are most familiar. All individuals are accustomed to pedagogical teaching strategies and automatically utilize these familiar patterns when teaching or instructing others. The pedagogical method presumes the learner to be dependent, in need of new knowledge. However, this approach is not necessarily a successful one with adults even though the adult may actually be dependent and in need of new knowledge. Knowles has identified four assumptions that must be recognized and dealt with if the education of adults is to be maximized.

   1 The adult's self-concept has moved from one of total dependency to one of increasing self-directedness.
   2 The mature adult has accumulated an expanding reservoir of experiences which becomes a rich resource for learning.
   3 The mature adult is ready to learn all tasks facilitating the performance of social roles.
   4 The mature adult has a problem-centered orientation to learning which is applied to immediate solutions.[35]

The points emphasized in the four assumptions are self-directedness, past experiences,

---

[32] Anne R. Somers, "Health Promotion and Consumer Health Education," in A Task Force Report, *Preventive Medicine USA*, Prodist, New York, 1976, p. 3.
   [33] Ian Newman and Richard Wilson, "Some Lessons Learned in Legislation," *Health Education*, November–December 1978, pp. 20–21.
   [34] Kay Kukowski and Betty Mathews, "A Framework for the Promotion of Health in King County," Health Promotion Committee, King County Health Planning Council, 1978.
   [35] Malcom S. Knowles, *The Modern Practice of Adult Education*, Follett Publishing Company, Chicago, 1970, p. 39. Copyright 1970 Malcolm S. Knowles. Used by permission of Association Press/Follett Publishing Company.

Table 3-1   A Classification of Levels of Health Promotion

Levels of health promotion	Spectrum of behaviors	Settings congruent for health teaching
1. Health Improvement	The practice of healthful lifestyle habits which lead to longer life expectancy and sense of well-being	Home and social/physical environment Business and industry Schools Community organizations (i.e., YWCA, YMCA, family fitness centers, wellness centers, senior citizen centers, etc.)
2. Health Maintenance	The practice of self-care and self-referral by individuals based on sufficient understanding of one's health to: 　Present one's self for appropriate screening to prevent illness 　Note changes in one's health status and take appropriate self-care and/or self-referral	Voluntary health agencies Health departments Medical association Hospital association Health maintenance organization Pharmacies Wellness centers Senior citizen centers Alternative health clinics Media health messages
3. Health Evaluation	Presentation of self for health evaluation	Primary care service: 　Physician's office 　Clinics, hospital 　Alternative health clinics 　Nurse practitioners' settings 　Self-care clinics
4. Health Restoration	The understanding by consumers of all aspects of the medical condition in order to: 　Prevent its recurrence 　Manage any limitations resulting from the condition	Hospitals Convalescent home care Rehabilitation programs
5. Rehabilitation	Coping with disabling conditions	Nursing homes Home care programs Friends and family Community agencies (i.e., blind, multiple sclerosis, etc.) Rehabilitation programs

readiness to learn new roles, problem-centered learning, and immediacy of solutions. When formulating teaching strategies for adults, the following precepts should serve as guidelines.

1　Behavior which is rewarded is most likely to recur.
2　Readiness to learn is promoted by a nonthreatening environment.
3　Participation in the learning plan promotes learning, the rate of learning, flexibility and motivation.

4 The best learning takes place when what is to be learned is immediately useful.

5 A nonautocratic atmosphere promotes initiative, creativity, self-confidence, and independence.[36]

Client participation in the teaching-learning process is essential. When nurses want to influence a behavior change in a client, it must be remembered that health problems frequently involve more than one health behavior. Persuading a client to change one health behavior is a *beginning* step in health promotion. The beginning step, even though it may be a minute one, is important toward building a health program that will be ultimately successful. The beginning step when attained by the client, demonstrates a successful effort and sense of satisfaction which serves as a solid base for additional behavioral change.

The client must perceive the attainment of each behavioral change to be important, and it helps to provide written instructions along with verbal instruction. Written instructions are best when they are brief, specific, readable, and organized. See Objective Evaluation of Outcomes at end of chapter.

Principles of Learning

Many principles of learning have been formulated by various schools of psychology. Some that apply to the work of the nurse are included here.

1 Learning takes place more effectively when an individual is ready, both physically and mentally, to learn.

2 Individual differences must be considered if effective learning is to take place.

3 Motivation, either from within or without the individual, is essential for learning.

4 What is learned in any given situation depends on the individual's perception of the situation.

5 An individual learns what she or he actually uses or what has relevance for her or him.

6 Learning takes place more effectively when the individual has a sense of satisfaction and when the learning is personal.

7 Evaluation by learner and teacher is essential in determining whether desirable changes in behavior are taking place.

These principles bear consideration as the nurse plans and conducts teaching and develops accompanying learning experiences. None of these principles functions alone, but they are interdependent. A consideration of these principles follows.

Tools for Educating Consumers

Tools can be considered as devices and procedures that facilitate the human's natural capacities. For nurses using tools, its intended function is more relevant than the use

[36] Malcom S. Knowles, *The Adult Learner: A Neglected Species,* 2d ed., Gulf Publishing Company, Houston, 1978, pp. 64–65. Copyright 1978 Gulf Publishing Company. Used with permission. All rights reserved.

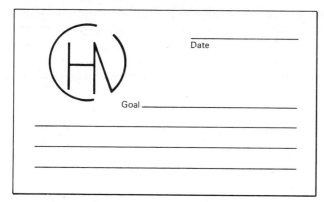

Date _____

Goal _____

_____

_____

_____

Figure 3-4   A nursing prescription.

of the tool itself.[37] Teaching tools need to be considered by nurses in terms of their potential applicability with specific clients. Instead of presenting a tool in its most perfect form, community health nurses need to realize that a selected tool can be modified so that it is understandable and serves as an incentive for each client. For example, when writing goals for clients, use the client's own words rather than nursing jargon. Give simple analogies that have concrete meaning for the client's understanding. Break down what appears to be a complicated tool into simple understandable parts. In this way tools can be fun to work with while educating clients.

Behavioral Objectives   After eliciting the health concerns of the client and family and discussing all feasible alternatives, the nurse must make a judgment regarding goals and/or objectives to which clients will be responsive. See Objective Evaluation of Outcomes below. When objectives are written specifically for the client in behavioral terms, they serve as a reminder of desired goals to be attained. See the example on p. 80.

Objectives written with clients can be considered an important tool for nurses to utilize while educating clients. To ease the actual procedure of writing objectives, the nurse can think of the behavioral objective as a "prescription for action." The piece of paper given to the client with the prescriptive activity and/or goals written on it serves as a concrete symbol of the contract or agreement between client and nurse and impresses the client regarding the professional nature of the transaction. It might help to have a nursing prescriptive pad with a community health logo printed on it for nurses to distribute to clients. See the suggested example (Fig. 3-4).

Protocols   By the nature of their practice, community health nurses frequently manage case loads and make decisions independently and with minimal guidance from others. When discussing a health regimen with clients, a helpful tool for the nurse to utilize is the teaching protocol. The word "protocol" has a variety of interpretations. For the purpose of health teaching, a *protocol* is defined as a stepwise guide using a teaching-learning behavioral change and contractual model leading to the education of

[37]Ralph E. Anderson and Irl Carter, *Human Behavior in the Social Environment,* 2d ed., Aldine Publishing Company, New York, 1978, p. 41.

a person about some aspect of health care.[38] Protocols are meant to serve as guides, not as "rigid cookbooks." They can be individualized to fit particular settings, situations, and clients. Essentially a protocol (1) provides a consistent database, (2) helps ensure thoroughness, (3) is convenient, (4) facilitates audit of care and performance, and (5) encourages continued learning.[39] Teaching protocols help nurses to educate clients, rather than giving information only.

The *teaching protocol* as advocated by Mitchell is primarily a tool for the nurse to provide the education needed by clients regarding specific health concerns, to encourage client questions, concerns, and perceptions regarding health concerns, and to facilitate the establishment of a contract or agreement toward goals agreed upon by client and nurse.

The basic outline of a teaching protocol can be structured as follows: Note that the client's knowledge of a health concern is assessed before eliciting the client's perceptions and feelings regarding the health concern.

1 Assess client's *knowledge* regarding a specific health concern.
2 Provide information, using visual aids as available.
3 Obtain feedback in the client's own words.
4 Apply knowledge, if feasible, using an actual or simulated situation.
5 Correct misinformation. Explain any errors or gaps in knowledge as indicated by the client's responses.
6 Assess client's *perceptions* and *feelings* regarding the health concern as it affects her or him.
7 Discuss perceptions and feelings, being sensitive to the client's unique situation.
8 Provide relevant information regarding related factors associated with the health concern.
9 Obtain feedback regarding the client's understanding of the additional related factors.
10 Correct misinformation. Explain any errors or gaps in knowledge as indicated by the client's responses.
11 Answer questions and ask if there is anything else about the health concern that the client wants to know or discuss.
12 Write on a prescriptive pad the contract or agreement which portrays the desired goals the client has agreed to work toward within a specific time frame.
13 Arrange for a return conference to evaluate the client's progress toward attainment of goals.[40]

An example of a teaching protocol for hypertension as written by Mitchell is published in the *American Journal of Nursing,* May 1977. Nurses can develop individualized teaching protocols on many subjects for which consumers need improved and more accurate education. The following example of an individualized teaching protocol is

---

[38] Ellen Sullivan Mitchell, "Protocol for Teaching Hypertensive Patients," *American Journal of Nursing,* 77:808–809, May 1977.
[39] Carolyn M. Hudak et al., *Clinical Protocols,* J. B. Lippincott Company, Philadelphia, 1976, pp. 4–5.
[40] Mitchell, op. cit., pp. 808–809.

for a client, Mr. D., who has an elevated blood pressure, is overweight by 15 lbs, has been started on the medication hydrochlorothiazide 50 mg/day for hypertension, and wants to change daily diet habits.

Teaching Protocol for Mr. D.

1 Client's knowledge regarding nutrition:
  a Knows the basic four
  b Realizes that an interrelationship exists between food intake and cardiovascular problems
  c Enjoys eating
  d Some preferred foods include steaks, french fries, potato chips, pizza, cheese, nuts, ice cream, cream pies, etc.
2 Information needed:
  a Foods high in potassium and sodium
  b Foods high in sugar
  c Foods high in fat content
  d The risk factor of foods high in fat leading to atherosclerosis
3 Feedback of client:
  a "I didn't realize red meat was so high in fat!"
  b "I'm willing to cut down on desserts."
  c "I'd like a list of foods high in potassium."
4 Use of concrete examples:
  Have the client identify which foods are high risk in the following dinner menu.
  a Fried chicken
  b Baked potato
  c Broccoli
  d Green salad with roquefort dressing
  e Chocolate cake with rum frosting
  f Coffee
5 Correction of misinformation: Discussion of fried chicken versus baked in terms of fat content, substitution of lemon juice or dressings advocated in low salt, low sugar diets in place of roquefort dressing, substitution of a baked apple or fruits instead of chocolate cake
6 Client's perceptions and feelings regarding a change in diet habits: "I want to change my eating habits, but feel that I am lacking in a great deal of knowledge about the best foods for me to eat. I think it will take time to change my eating patterns, but I want to try. I know I'll feel better and have more energy."
7 Adaptations needed for client's situation:
  a Provide a diet plan acceptable to the client
  b Provide a list of foods high in potassium
  c Encourage client not to salt foods at the table
  d Encourage client to substitute fruit for dessert whenever possible
8 Feedback of client:
  a "I'd like a diet plan for a week and I'll see if I can follow it."
  b "I think I can gradually reduce my salt intake."
  c "Maybe I'll substitute fruit for dessert once a week to start."
9 Questions:
  a "What are some good books I can read?"

    b Suggest books that are accessible and within the interest of the client, for example:

      (1) Nathan Pritikin, *The Pritikin Program for Diet and Exercise,* Bantam Books, New York, 1979.

      (2) Norma M. MacRae, *Mushroom 'n Bean Sprouts,* Pacific Search Press, Seattle, Wash., 1979.

10 Contract and/or agreement: By the end of 2 months (date: ___) I will be able to:

    a Name foods I eat regularly that are high in potassium

    b State that I rarely salt foods at the table

    c Report that I eat fruit for dessert at least 3 times a week

Signature _____

11 Return conference time: Every 2 weeks agreed upon by client and nurse

Teaching Protocol Outline

   1 Client's knowledge of health concern

   2 Information needed

   3 Feedback of client

   4 Use of concrete examples

   5 Correction of misinformation

   6 Client's perceptions and feelings regarding health concern

   7 Adaptations needed for client's situation

   8 Feedback of client

   9 Questions

 10 Agreement and/or contract

 11 Return conference time

Teaching protocols also can be written for self-care of clients at the health improvement and health maintenance levels of health promotion. These protocols can include recommended guidelines for healthful lifestyle habits and self-appraisal of health status as a basis for self-care and self-referral. A suggested outline for a self-care protocol which can be distributed to consumers is shown below.

Protocol for Self-Care

   1 Identification of a health concern.

   2 Description of common signs and symptoms that arouse the attention of consumers.

   3 Ordering of signs and symptoms from low risk to high risk in terms of seriousness and urgency.

   4 Identification of recommended behaviors for each sign and symptom, using a visual scheme easy to follow.

   5 Listing of recommended services of health providers and community resources as signs and symptoms become high risk in seriousness and urgency.

An example of a self-care protocol for burns is given in Table 3-2.

As consumers become responsible for maintaining health through the use of teaching and/or self-care protocols, it might be anticipated that irrelevant telephone calls or visits to health providers may be reduced.

Table 3-2 Self-Care Protocol for Burns

Signs and symptoms	Recommended behaviors
First-degree burns 1 Red, no blisters 2 Increased warmth and sensitivity 3 Pain	1 Immerse burn in tepid or cold water or put soft cloths soaked in ice water on burn 2 Repeat, if painful 3 Aspirin, if necessary, for pain 4 Do *not* use butter, oils, creams, grease on burn 5 *If pain lasts over 48 hours, call doctor*

Second-degree burns
1 Red with blisters
2 Swollen, puffy, weepy
	1 Immerse burn in tepid or cold water
	2 See recommended behaviors for first-degree burns
	3 Wash off dirt and grease *gently* with soap and water
	4 Leave blisters intact!
	5 Cover burned area with clean gauze dressing loosely—if burn area is rubbing against clothing, tape gauze well away from burn area
	6 Change gauze dressing as necessary or every 2 to 3 days; Wash hands well before changing dressings
	7 *If burn is extensive, or on hands and face:*
	  a *See doctor,* or
	  b *Go to emergency room of nearest hospital*

3 If patient goes into shock:
  a Cold, clammy skin
  b Fast, weak pulse
  c Pale, dizzy
  d Nausea
  e Dilated pupils
4 If burn becomes infected:
  a Fever
  b Increased pain and swelling
	8 If patient goes into shock:
	  a Have patient lie down
	  b Elevate legs a few inches
	  c Keep patient warm
	  d Check pulse regularly
	  e Reassure patient
	9 If burn becomes infected, *see doctor*

Third-degree burns 1 Raw, white, charred black 2 No pain	1 *See doctor,* or 2 *Go to emergency room of nearest hospital* 3 Protect burned area with clean cloths; Cut away burned clothing; Remove rings and bracelets (if easily accomplished); *Be calm* 4 Give fluids

The Decision Tree[41] When faced with a complex decision and uncertain about what to do, a decision tree is an effective tool for outlining choices, alternatives, risks, objectives, rewards, and information needs. A decision tree is as it sounds; it has branches and nodes. When diagrammed, the tree shows routes by which various possible alternatives and outcomes are pictured. The nurse can use the decision tree when feeling uncertain about what course of action to take. For example, while driving to

[41] John F. Magee, "Decision Trees for Decision Making," *Harvard Business Review*, 42(4) 126–138, July–August 1964.

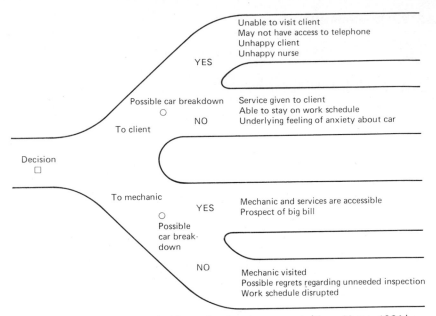

Figure 3-5 Decision tree. □ = decision point; ○ = chance event. (*From Magee, 1964.*)

work in the morning, the nurse notices a different and somewhat alarming noise in the motor of the car. A decision has to be made about the car since it affects the nurse's schedule for the day. Should the nurse visit the client needing a colostomy irrigation as scheduled at 9 A.M. and drive 10 miles to the client's home, or should the car be taken to a mechanic immediately to forestall a breakdown? What are the payoffs for either course of action? The decision tree can be pictured in Fig. 3-5.

The illustration shows the choices available for the nurse: visit the client as scheduled, or visit the mechanic for an automobile inspection. Each branch represents a course of action relating to a decision. Each node represents a chance event—the car will or will not break down. Associated with the chance event are alternative forks through the tree which show the payoffs at the end of each terminal branch. In the illustration the decision and action points are symbolized by a square and the chance events by circles. The decision tree provides a visual image of the problem, choices, and payoffs. It shows action choices with different possible events or results of action which are partially affected by chance or other uncontrollable circumstances.[42] It also deals only with those decisions, events, or results that are important in the situation under study. For the nurse who likes to work with visual tools, a basic background pattern of a decision tree can be lightly drawn and photocopied on blank sheets of paper so that when utilized with a client, the nurse only has to fill in the pertinent material for the specific decision confronting the consumer. The nurse and consumer can work together in developing the alternatives and payoffs associated with every course of action. The decision tree tool can be left with the consumer to study until the final conclusion is reached.

[42] Ibid.

OBJECTIVE EVALUATION OF OUTCOMES

If you don't know where you are going, you will end up somewhere else.[43]

Behavior is basically goal-oriented. When the nurse examines behavior of self or that of consumers, recognition must be given to the appearance of most behaviors as being goal-oriented, whether there is conscious acknowledgement of such or not. The goal may be anticipation of a reward, the approval of a significant other, the vision of a pleasure, a feeling of innate satisfaction, gratification of one of the senses, etc.

To assist clients in formulating desired health outcomes, written goals or objectives are helpful in crystallizing the extent and parameters of the results desired. The nurse can write a rough draft of tentative goals for the client and encourage examination of the written goals in terms of their attractiveness and desirability, ease of accomplishment, challenge to the client, and potential satisfaction when goals are achieved. Or the nurse may write one goal on a pad that simulates a prescription, and the client will be expected to follow through with the goal similarly to following through with a prescriptive activity. See example under Tools for Educating Consumers.

In order to make written goals appear attractive and comprehensible to clients, they should be written as behavioral objectives. *Objectives* are defined as being goals or outcomes sought. Or put another way, an objective is a description of what things will be like when a goal has been achieved. It is a statement identifying the intended conditions for the conclusion of an activity. An objective is a destination.[44] Behavioral objectives are explicitly written to describe specific behaviors that clients have agreed will demonstrate their accomplishment of desired health results. A good behavioral objective communicates where the learner is going and when the desired behavior has been reached.

When writing objectives for or with clients, utilize the following three suggestions as advocated by Hogue:

1 Think about the regimen from the client's point of view. Use words that are familiar and have meaning for the client. Acknowledge specific competencies and strengths of the client which promise that accomplishment of the objectives can be achieved. Recognize and adapt for other factors which compete for the client's time and energy such as family responsibilities, social roles, working commitments, etc.

2 Use the power of existing natural client support systems such as family, friends, neighbors, or significant others. Ask the client who provides help when it is needed. Discuss or review the regimen with the support person if this is feasible and agreeable with the client.

3 Collaborate and communicate with others interested in the client's progress such as other health care providers (nurses, physicians, community clinic personnel, etc.).[45]

---

[43]Laurence J. Peter, *The Peter Prescription,* William Morrow & Company, Inc., 1972, New York, p. 141.

[44]Ibid., p. 141.

[45]Carol C. Hogue, "Nursing and Compliance," in R. Brian Haynes, D. Wayne Taylor, and David L. Sackett (eds.), *Compliance in Health Care,* The Johns Hopkins University Press, Baltimore, Md., 1979, pp. 255–257.

Three taxonomies categorizing levels of knowledge, attitudes and beliefs, and psychomotor skills have been developed to facilitate the writing of explicit behavioral objectives. A *taxonomy* is an organizational process for classification of objectives. Its purpose is to categorize gradations of learning sequentially from a beginning level to more complex levels. It classifies and describes client behaviors which represent intended outcomes of teaching endeavors. Bloom, Krathwohl, and Harrow have published taxonomies for cognitive learning, affective learning, and psychomotor learning. *Cognitive learning* deals with knowledge and understanding and consists of six graduated levels or domains. Descriptions of the domains are as follows:

1 *Knowledge* Knowledge is defined as the remembering of previously learned material. This may involve the recall of a wide range of material, from specific facts to complete theories, but all that is required is the bringing to mind of the appropriate information.

2 *Comprehension* Comprehension is defined as the ability to grasp the meaning of material. This may be shown by translating material from one form to another, by interpreting material, and by estimating future trends.

3 *Application* Application refers to the ability to use learned material in new and concrete situations. This may include the application of such things as rules, methods, concepts, principles, laws, and theories.

4 *Analysis* Analysis refers to the ability to break down material into its component parts so that its organizational structure may be understood. This may include the identification of parts, analysis of the relationships between parts, and recognition of the organizational principles involved.

5 *Synthesis* Synthesis refers to the ability to put parts together to form a new whole. This may involve the production of a unique communication, a plan of operations, or a set of abstract relations.

6 *Evaluation* Evaluation is concerned with the ability to judge the value of material for a given purpose. The judgments are to be based on definite criteria. These may be internal criteria or external criteria.[46]

Affective learning deals with attitudes and beliefs and involves the study of one's value system on behavior. Five levels or domains are identified as follows:

1 *Receiving* Receiving refers to the person's willingness to attend to particular phenomena or stimuli. Learning outcomes range from the simple awareness that a thing exists to selective attention on the part of the learner.

2 *Responding* Responding refers to active participation on the part of the learner. At this level the learner not only attends to a particular phenomenon but also reacts to it in some way. Learning outcomes in this area may emphasize acquiescence in responding, willingness to respond, or satisfaction in responding.

3 *Valuing* Valuing is concerned with the worth or value a learner attaches to a particular object, phenomenon, or behavior. This ranges in degree from the more simple acceptance of a value to the more complex level of commitment. Valuing is based

[46]Benjamin S. Bloom et al. (eds.), *Taxonomy of Educational Objectives: The Classification of Educational Goals: Handbook I: Cognitive Domain,* Longman, Inc., New York, 1956, pp. 201–207. Copyright 1956 Longman, Inc. Reprinted by permission.

on the internalization of a set of specified values, but clues to these values are expressed in the learner's overt behavior. Learning outcomes in this area are concerned with behavior that is consistent and stable enough to make the value clearly identifiable.

4 *Organization* Organization is concerned with bringing together different values, resolving conflicts between them, and beginning the building of an internally consistent value system. Thus the emphasis is on comparing, relating, and synthesizing values. Learning outcomes may be concerned with the conceptualization of a value or with the organization of a value system.

5 *Characterization by a value or value complex* At this level of the affective domain, the value system has controlled the individual's behavior for a sufficiently long time to have developed a characteristic lifestyle. Thus the behavior is pervasive, consistent, and predictable. Learning outcomes at this level cover a broad range of activities, but the major emphasis is on the fact that the behavior is typical or characteristic of the learner.[47]

Psychomotor learning deals with motor skills, dependent upon physical ability and coordination. Six levels or domains are identified as follows:

1 Reflex movements
2 Basic fundamental movements
3 Perceptual abilities
4 Physical abilities
5 Skilled movements
6 Nondiscursive (movement) communication[48]

The purpose for studying the taxonomies prepares the nurse with a knowledge base for writing explicit, distinctive, and appropriate objectives for clients. If the intended outcome is knowledge or understanding alone, the cognitive domains should be studied to determine the level of learning most suitable for the client. The cognitive domains are associated predominantly with most methods of formal and informal education. Attitudes and beliefs are concomitant with cognitive learning, but generally receive much less attention in formal and informal educational settings. Changing attitudes and beliefs tend to require longer periods of time than instructing about new phenomena. Familiarity with affective domains is important for the nurse to determine the level at which the client is behaving. When the nurse wants more than simple compliance from a client, clues must be sought that indicate that the third level, valuing, has been reached by the client. The domains for psychomotor learning deal mainly with physical ability and coordination and are useful primarily for nurses teaching motor skills.

When preparing objectives for clients it is best to write goals that are realistic, appropriate, achievable, specific, and measurable (if possible). Beginning objectives should aim toward *slight* improvements to ensure successful achievement by the client.

[47]David R. Krathwohl et al., *Taxonomy of Educational Objectives: The Classification of Educational Goals: Handbook II: Affective Domain,* Longman, Inc., New York, pp. 176–185. Copyright 1964 Longman, Inc. Reprinted by permission.
[48]Anita J. Harrow, *A Taxonomy of the Psychomotor Domain,* Longman, Inc., New York, 1972, pp. 46–93.

As client competencies are demonstrated, self-esteem increases. When objectives have a defined time frame for achievement, the client is motivated or challenged to meet the deadline. Numbers represent concrete manifestation of achievement, and if possible they should be evident in the objective statement as additional motivator.

An example of behavioral objectives written in recognition of the three taxonomies is given below. It is for the client who wishes to remember to take medication for hypertension daily without fail. The written objectives which describe desired outcome behaviors may be written as follows:

1 *Cognitive domain* (knowledge level) Describes accurately the daily procedure used for taking hypertension medication, including:
   a The number of tablets
   b The color and appearance of tablets
   c The time of day taken
   d The method for reminding
2 *Cognitive domain* (application level) Shows by marks on a flow sheet or calendar the daily administration of hypertension medication for a period of 1 week
3 *Affective domain* (valuing level) Values ability to assume responsibility for current administration of hypertension medication, as determined by
   a Self report in 1 week
   b Rating of satisfaction on a scale of 1 to 10 (1 = poor and 10 = excellent)
4 *Psychomotor domain* (basic fundamental movements level) Demonstrates basic fundamental movements in oral administration of current hypertension medication

It will be noted that each objective is written from the perspective of the client's learning, begins with a verb that specifies observable or measurable behavior, describes the terminal performance that is anticipated as an outcome, states one learning outcome rather than a combination of ideas, and is written at a level that can be attained realistically by the client.[49] For accomplishment objectives, it is important to involve the client in determining what can be done and what the client agrees to do. When others participate in the setting of an objective, understanding and acceptance will result.[50]

Nurses must get into the habit of writing objectives for activities or programs in which they are engaged. The writing of objectives clarifies the purpose of the activity or program, sets boundaries of expectations regarding outcomes, provides consistency of direction toward the goal, and acts as guidelines for anticipated performances. The actual composition and writing of useful behavioral objectives is difficult initially, but the process becomes easier with practice. Questions to think about while writing objectives that are designed for clients are:

1 Are learning outcomes appropriate for this client?
2 Are all possible learning outcomes remembered?
3 Are the objectives attainable for the client?

[49]Norman E. Gronlund, *Stating Behavioral Objectives for Classroom Instruction,* The Macmillan Company, New York, 1970, p. 11.
   [50]Peter, op. cit., p. 146.

4 Are the objectives in harmony with the basic principles of learning?
   a Is the client *ready* to proceed successfully with the objective?
   b Is the client *motivated* or does the client want to work toward the attainment of the objective?
   c Is the client apt to *retain* the terminal behavior as something for continued use?
   d Is the client apt to *apply* the terminal behavior in other new situations?[51]
   e Does the client understand and accept the intent of the objective?

Before being able to work effectively with the client, the nurse must know the learner. What are the client's goals and objectives in relation to health? or does the client have any? Those who live close to the poverty line and move from one family crisis to another frequently have no objectives. The nurse will sense the lack of motivation toward optimal health in many low-income families, where there is the constant threat and fear of unemployment with resulting inability to pay the rent or buy sufficient food and clothing. The lack of independence engendered by welfare may be another reason for low motivation. These families are more concerned with their critical situations than with long-range problems of health. A practical approach is usually the wisest one in working with low-income groups.

Behavioral objectives that show tangible movement toward desired outcomes are readily attainable, are written at a level understandable and achievable, and are acceptable to the family will be successful, particularly if the nurse has taken the initiative to elicit the interests and desires of the family before writing and interpreting the meaning of the objectives to them.

SUMMARY

Before interacting with consumers who are functioning as well individuals in community settings, community health nurses must take inventory of their own skills in meeting strangers and communicating as professional nurses in a teaching, counseling, or helping role. To understand and appreciate consumer behavior in its many forms, a model by Engel, Kollat, and Blackwell is provided for the purpose of showing the many variables influencing and constraining consumer decisions. Because consumers have great need for accurate health information, a variety of tools are suggested for use in educating clients according to their health needs.

Health outcomes are best evaluated based on goals agreed upon by the client and nurse early in their work with each other. When the goals are written as behavioral objectives they supply the extent and parameters of results desired. A taxonomy of behavioral objectives is presented for cognitive learning, affective learning, and psychomotor learning.

SUGGESTED READING

Anderson, Ralph E., and Irl Carter: *Human Behavior in the Social Environment; A Social Systems Approach,* 2d ed., Aldine Publishing Company, New York, 1978.

[51] Gronlund, op. cit., pp. 29–30.

Beier, Ernest G.: *The Silent Language of Psychotherapy,* Aldine Publishing Company, Chicago, 1966.

Bloom, Benjamin S. et al.: *Taxonomy of Educational Objectives: The Classification of Educational Goals: Handbook I: Cognitive Domain,* Longman, Inc., New York, 1956.

Brammer, Lawrence M.: *The Helping Relationship: Process and Skills,* Prentice-Hall, Inc., Englewood Cliffs, N.J., 1973.

Branden, Nathaniel: *The Disowned Self,* Bantam Books, Inc., New York, 1971.

Caplan, Gerald: *Principles of Preventive Psychiatry,* Basic Books, Inc., Publishers, New York, 1964.

Carkhuff, Robert R.: *Helping and Human Relations: Volume I,* Holt, Rinehart and Winston, Inc., New York, 1969.

Carkhuff, Robert R.: *Helping and Human Relations: Volume II,* Holt, Rinehart and Winston, Inc., New York, 1969.

Carlson, Carolyn E. (ed.): *Behavioral Concepts and Nursing Intervention,* J. B. Lippincott Company, Philadelphia, 1970.

Combs, Arthur W., Donald L. Avila, and William W. Purkey: *Helping Relationships,* Allyn and Bacon, Inc., Boston, 1971.

Craig, James H., and Marge Craig: *Synergic Power Beyond Domination and Permissiveness,* Proactive Press, Berkeley, Calif., 1974.

Engel, James F., David T. Kollat, and Roger D. Blackwell: *Consumer Behavior,* 2d ed., Holt, Rinehart and Winston, Inc., New York, 1973.

Ferguson, Tom: "The New Medical Consumer," *Medical Self-Care,* No. 9, Summer 1980, pp. 4–8.

Frankl, Viktor E.: *Man's Search for Meaning,* Washington Square Press, New York, 1963.

Gartner, Alan, and Frank Riessman: *Self-Help in the Human Services,* Jossey-Bass Publishers, San Francisco, 1977.

Gronlund, Norman E.: *Stating Behavioral Objectives for Classroom Instruction,* The Macmillan Company, New York, 1970.

Harrow, Anita J.: *A Taxonomy of the Psychomotor Domain,* Longman, Inc., New York, 1972.

Haynes, R. Brian, D. Wayne Taylor, and David L. Sackett (eds.): *Compliance in Health Care,* The Johns Hopkins University Press, Baltimore, Md., 1979.

Hudak, Carolyn M. et al.: *Clinical Protocols,* J. B. Lippincott Company, Philadelphia, 1976.

Knowles, Malcolm S.: *The Adult Learner: A Neglected Species,* 2d ed., Gulf Publishing Company, Houston, 1978.

Knowles, Malcolm S.: *The Modern Practice of Adult Education,* Association Press/ Follett Publishing Company, New York, 1970.

Krathwohl, David R. et al.: *Taxonomy of Educational Objectives: The Classification of Educational Goals: Handbook II: Affective Domain,* Longman, Inc., New York, 1964.

Lazes, Peter M. (ed.): *The Handbook of Health Education,* Aspen Systems Corporation, Germantown, Md., 1979.

Magee, John F.: "Decision Trees for Decision Making," *Harvard Business Review,* July–August 1964, 42(4):126–138.

Mager, Robert F.: *Preparing Instructional Objectives,* Fearon Publishers Inc., Palo Alto, Calif., 1962.

Mayeroff, Milton: *On Caring,* Harper & Row, Publishers, Inc., New York, 1972.

Mayers, Marlene: "Home Visit—Ritual or Therapy?" *Nursing Outlook,* **21**(5):328–331, May 1973.

Metsch, Jonathan M., and James E. Veney: "Consumer Participation and Social Accountability," *Medical Care,* **14**(4):283–293, April 1976.

Mitchell, Ellen Sullivan: "Protocol for Teaching Hypertensive Patients," *American Journal of Nursing,* **77**:808–809, May 1977.

Moustakas, Clark: *Personal Growth,* Howard A. Doyle Publishing Company, Cambridge, Mass., 1969.

Mushkin, Selma J. (ed.): *Consumer Incentives for Health Care,* Prodist, New York, 1974.

O'Neill, Nena, and George O'Neill: *Shifting Gears,* M. Evans & Co., Inc., New York, 1974.

Otto, Herbert A., and John Mann: *Ways of Growth,* Grossman Publishers, New York, 1968.

Peter, Laurence J.: *The Peter Prescription,* Bantam Books, Inc., New York, 1972.

Pohl, Margaret L.: *Teaching Function of the Nursing Practitioner,* Wm. C. Brown Company Publishers, Dubuque, Iowa, 1968.

Rogers, Carl R.: *Freedom to Learn,* Charles E. Merrill Publishing Company, Columbus, Ohio, 1969.

Rokeach, Milton: *Beliefs, Attitudes, and Values,* Jossey-Bass, Inc., Publishers, San Francisco, 1970.

Somers, Anne R.: "Health Promotion and Consumer Health Education," in a Task Force Report, *Preventive Medicine USA,* Prodist, New York, 1976.

Towle, Charlotte: *Common Human Needs,* National Association of Social Workers, Inc., New York, 1965.

Vickery, Donald M., and James F. Fries: *Take Care of Yourself: A Consumer's Guide to Medical Care,* Addison-Wesley Publishing Company, Inc., Reading, Mass., 1976.

Chapter 4

Becoming Oriented to Communities

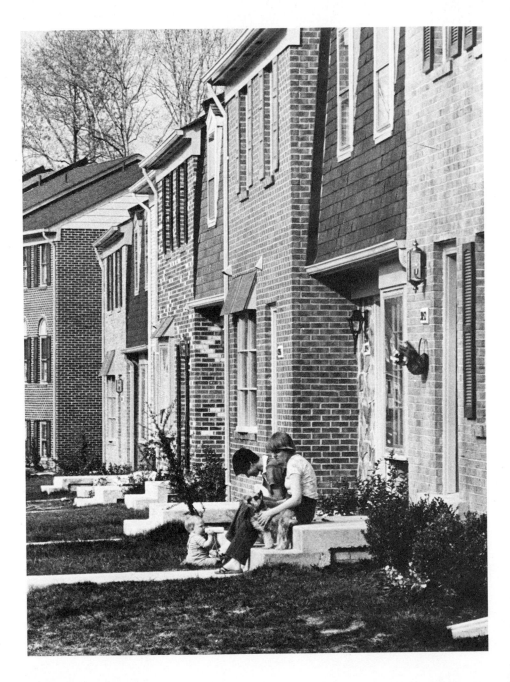

Since community health nurses are practicing in a variety of geographical locations, the setting of the local community and factors affecting it must be studied in addition to the health needs of the local residents. Each community, whether urban, suburban, or rural, has its own unique characteristics, strengths, and limitations. As knowledge is gained about a community, the nurse is better able to play a significant role in developing awareness of and improving the health practices of its people. As stated by Remillet and Reading, the community health nurse must know the community being served. The nurse must have accurate knowledge of the age-group percentages, ethnic differences, the dominant culture and subcultures, sociological factors that spawn health problems, and the resources for finding solutions once problems have been differentiated from cause. Accumulation of data is only the beginning; application of the findings in order to assess needs further and to participate in realistic decision making to improve the environment for better living follows in logical sequence.[1]

By looking at the field of health as a generalist in nursing, the community health nurse must be prepared to know multiple facets of the community; the health problems, needs, and desires of consumers; health resources, personnel, and facilities; and methods for integrating the health-care system so that all parts complete a whole. When viewed as wholeness of individuals, families, and groups, health opens up many new avenues of approach and responsibility which the community health nurse can meet with creative, ingenious, and enterprising action and by seeking to act as a coordinating, facilitating agent. In these times of rapid change, the role of the community health nurse must also reflect change to keep up with the requirements of our progressive society.

THE COMMUNITY

The term "community" is an elusive concept because of the variety of meanings it suggests. Many definitions for community have been proposed in literature and the perspective that is most easily adapted to the needs of the investigator is the one usually selected. For the purposes of this book, a *community* as defined by Anderson and Carter is a consciously identified population with common needs and interests; it may occupy a common physical space, engage in common activities, and have some form of organization that provides for differentiation of functions, making it adaptive to its environment as a means of meeting common needs. Its components include the individuals, groups, families, and organizations within its population, and the institutions it forms to meet its needs. Its environment is the society within which it exists and to which it adapts, and other communities and organizations outside itself that impinge on its functioning.[2]

When the community health nurse prepares to study a community, the consciously identified population that is selected may be living in a common physical space or

---

[1] June Remillet and Sadie Reading, "Adapting to Changing Community Health Needs," *Nursing Outlook,* 18(10):47, October 1970.

[2] Ralph E. Anderson and Irl Carter, *Human Behavior in the Social Environment,* Aldine Publishing Company, New York, 1978, pp. 53–54. Copyright © 1978 Ralph E. Anderson and Irl Carter. Reprinted with permission.

geographic area, may have common needs and interests, engage in common activities, may have organized themselves as a visible and effective means for designating their needs, and may have established buildings or customs and practices that promulgate their interests. For example, a retirement home, a hospital, a school, an industrial plant, a small town, a group of surgical nurses, a group of residents living in low-income housing, a jogging club are some examples of communities. For any citizen, communities can be represented in a variety of perspectives dependent on that individual's interests, needs, memberships, and location. Some functions which communities perform are

1 Maintenance of a way of life
2 Satisfaction of common needs, interests, and ambitions
3 Maintenance of a social consciousness or "sense of community"
4 Organization in pursuit of common goals[3]

The nurse can focus on all behavior within a community from three points of view: (1) maintenance of the physical and social environment; (2) securing of help and support at times of stress; and (3) strengthening of individuals to gain a sense of self and social worth.[4] The nursing emphasis will be gauged by the nurse's perception of the diverse needs of the community citizens. For example, from the first point of view, the nurse may work mainly with the elementary school population in terms of safety and immunizations. The second point of view will be directed toward young married couples with newborn infants who are entering the family system. Low-income families living within a specified housing project may be responsive to the emphasis on the third point of view, particularly when they are ready to participate in community planning and action directly affecting them.

THE COMMUNITY HEALTH NURSING PROCESS

Community health nursing is a synthesis of nursing practice and public health practice applied to promoting and preserving the health of populations. In community health nursing practice the consumer is the client. Consumers include individuals, groups, and the community as a whole. To become acquainted with a given community or selected populations, the nurse must determine the factors for which more data needs to be secured in order to make an adequate assessment. A realistic assessment of the health and status of the community is systematic and continuous. It takes note of the present and future health of individuals, families, and communities in terms of human-environment interrelationships. An assessment is done for the purpose of deciding the efficacy of a nursing action. If the health status data provide a basis for believing a nursing action will promote beneficial growth or change in the community, then a nursing diagnosis derived from the health status data is determined. The nursing

[3]Ibid., pp. 53–54.
[4]Donald C. Klein, *Community Dynamics and Mental Health,* John Wiley & Sons, Inc., New York, 1968, p. 10.

diagnosis delineates the kind of nursing action considered to be appropriate in the selected community. Planning is essential for engineering actions which will produce desired outcomes. Implementing the plan means "doing it." Evaluation determines how well objectives were accomplished, if outcomes demonstrated success, if omissions or unanticipated factors were disclosed, if satisfaction of consumer groups was gained, and if a need was revealed for continuing study and community involvement.

Assessing the Community

Data collection is prerequisite to a realistic assessment of a community and establishment of a proposed nursing diagnosis. Accomplishing a needs assessment of a community requires an exploration of a variety of approaches to be utilized in the pursuit of desired data. As described by Warheit, Bell, and Schwab, the following approaches can be used independently or as parts of an integrated sequential program.

1 Key informant
2 Community forum
3 Rates under treatment
4 Social indicators
5 Field survey[5]

First, however, informal observations of a new community provide an overview which serves to guide the nurse in the appraisal for indications of health status and in the questioning of factors leading to possible selections of consciously identified populations. Sociodemographic information about a community can be obtained from census reports, U.S. Department of Health, Education, and Welfare (DHEW) publications, planning departments, health planning councils, state, county, and city agencies, chambers of commerce, colleges and universities, and other organizations involved in collecting and utilizing population information. Data on age, race, sex, ethnicity, family income, per capita income, marital status, family structures, housing characteristics, population density, mobility, migration and distribution, labor force characteristics and educational levels can be obtained from census reports. From health and welfare agencies one can secure information on morbidity, mortality, and treatment patterns; and from planning councils, information can be found on land use and population changes. In addition, a list of human service agencies functioning in the community can be obtained from councils of social agencies or similar groups.[6]

Before doing a needs assessment of a community, the purpose must be clarified in words that seem reasonable and acceptable to respondents. What information is wanted? Why is it important? How will the information be used? Questions must be devised in advance of interviews or questionnaires so that the important issues are addressed and time is utilized advantageously.

[5] George J. Warheit, Roger A. Bell, and John J. Schwab, *Needs Assessment Approaches: Concepts and Methods,* U.S. Department of Heath, Education, and Welfare Publication ADM-79-472, 1977, p. 19.
[6] Ibid., pp. 16–17.

Observation of a Community   To study unofficially a new community, a nurse should first obtain a map and drive around the local community to gain impressions of the housing, spacing of residences, environmental conditions, business and industrial establishments, neighborhood services (e.g., grocery stores, transportation facilities, shopping centers, educational facilities), recreational facilities (e.g., parks or playgrounds), health facilities (e.g., hospitals, physicians' offices), community resources, safety of the environment, number of churches, and the faces of the people. Some of the questions that may come to mind are: How do the people support themselves? Is there evidence of pride in the community? How did this community come into being in the first place? Is there a "mix" of population such as several nationalities and races, extremes of wealth and poverty, extremes of young and old? Do the people seem preoccupied, busy, impersonal, friendly, prosperous, poor, old, young? Since impressions change as more is learned about the community, the nurse may wish to record the first impressions of the area which can serve as a comparison tool in the future.

After gaining early impressions, a suggested second activity is to purchase a local newspaper and scan the contents. Does it reflect national, state, and local news or does it concentrate on folksy items? What is the nature of the advertisements in the paper? Are there editorial comments that give a sense of the attitudes of the residents? Are there any health items reported? Are there announcements of local meetings or reports of local agency activities? Are there meetings or facilities that the nurse may want to visit?

By getting a feel of the appearance and interests of the community, the nurse can map out subsequent activities to engage in. Questions can be formulated for which the answers will help the nurse to reach the ultimate goal of getting well acquainted with the community. A well-informed community health nurse must know the characteristics, idiosyncrasies, and attitudes of the community. It takes time for a new nurse to become well informed, but a carefully planned, informal study facilitates the process.

Needs Assessment: Key Informant Approach   Every community has formal and informal leaders who hold positions of power, influence, or status in terms of facilitating or hindering community actions. The key informant approach is based on the selection of individuals who are in a position to know the community's needs and health utilization patterns. The people normally sought as key informants are public officials; administrative and program personnel in the health and welfare organizations of the community; health purveyors from both the public and private sectors, including physicians and nurse practitioners; the program clinical staff of agencies such as community mental health centers, vocational rehabilitation organizations, guidance clinics, and others engaged in either the delivery of primary care or the administration of health programs. Other influential leaders who are not necessarily health oriented may be found in professions and occupations such as industries, banks, clergy, and law. Associations representing service clubs, labor unions, political party organizations, communication media, community councils or boards, voluntary health organizations, housing authorities, fraternal groups, cultural groups, and minority groups are additional sources for finding key community leaders.

The advantages of the key informant approach are its simplicity and inexpensiveness. Input is gained from many different individuals, each having a personal perspective, and the opportunity is provided for a broad discussion of needs and services important to the community. The disadvantage of the approach is the existence of individual bias. These perspectives, even collectively, may not represent an accurate appraisal of the total needs or types of needs existing in the community.[7]

Needs Assessment: Community Forum Approach The community forum approach relies on individuals who are asked to assess the needs and service patterns of those in the community. A forum is designed around a series of public meetings to which all residents are invited and asked to express their beliefs about the needs and services of the community. The approach is a flexible one in that it can elicit information from any member of the community willing to attend a public meeting. It can also include input from specific age, racial, ethnic, or other groups with special needs.

A concerted effort to publicize the meetings and to encourage attendance from all segments of the community's population is necessary. Letters urging attendance can be mailed to individuals, families, and selected organizations. Posters, fliers, and personal invitations can be utilized in the effort to reach concerned residents.

The advantage of community forums is the relative ease of arranging and conducting inexpensive meetings. Many segments of the community are given the opportunity to provide input, often identifying areas of previously undefined need. Disadvantages of community forums include locations of meeting sites which must be strategically placed. Sometimes attendance of individuals at meetings are not representative of the community's population. For best results, the meetings must be well attended by a cross section of knowledgeable persons who are articulate in expressing their beliefs and sharing information.[8]

Needs Assessment: Rates under Treatment Approach The rates under treatment approach is based on a descriptive enumeration of persons who have utilized the services of the health and welfare agencies of the community. The underlying assumption is that the needs of the community (population) can be estimated from a sample of persons who have received care or treatment.

When rates under treatment approaches are used, information about clients of selected agencies provide data which are descriptive of the services of that agency. Data which are generally solicited include:

1 The sociodemographic characteristics of the clients, i.e., age, race, sex, ethnicity education, place of residence
2 The presenting problem or problems
3 The characteristics of care and services provided
4 The frequency and duration of the care and treatment process
5 The sources of referral
6 Where possible, the outcomes of treatment or services provided

[7] Ibid., pp. 20–21.
[8] Ibid., pp. 22–24.

To secure information about health and welfare agencies existing in the community, directories are generally available. These directories have been compiled by a coordinating or planning agency, and they list the names, telephone numbers, and addresses of a wide variety of community resources, the purpose for which they were formed, the services they offer, the source of financial support, the eligibility requirements for consumers, and the fees. Such a booklet or carefully compiled handbook organized with health-services information is essential data for the community health nurse to have at all times. Frequently the directories have a classified index, which assists in locating needed services according to a given category, such as welfare assistance, services for unmarried mothers, handicapped children and adults, vocational training, special education for special conditions, services for the aging, and many more categories. The classification is done to facilitate the location of needed information within a minimum of time.

For nurses utilizing the rates under treatment approach, a careful plan of how agency records will be handled to assure complete confidentiality and/or anonymity of record contents is absolutely necessary. If the procedure for maintaining anonymity and/or confidentiality of clients is not carefully conceived, few agencies will allow their records to be perused. The focus of the rates under treatment approach is on broad sociodemographic and geographic information and on the types and duration of services provided, not on individual persons. When this is made evident to those being asked for data, the likelihood of receiving cooperation is increased.

The advantage of the rates under treatment approach is the availability of data and the relatively low cost of securing and examining them. Disadvantages of the rates under treatment approach include the problems associated with guaranteeing anonymity and confidentiality of records satisfactorily, and determination of community needs based on a sample of clients utilizing services provided by selected health providers in the community.[9]

Needs Assessment: Social Indicators Approach   The social indicators approach is based primarily on inferences of need drawn from descriptive statistics found in public records and reports. The underlying assumption of the approach is that it is possible to make useful estimates of the needs and social well-being of those in a community by analyzing statistics on factors found to be highly correlated with persons in need. These statistics are regarded as indicators of need. Some factors commonly used as indicators include the spatial arrangements of the community's people and institutions; the sociodemographic characteristics of the population, i.e., age, race, sex, income; the social behavior and well-being of people, particularly as it relates to crime, substance abuse, family patterns, and morbidity and mortality rates; and the general social conditions within which people live, i.e., substandard housing, overcrowding, accessibility to services, and economic conditions. These and other social indicators can be analyzed as constellations, providing important information about a community and its needs.

Typical data which serve as indicators of need are:

[9] Ibid., pp. 26–29.

1 Population characteristics—density, race, ethnicity, national origin, marital status, age, sex, and family status
2 Housing characteristics—type of structure, owner- or renter-occupied dwellings, persons per dwelling, and substandard indices
3 Mortality and morbidity rates—tuberculosis, infant mortality, venereal disease, or suicide
4 Crime patterns and arrest records—those dealing with substance or personal abuses
5 Education
6 Income
7 Fertility and fecundity rates

These data can be obtained from the U.S. Government Printing Office; the U.S. Department of Commerce, Bureau of Census; county health departments (vital statistics); community mental health centers; private medical practitioners; comprehensive health planning agencies; and local community colleges and universities.

Advantages of the social indicators approach is the presence of vast data pools already existing in the public domain, i.e., census reports, government agency statistics, etc. In addition to ready access, most social indicators can be secured at relatively low cost. Data can be obtained in amounts best fitting the purposes of the needs assessment. Disadvantages of the use of social indicators data is that they represent indirectly the needs of the community. Conclusions about community needs based on spatial characteristics of areas, or on indicators reflecting social class values rather than genuine human conditions should be regarded with caution. To be reliable and useful, social indicators data should be obtained from a wide variety of sources.[10]

Needs Assessment: Field Survey Approach The survey approach is based on the collection of data from a sample or entire population of a community. The most common methods used are interview schedules or questionnaires. These are composed of items designed to elicit information from respondents regarding their health, social well-being, and the patterns of care or services being received.

The three most common techniques for gathering information in surveys are (1) the telephone interview, (2) the mailed questionnaire, and (3) the person-to-person interview. Although the methodology of each is somewhat different, their basic format is the same. Each employs questions which ask respondents about health status, health history, use of health service agencies, self-perceptions of health and social needs, etc.

Advantages of survey approaches are that they provide specific information from individuals regarding their needs and utilization of health services. Information gained from one member of a household about the needs and utilization of health services of all family members is acceptable. Disadvantages of surveys are their tendency to be expensive, particularly if a great many questions are asked, and the population is widely dispersed. Some individuals are reluctant to supply information about themselves and family members.[11]

[10] Ibid., pp. 30–38.
[11] Ibid., pp. 39–47.

The Health System within the Community

In many communities, according to Sanders, there are five types of health structures found within the health care system.[12] However, a sixth type has emerged in recent years which is designed to meet the needs of consumers who have not been serviced adequately by the five existing systems. The sixth structure includes the proliferation of neighborhood clinics, community service centers, and neighborhood health stations which have come into being, often with the assistance of the Office of Economic Opportunity, and focus primarily on the needs of minority or low-income groups. The six health structures are closely intertwined, yet distinct enough to be studied separately by those nurses who wish to serve as coordinators and collaborators with all the structures. The five health structures described by Sanders are (1) private office practice of professionals, namely the physician or group of physicians working in the office or clinic setting; (2) group health care, in which consumers buy medical and health services by becoming members of facilities set up for that specific purpose; (3) large hospital and clinics with their own boards and clientele; (4) public health agencies that protect, administer, and perform more preventive than curative health services for the consumer; and (5) those facilities and personnel who sell treatment products and appliances required, such as pharmacists, orthopedic supply houses, and similar establishments. Each of the health subsystems requires a different network of organized activity and therefore operates within an individualized organizational structure, which may be loose-knit or tightly coordinated.

Each health structure fulfills community expectations of a specified sort and conducts its affairs within certain codes of operation.[13] Nurses work in most of the health subsystems and give special services concurrent with the health structure and abide by the code of operation expected within that particular structure. Each health subsystem has basically similar expectations for the functioning of the nurse, but the manner in which nursing tasks are performed varies according to the structure and setting. In the sixth health structure, which was described as a burgeoning number of community health centers, neighborhood multiservice centers, free clinics, or similarly named stations which have come into existence because of needs of consumers, nurses either volunteer their time or are employed by organizations or consumers who receive funding from governmental sources. In the centers in which consumers are participating actively in the determination of health services, nurses play a different role than in any of the other five health structures. Primarily they are working *with* rather than *for* the consumer of health services, and this entails a redirection in focus in many ways, As described by Milio, the nurse sometimes must play a subtle role, or nonvisible one, in order to accomplish a desired objective.[14] Or the nurse must be able to account for the nursing activities in a way that makes sense and is relevant to the consumer.[15]

---

[12] Irwin T. Sanders, "The Community: Structure and Function," *Nursing Outlook,* 11(9): 642-643, September 1963.

[13] Ibid., p. 643.

[14] Nancy Milio, *9226 Kercheval: The Storefront that Did Not Burn,* The University of Michigan Press, Ann Arbor, 1970, p. 31.

[15] Kate R. Lorig, "Consumer-Controlled Nursing," *Nursing Outlook,* 17(9):52, September 1969.

It is an important task of the community health nurse to be cognizant of all facets operating within the health-care system in the given community, to be knowledgeable about coordination practices and procedures with other nurses and professional personnel working in the health structures, and to be able to interpret and link all six health structures in an understandable and intriguing way to the consumer.

An Experiential Exercise for Getting Acquainted with a New Community

Initially, nursing students tend to feel shy about entering a new community as a community health nurse. They fantasize an image in which they see themselves as imparting "pearls of wisdom" to clients—speaking with authority and great knowledge! Obviously, upon entering a community for the first time, students do not possess the essential knowledge which is implied in the fantasy. An exercise which propels students to enter the new community on a "discovery" basis has been found to be helpful in broadening their knowledge base, securing data about the community and its resources, experiencing the climate of a given setting, and building confidence in self to perform independently and assertively. The exercise is an experiential one, whereby students are asked to pretend to *be* a described person in need of particular services. For example, students may be given a written situation and assignment which give a general direction for their exploration of community resources. Suggestions of situations which can be given to students are described briefly as follows.

> You are a young wife and mother who recently arrived in the local community. Your husband is out of work but is making the rounds regarding job possibilities. Your child is 16 months old, is developing normally, but tends to have too many bouts of upper respiratory infections. You wish to rent an apartment or home and want to find one today. According to the welfare worker, you can pay up to —— a month for a place.

> You are a 70-year-old widow who is hardy, curious, and full of energy. You want to volunteer your services wherever there seems to be a need. You want to visit community facilities that may be interested in receiving volunteer services from an elderly lady.

After reading the situations, students are encouraged to work in pairs or trios and venture forth into the new community as explorers. Providing the students with local directories of community resources, a people's yellow pages directory, the telephone book, the local newspaper, and maps will give them basic reference sources from which to draw a plan of action.

Students are amazingly resourceful and learn about a variety of valuable community facilities while doing this exercise. By working in pairs or trios, they support each other in taking the initiative to enter new agencies, make purposeful inquiries, and enact a pretended role. They tend to like to discover by themselves! They sometimes learn that if they present themselves as described by their situation, they are treated differently than if they introduce themselves as nursing students. They learn about the reality of supply and demand of low-cost housing, adequacies and inadequacies of community facilities, and concern for prospective clients. As a consequence of this exercise, students serve as reference persons for each other as they work with families and ask each other for information about available resources for specific health problems. Secondary to this experience, and far more valuable, is the knowledge the students learn about their own values and sanctions, social expectations, and family norms. They are confronted with various lifestyles and social situations that facilitate a greater understanding of the health care delivery system in this country.

Commentary by students about their experiences give some idea of diversity of reactions and viewpoints:

> Today has helped us to see more realistically some of the problems of low-income families and alternatives for assistance. Coming from a middle-class suburban background, frankly, I never really considered the problems of this population. Until now it had no personal relevance for me.

> If I learned nothing else today, I experienced the frustration the family in question would feel in being homeless after a day's search. I'm also 3 times as glad for the roof over *my* head tonight.

> We presented our 70-year-old widow as though she were flesh and blood, which, of course, she is—though we haven't met her yet—and she was soon as real to us as she was to those who were so anxious to give her a niche to fill. When on a couple of occasions we thought it best to admit we were nursing students with a hypothetical case, we were just as warmly received.

> After spending the entire day on my feet, I have to say I am really impressed with my community. I was met with consideration and kindness wherever I visited. Of course, I am prejudiced toward one particular facility—the senior citizens center of ____. I took a nice long look around before ever going up to the building. Was I ever suprised to see tables full of old women making quilts as fast as their hands would travel. I wanted to sit right down and get started working with them.

HEALTH CARE DELIVERY IN THE UNITED STATES

The health care delivery as it exists in the United States today is made up of providers of care from the public and private sectors. Health care providers represent public health agencies and/or city or county health departments, voluntary and proprietary hospitals, medical schools, physicians, health maintenance organizations, philanthropies, and public and social service organizations. They provide care and treatment for the population dependent on the ability to pay a fee for service. Traditionally, there has always been a dual system of health care in the United States. The private sector has provided care for those who have been able to pay for services in either an out-of-pocket way or a third-party prepayment plan. The public sector has provided care for those who are classified as medically indigent. Up to the present, these people have been characterized as welfare, medicare, and medicaid recipients. They have come predominately from the lower socioeconomic levels of income.[16]

[16] Herbert Harvery Hyman (ed.), *The Politics of Health Care,* Praeger Publishers, New York, 1973, p. 160.

It is important for the community health nurse to be cognizant of the present system of health care delivery. At the same time, it is vital to keep up-to-date and knowledgeable about pending health care legislation which may be in the process of being authorized and funded by national and state legislative bodies. Decisions about health care delivery are influenced increasingly by national and governmental policy. New directions for health care, health standards, accessibility, and financing of health care are all subject to changes which will have direct consequences for the consumer and health professional. The community health nurse who keeps current with legislative news and proposals is in the position of preparing for health care delivery as changes occur, of devising health-supporting patterns of living, and raising the consciousness of consumers about access to health services.[17]

SOCIOECONOMIC LEVELS IN THE COMMUNITY

Many specific health problems in the United States are thought to be related directly to poverty, yet affluence also contributes to unhealthy conditions. Socioeconomic levels have a bearing on health status and must be studied in terms of the effect that money, education, living patterns, and lifestyles have on the well-being of consumers. For example, conditions of poverty such as poor housing, inadequate nutrition, and frustration of unemployment can set the stage for pneumonia, influenza, tuberculosis, obesity, apathy, depression, accidents, and chronic disabilities. Affluent individuals who succumb habitually to self-indulgent attributes are vulnerable candidates for coronary heart disease, diabetes, alcoholism, and diagnosed psychiatric maladies.

The composition of each community has its own structure and personality which is not duplicated by any other community. Citizens generally have a vague awareness of the composition of their community but, upon questioning, reveal a lack of specific knowledge about any aspect under inquiry. They often will deny the existence of social classes yet acknowledge the presence of families of different socioeconomic levels residing in segregated neighborhoods, either voluntarily or without choice. Socioeconomic levels are differentiated by their degrees of prestige, education, income, residence, and access to products and services in the community. They are unorganized groups. People are born into them, marry into them, or otherwise enter them from adjacent socioeconomic levels. Within them, people tend to associate with each other more than with others outside their socioeconomic level. On the average, people of different socioeconomic levels vary in aesthetic tastes, in the type of books and magazines they read, the way they vote, the size of their families, the way they spend their leisure time, and even in their sex morality.[18]

In our changing society, the characteristics identifying socioeconomic levels are constantly fluctuating, and clearly defined criteria for determining socioeconomic levels are becoming less distinct. For the purposes of community health nurses, it is valuable to maintain a curiosity about the changing nature of the social-class system, to keep up to date with current events, happenings, and research studies, in order to

[17]Nancy Milio, *The Care of Health in Communities: Access for Outcasts,* Macmillan Publishing Company, Inc., New York, 1975, p. 298.

[18]Roland L. Warren, *Studying Your Community,* The Free Press, New York, 1965, p. 351.

meet health needs of new groupings of citizens as they occur and to relate with understanding, acceptance, and readiness to the wants of the consumer.

It is important to be aware of (1) one's own method for classifying families in terms of socioeconomic level and avoiding the stereotyping based on unvalidated data, (2) one's own feelings of withdrawal and superiority based on past personal experiences, and (3) the family's receptivity cues to general services. When the nurse is cognizant of general behaviors and attitudes representative of each socioeconomic level and of personal reactions to a social-class image, then there is greater ability to identify strengths and weaknesses of a given family with objectivity and to work in an effective, understanding, and facilitative manner. By recognizing the family as possessing characteristics representative of an identified socioeconomic level, but also exhibiting unique characteristics which cannot be classified, the nurse is helped to view the family as a distinct entity rather than squeezing it into a poorly fitting stereotype.

Community health nurses are commonly thought to come from a middle-class orientation and do much of their health practice with people of lower socioeconomic levels. Of interest are the great variety of studies that have focused on the nurse image as seen in the context of social-class perspective. Simmons reported that in general the evaluation of nurses becomes consistently more favorable as the opinions move from higher to lower socioeconomic groups.[19]

Watts compared selective characteristics of people of lower and middle socioeconomic levels and described the person of lower socioeconomic level as being oriented to the present rather than the future and taking pleasures as they are available rather than planning for the future. The person of middle-class orientation looks to the future and is willing to defer gratifications by planning ahead and saving for desired goals. Middle-class individuals value cleanliness, work, and self-discipline.[20]

In regard to health activities, studies have been reported in professional health journals and books indicating that members of the lower socioeconomic levels have a high percentage of illnesses and are dissatisfied with the medical care available to them.[21] They have less information and knowledge about disease and are more likely to hold irrational ideas about illness, rely on folk medicine and fringe practitioners, and delay seeking medical treatment.[22] It is generally accepted that medical care is not as readily accessible to persons of the lower socioeconomic levels in the present health care system. Members of the middle and upper socioeconomic levels know more about the dynamics of illness and health and are more aware of medical care resources for prevention and treatment of sickness. They make use of available resources in a climate of social acceptance.[23]

There are general differences of behavior required of the nurse when associating

[19] Leo W. Simmons and Virginia Henderson, *Nursing Research, a Survey and Assessment,* Appleton-Century-Crofts, Inc., New York, 1964, p. 179.

[20] Wilma Watts, "Social Class, Ethnic Background, and Patient Care," *Nursing Forum,* 6(2): 155–162, Spring 1967.

[21] Evelyn Millis Duvall, *Family Development,* 2d ed., J. B. Lippincott Company, Philadelphia, 1962, pp. 85–86.

[22] David Mechanic, "Illness and Cure," in John Kosa, Aaron Antonovsky, and Irving Kenneth Zola (eds.), *Poverty and Health,* Harvard University Press, Cambridge, Mass., 1969, p. 207.

[23] Duvall, op. cit., p. 85.

with the different socioeconomic levels of people. Some of the perceptions of the nurse are described as follows. When working with people of lower socioeconomic levels, nurses often prefer the families who are responsive to suggestions, seem to value the nurse's teaching and friendship, and demonstrate changes in health practices concurrent with the nurse's influence. The apathetic families described in Chap. 5, such as low-income families, tend to be frustrating to the nurse because it is so difficult to determine if there has been any nursing influence whatsoever. A greater, more intensive effort must be made by community health nurses to study families of lower socioeconomic levels and having multiple problems because the health needs are so great and new, innovative methods for giving nursing services to these families are so greatly needed. The use of role-playing techniques has been strongly recommended by many professional workers because it is appropriate to the style of this population. Role playing is action-oriented, concrete, visual, and sometimes gamelike.[24] It is certainly a method with which nurses are acquainted, yet it is used little with families. In Chap. 5 an elaboration of ways for working more effectively with low-income families is given. When working with families of middle socioeconomic levels, nurses again prefer the responsive families who are interested in health information and teaching on a curing and prevention basis. The fact that these families are often better educated than families of lower income requires the nurse to be prepared insofar as possible to give an intellectual explanation of any symptom about which there is an inquiry. When a family member of middle-class orientation is better educated than the nurse, this sometimes causes the nurse to feel anxious, thereby inhibiting the presentation of a professional image. With families of upper socioeconomic levels, the nurse is sometimes relegated to the status of servant or domestic and responds according to her or his perception of this station in life. With all socioeconomic levels, it helps to be thoughtfully prepared before making a contact, so that the best approach is used. If alternative options are ready, in case a change of plan is required, the nurse feels prepared and comfortable in giving the needed health services.

DIAGNOSING A COMMUNITY HEALTH PROBLEM

After an initial appraisal of a selected community, the nurse is cognizant of the presence of many health facilities, resources, assets, and concerned leaders. Gaps and inadequacies are recognized as existing in conjunction with some health resources and neighborhood settings. When health needs are apparent, what can the community health nurse do to remedy the problems that are seen?

First, a conceptualization of the meaning of community health must be internalized. By viewing health as a total life process, including the adaptation of the individual to the stresses in internal and external environments, one inevitably recognizes that societal forces or social problems have a strong influence on the health of individuals and communities. One is led to conclude that to improve the health of communities, correction of adverse social factors which perpetuate or accentuate maladjustment in

[24] Salvador Minuchin, Braulio Montalvo, Bernard G. Guerney, Jr., Bernice L. Rosman, and Florence Schumer, *Families of the Slums,* Basic Books, Inc., Publishers, New York, 1967, p. 37.

the environment is required.[25] Some community health problems that generally and profoundly affect well-being include poverty, urban crowding, inadequate sanitary and waste disposal, pollution, insecurity, and food shortage. In addition, as described by Milio, when a full array of health services are not located where people (the intended consumers) are or when prices or other program characteristics intervene as barriers, people become outcasts of health care. Social groupings who are identified as outcast are those of low income, poor living areas, old age, minority race, or majority sex.[26]

Secondly, the nurse must seek an "outcast" group or health conditions revealing inadequacies. In most communities, there are several consumer groups or health deficiency areas which can be identified by the nurse. It is only a matter of personal preference and selection. Some questions the nurse might consider are:

What do the people of this community identify as health needs?

Do all people in this community have equal access to health care? If not, who are the ones who do not have easy access? What are the barriers preventing easy access?

Does the health care delivery system in this community give preventive services? If not, are there strategies that might change or improve the system?

Are low-income people in this community concerned about health problems? If not, can they be motivated to become active participants for improved conditions?

Are consumers in this community responsive to health education programs? If not, how might health education programs be made to seem more stimulating and get more attention?

Is there malnutrition in this community? If so, where does it exist? Is it due to lack of education, inadequate funds, personal beliefs and values?

Do people in this community see nurses as community organizers, facilitators, consumer advocates, or social activists?

Some statements about health conditions in the United States are offered for the purpose of stimulating investigation whether these same conditions exist in the local community. Even though the United States is an affluent nation, infant mortality is high statistically, particularly for races other than Caucasian. There is evidence of malnutrition, particularly among blacks and persons of Spanish origin living in low-income neighborhoods. The poor have more disability and limitation of activity because of chronic disease. Even though the overall death rate in the United States has changed little since the 1950s, increased deaths in the middle years (ages 15 to 65) have occurred. Young adults are dying primarily from accidents, homicide, and suicide; and older adults are dying from the diseases of affluence—heart disease, cancer, and stroke.[27] Two-thirds of all accidental deaths occurring from ages 1 through 35 involve automobiles.[28] Eating patterns for citizens in the United States emphasize high con-

---

[25] Lee M. Howard, *Key Problems Impeding Modernization of Developing Countries,* Agency for International Development, Washington, D.C., 1970, p. 50.

[26] Milio, op. cit., p. 63.

[27] Ibid., pp. 43–50.

[28] Committee on Ways and Means, *National Health Insurance Resource Book,* Government Printing Office, Washington, D.C., 1974, p. 82.

centrations of refined sugars and starches which lead to conditions such as dental caries, diabetes mellitus, gastric ulcers, and obesity. Occupationally induced diseases kill 100,000 persons annually.[29]

Any of the above named problems, to cite only a few, can be selected for study by the nurse and preventive measures of some type instituted. Any effort, no matter how small, is worth the energy expended. In-depth exploration and analysis of any selected community health problem in relationship to existing social conditions and the health care delivery system as practiced in the United States is essential in order for the nurse to acquire a knowledge base sufficient for making a diagnosis and deciding future strategies for action.

The following example illustrates how nursing students can assess a selected community, identify a problem area, and diagnose a nursing activity. On a visit to the kindergarten rooms of the local school, a nurse noted obvious dental caries and poor oral hygiene practices of the children. In a subsequent conference with the principal of the school, the nurse obtained the addresses of the kindergarten children and learned that a high proportion of families were low-income. The nurse ascertained that no health screening was done routinely at this school and was informed that health education sessions were wanted. They were not always carried out, however, because the teacher felt unprepared in teaching about health practices. The nurse's thought process went like this: (1) My selected community is this kindergarten. (2) I must look into the mouths of all the children and assess the extent of dental caries. (3) I must talk with the teacher to find out her interest in oral hygiene and health practices. (4) I must determine if parents will support a program promoting dental services of some kind. (5) I must decide on an activity that will be most beneficial—finding dentists for the children, finding methods of payment for dental care, teaching good oral hygiene and prevention of caries, promoting a fluoride program in this school, having a dental clinic made up of volunteer dentists and dental hygienists. At this point the nurse was ready to assess the selected problem area in depth, determine alternatives which would be most appropriate and acceptable for the kindergarten, consumers, and school population, and decide on an appropriate nursing diagnosis.

INTRODUCTION TO COMMUNITY ACTION

Involvement in any kind of community action is a learning experience. A nursing student may start with a simple idea of improving health conditions in a local neighborhood, such as eliminating safety hazards from a playground for children. However, as suggestions for change are offered to individuals presumed to have control of the playground, the student soon learns that the mechanism for instituting change is complex, slow, and oftentimes frustrating. The student who persists with the idea soon learns about the existence of power, authority, influence, leadership, organizational structures, politics, vested interests, and strategies. The importance of accumulating and documenting the necessary data during the assessment period becomes apparent. Also

[29] Milio, op. cit., p. 51.

Table 4-1   Interrelating the Community Health Nursing Process with the Community Organization Process

Community health nursing process	Community organization process

1 Assessing
  a Diagnosis
    (1) Documentation of a health need
2 Planning
  a Goals and objectives to be attained
  b Theoretical rationale
	1 Identifying needs or objectives
	  a Discontent with existing conditions
	2 Ordering or ranking of needs or objectives
	3 Developing the will and confidence to work at the needs or objectives
	4 Finding the resources (internal and external) to deal with the needs or objectives
	  a Finding acceptable leaders (formal and informal)

3 Implementing
  a Strategy
	5 Taking action
	  a Activities with emotional content
	6 Extending and developing cooperative and collaborative attitudes and practices in the community
	  a Utilize goodwill existing in the community
	  b Active and effective lines of communication
	  c Positive reinforcement of strengths

4 Evaluating a Criteria for evaluating terminal objectives	7 Evaluating

learned are how expeditiously an influential person can secure results; how chances for success are greater if a group of concerned citizens are involved, rather than one lone individual seeking to be heard; how necessary it is to know how the "local system" works, communicates, and operates.

For purposes of assisting the beginning student in entering the complex community arena, guidelines, as proposed by Ross, are presented. The guidelines are easily grasped and give one perspective for comprehending community action "as we would like it to be" compared with "what it turns out to be." The guidelines also are analogous with the community health nursing process, yet offer broader dimensions for exploration. Table 4-1 shows the interrelatedness of the community health nursing process with the community organization process.

Community Organization Process

Community organization, as defined by Ross, is a process by which a community identifies its needs or objectives, orders these needs or objectives, takes action in respect to them, and in so doing, extends and develops cooperative and collaborative attitudes and practices in the community.[30] One primary purpose for engaging in the community organization process is to build and strengthen community integration. When the

[30] Murray G. Ross, *Community Organization,* Harper & Row, Publishers, Incorporated, New York, 1955, p. 39.

process is separated into steps and essential principles are clarified in conjunction with each step, the process is easily understood and translated into practice.

1 *To identify health needs* there must be evidence of discontent with existing conditions. This discontent must be focused into specific concerns which are shared by many in the community and for which factors can be explored regarding possible solutions. When exploring ideas with citizens, it is advisable to discern their health *wants*, as opposed to their health *needs*, so that support from a substantial number of citizens is gained regarding any potentially selected health issue. Ideally, the movement toward a health objective should be instigated by the citizens or at least receive their enthusiastic endorsement, so that motivation toward action is already inherent.

2 *The ordering of needs or objectives* is primarily setting priorities and focusing on the most urgent health need or desire first. When a health issue is selected that represents the citizens' wants, commitment and action will be secured early with minimum prompting from any health expert. People have always known of health *needs* that would be beneficial for them, but few individuals respond to "You should have this" or "You need this" unless they *want* it. For example, a community may tend to be apathetic and unconcerned about the general drug traffic problem on which the communication media is concentrating until several local high school students from respectable homes in their own community are picked up and jailed for possession of illegal drugs. Then the citizenry is truly alerted, aroused, and ready to take action in any advised direction that will resolve the problem. Progress cannot be made in the community any faster than the understanding and consent of the concerned group of citizens.[31]

3 *To develop the will and confidence* to work with a selected health concern, leaders (either formal or informal) from the community must be found and utilized. These leaders must be regarded as acceptable representatives of the interests or participating community subgroups. When local community leaders work actively with an identified health issue, participate in gathering data and planning action, their influence spreads, and other interested citizens are drawn into the work force.

4 The core of persons who are recognized and accepted as members of a citizens' committee working on a selected health issue represent the *human resources* in the community who are held accountable by the local population. It is advisable that the concerned group represent a valid cross section of citizens and agencies in the community, that some key influential persons be included, and that a professional individual with expertise in knowledge about the selected health issue be asked to serve as a consultant when needed. By expecting committee members to be involved, the gathering of a wide variety of resources within and without the community evolves in surprising directions when the group is allowed to be innovative and creative. The capacity of local citizens to solve problems and help themselves has unlimited potential, and the task of the chairperson and/or facilitator need only be aimed at exerting indirect leadership and giving support whenever required by the group. An early action of the committee is the determination of goals or objectives to be achieved. The nurse who is a member of the committee can be instrumental in assuring that the objectives are written behaviorally, are attainable, and are acceptable to the local citizenry. (See Chap. 3 for guidance in writing behavioral objectives.) When everyone on the committee is

[31] Clarence King, *Working with People in Community Action*, Association Press, New York, 1965, p. 82.

well acquainted with, understands, and accepts the goals and/or objectives of their common endeavor, a frame of reference which serves as a basis for providing consistent direction is established.

5 Members of the citizens' committee will decide on the *action* necessary and most appropriate in order to attain their objectives. To develop strength and cohesion as a working group, activities with emotional content must be recognized as essential for developing an integrated spirit. The committee will have times of hard work, serious discussions, arguments, and problem-solving endeavors, but it is hoped that they will also have times of laughter, friendship, and celebrations. If a light touch and festive spirit is maintained when the occasion warrants it, members of the committee will remember the fun along with the hard work and associate the whole endeavor as purposeful and valuable. When unforeseen events occur requiring changes of plan and adaptation of action, a committed and integrated citizens' committee is able to provide flexible alternatives with minimal internal opposition.

6 It is important that *collaborative and cooperative attitudes and practices* in the community be in operation during the entire community organization process. The requirement that lines of communication remain active, open, and effective is more easily stated than accomplished. The citizens' committee should aim toward utilizing the goodwill that exists in the community. This can be done in a variety of ways such as person-to-person contacts, sharing information informally, and utilizing strengths and resources within the community. With an active and open communication system existing within the committee and with representative community citizens, it is probable that differences of opinions, tensions, and conflicts will occur. However, this lends life and vitality to a movement as opposed to easy consensus or "groupthink." *Groupthink* refers to the mode of thinking that individuals engage in when concurrence-seeking becomes so dominant in a cohesive in-group that it tends to override realistic appraisal of alternative courses of action.[32] Members of cohesive groups must guard against groupthink characteristics such as amiability, avoidance of harsh statements in opposition to a colleague's or leader's ideas, and concurrence with all major decisions by the group, instead of voicing inner misgivings regarding an idea. Open conflict or disagreements should be allowed to occur within a citizens' committee, and when this happens, resolution of the conflict must be handled, whether constructively or destructively. If constructively handled, increased understanding, tolerance, and strength are developed in the committee. When the attitudes of persons allow for cooperative and collaborative work, they learn to endure, welcome, and move comfortably with diversity and tension.[33]

An effective activity and communication device is the employment of a pilot project. When a problem is worked out on a small scale, it provides the opportunity to see and hear how an idea, technique, or operation will work. It also brings out obstacles or oversights that had not been considered in the initial plan. Clarification of procedures and outcomes also is facilitated as individuals asked to participate in the pilot study give feedback regarding their responses and interpretation of the instructions.

7 Throughout the entire community organization process, mechanisms for *evaluation* of each step are essential. This can be the task of a health professional or a nurse. Gathering essential data, requesting feedback at each step, presenting a rationale or argument for the inclusion of each step, and suggesting alternative ideas are all proce-

[32] Irving L. Janis, "Groupthink," *Psychology Today*, 5(6):43–46, November 1971.
[33] Ross, op. cit., p. 49.

dures facilitating ongoing evaluation as each step of the process is examined. Success of a project is more easily assured if evaluative means are utilized throughout the process.

The role of the health professional who is facilitating the community organization process in regard to a specific health issue is one of working *with* the citizens, encouraging the development of all the essential elements in the process, making use of consultation as necessary, serving as a worker in the background rather than the forefront, and strengthening the capacity of the local citizenry to function as a team toward accomplishment of the goals and objectives to which they have committed themselves.

It must be pointed out that the steps of the community organization process are not necessarily followed in order. Sometimes early action will hasten the development of the other elements in the process. What is essential is that all activities have a purpose, that the positive and negative alternatives are considered before acting upon them, and that the community group is continuously evaluating or judging the evolving events that occur as movement progresses toward the established goals.

THREE MODELS OF COMMUNITY ORGANIZATION PRACTICE

According to Rothman, there are three models of community organization practice designed for making change in a community. The three approaches or models can be used in pure form or can be combined. The essentialities of each approach are summarized in order for nursing students to be consciously aware of the strategies for selection in community organization practice and the roles students will utilize, contingent upon the model selected.

The Community Development Approach

The *community development approach* is a process designed to create conditions of economic and social progress for the whole community with its active participation and the fullest possible reliance on the community's initiative. This approach uses democratic procedures, seeks voluntary cooperation of consumers, encourages self-help measures by citizens, seeks to develop indigenous leadership of the local residents, and utilizes identified educational objectives. The change strategy may be characterized as, "Let's all get together and talk this over." If a wide range of community people are involved in determining their needs or wants, it is felt that consumers will be more inclined to participate in solving their own problems.[34] The community organization process, as described by Ross, is an example of a community development approach.

For nursing students who are getting started in community action, this approach is challenging and offers an opportunity to try many leadership and group development skills. Nursing students have utilized the approach on a small scale and have successfully implemented change in small, circumscribed communities. For example, after conducting a door-to-door survey of elderly citizens living in a low-income apartment

[34] Jack Rothman, "Three Models of Community Organization," in *Social Work Practice,* Columbia University Press, New York, 1968. Copyright 1968 National Conference on Social Welfare.

complex in which questions were asked about unmet health needs, it was found that the citizens expressed a variety of needs. A meeting of the residents was arranged to determine their responsiveness to the idea of a social and health center in the apartment building. During this community meeting, it was the intent of the nursing students to identify leaders among the residents, discuss the results of the survey about unmet health needs, elicit other areas of needs, and decide on goals as agreed upon by the residents and nurses. A health clinic subsequently was initiated in which services offered by nursing students consisted of taking comprehensive health histories, blood pressure readings, vital signs, and temperatures. Simple foot care was given, health counseling was offered based on the data secured in the health history, and referrals to appropriate resources were made. Weekly meetings of the residents and nurses led to a camaraderie that was warm and freely expressed. Social needs, as well as health needs, were given attention. When new problems arose, the residents felt comfortable in talking about their concerns during the weekly meeting and, upon encouragement from the nursing students, succeeded in finding acceptable solutions. The informal leaders who evolved showed pleasure in being instrumental toward effecting desired change and realizing their newfound capabilities.

The Social Planning Approach

The *social planning approach* emphasizes a technical process of problem solving with regard to substantive social problems. Agencies and organizations frequently utilize this approach as they seek to bring about desired changes according to their perspective of the area of need. Planning is rational and deliberate, and controlled change is involved. Community participation may be great or small. Proposed health bills that are designed to be introduced into the legislative process may be an example of the social planning approach. The change strategy utilized can be exemplified by, "Let's get the facts and proceed logically step by step." Appropriate and pertinent data are considered essential before decisions can be made about a rational and feasible course of action.[35]

The social planning approach is comprehended by nursing students as they participate actively with specific agencies studying data about existing social problems. For example, a multiservice center in a small community incorporated two nursing students in their planning process for gathering specific health data from residents living in the surrounding housing project area. The purpose of the center was to provide a variety of social services for any low-income person, regardless of race, creed, color, sex, or national origin. The plan was to construct a questionnaire which inquired about the needs of the low-income people and, at the same time, explain about the services available at the center. At the planning meetings, which were composed of individuals representing a variety of services, the students added their ideas to the design of the questionnaire and, at the same time, became conscious of the priorities, focus, and desires of personnel representing other disciplines. When the time came for the collection of data, the students realized with some surprise that the personnel at the center wanted the findings to bring out a need and desire for a cooperative day-care program.

[35] Ibid.

As it happened, the findings of the survey showed that the residents predominately supported the idea of a health clinic. Only 23 percent of the clientele wanted a day-care program. With the passage of time, it was noted that follow-up was done selectively on health needs as expressed by the residents. The findings of the questionnaire contained valuable data and were used as a basis for planning specific health services concurrent with the goals of the center.

The Social Action Approach

The *social action approach* aims at making basic changes in major institutions or in community practices which are presumed to be in need of correction. For example, if disadvantaged segments of the population were organized and made their desires known through group action, it is possible that necessary and additional resources would be made available to these people. Social action seeks redistribution of power, resources, or decision making in the community and/or changing of basic policies of formal organizations. The change strategy takes the direction of, "Let's organize to destroy our oppressor." By organizing a group of citizens and talking about easily identified problems, issues are crystallized and the means for bringing pressure on selected targets by mass action are devised. In the social action approach, clients are often considered victims of "the system," or "underdogs." The action mode is direct and sometimes confronting.[36]

An example of nursing students spontaneously employing the social action approach for themselves has occurred in the past and continues to be utilized whenever they become aroused. It happens when students become greatly dissatisfied with the teaching style of a selected instructor, start criticizing all aspects of the nursing course among themselves, and insidiously build an emotional climate which eventually reaches a passionate crisis level. At that point, small groups of students organize, decide to go to the dean of the school of nursing to complain, and demand a change of conditions in the classroom. The students feel "oppressed" and seek to have a voice in the system by applying pressure on the persons with authority. Their method generally is direct and confronting as they seek change of their untenable position. Depending upon the response of the person with authority, the students are satisfied, mollified, or offended, and through the experience learn the meaning of a social action approach from a personal perspective.[37]

When social reform in our society is the goal of the change agent, a mixture of social action and social planning is utilized. The reformer is faced with three tasks which must be considered. A coalition of power sufficient for the purpose must be formed; the democratic tradition, which expects every citizen to be not merely represented but to play an autonomous part in self-determination, must be respected; and the policies must be demonstrably rational.[38] Social reform involves activity by a group or coali-

[36] Ibid.
[37] Mary C. Jones, "Confrontation in a Classroom," *Nursing Outlook,* 18(11):47–49, November 1970.
[38] Peter Marris and Martin Rein, *Dilemmas of Social Reform,* Aldine Publishing Company, Chicago, 1967, p. 7. Copyright 1967 Peter Marris and Martin Rein. Reprinted by permission of Aldine Publishing Company.

tion of interests which acts vigorously on behalf of some outside client group which is at risk. The change strategy uses employment of facts and persuasion to apply pressure on decision-making bodies and/or campaign tactics.[39] An example of an organization involved with social reform is the League of Women Voters.

The major purpose for becoming acquainted with and studying the community organizations' models leads the nurse to be prepared in making situational diagnoses and analyses that will assist in choosing the appropriate and most effective community organization method. Regardless of the method chosen, when involved in community organization practice, the nurse eventually will see all types of action—the polite formality of community committees, deliberated by Robert's rules of order; protest marches; education of client groups regarding methods for getting the attention of power organizations; use of a "cause" or client group to promote personal gain. The nurse who considers community organization practice as a learning experience recognizes the opportunity for (1) learning to speak in public about an issue, (2) learning about various means for gaining attention, (3) knowing the importance of pertinent and appropriate facts, (4) planning strategy, (5) knowing the importance of timing, (6) gathering essential support from groups and/or organizations, rather than working alone, and (7) perceiving the advantageous role of persons in power.

When seeking the ear of a person of authority, it helps to be cognizant that communication and power cannot be divorced. Information implies action.[40] When a person agrees to listen she or he becomes committed to a response. It can be a response of agreement, a counter argument, other information, or selective inattention to the content of the message. The person with authority holds the inimitable position of governing the direction of messages people are communicating at that time. However, when attention is gained and messages truly heard, the potential of a realignment of power is possibly created. It is important to remember that seeds of ideas can be planted, regardless of immediate reactions of persons with authority, and that ideas can and do germinate even though dormant for a period of time.

KENT MODEL OF COMMUNITY ORGANIZATION

Kent has worked extensively with poor and disadvantaged people and has developed a community organization model which is effective with these populations. He believes that lack of opportunity, discrimination, and an unresponsive society have forced the disadvantaged person into an inflexible mold in which values and behaviors necessary for effective participation in society are discouraged. He advocates that poor and disadvantaged populations can be reached and motivated by assessing positive characteristics or strengths. For example, identified strengths of persons in poverty include the following methods of interaction: (1) They meet and talk personally and intimately in specific locations or geographical areas. (2) They are loyal to neighbors and friends. (3) Physical contact is a characteristic ingredient of interpersonal communication. (4) They maintain close contact with the extended family, particularly in certain ethnic

---

[39] Rothman, op. cit.
[40] Marris and Rein, op. cit., p. 281.

groups. Some groups place a higher value on having a number of children rather than acquiring material goods. (5) The lifestyle often consists of dependency on helping persons such as a member of one's family or a friend.[41] By recognizing and accepting the existence of the above characteristics or strengths, a beginning step is taken toward working effectively with disadvantaged persons.

Kent advocates looking at situations in disadvantaged areas in a "natural" way— including the minute and seemingly unimportant facts of life. In other words, the individual must be prepared to examine the real and natural situation of poverty from the perspective of poverty persons, consider ways for change, discover existing resources, and identify paths toward independent action by the poor. In taking a descriptive or "discovery" approach to the disadvantaged community, the student must be cognizant of being a stranger in an unfamiliar environment and attempt to observe "what's going on in the community." Helpful questions to keep in mind are:

What are the people doing?
What kind of games are the children playing?
Are there natural paths that most people are using?
What is the housing like?
What is the prevalent mode of transportation in this community?
What is the movement of people at certain time frames of the day?
Do people congregate at specific places at certain times of the day?

By getting a natural "feel" of the neighborhood through the senses and realizing that the neighborhood belongs to its residents, the beginning step toward assimilation into a new environment is initiated.[42] Natural problems of concern to the residents are the ones for which to look. Frequently, the optimal time for helping disadvantaged persons is during a crisis period, whether the crisis is health-related or not. If concrete, constructive assistance is given to a person during an immediate crisis, her or his capacity for learning experientially is at an optimal level. Action toward resolution of the problem creates an acceptance and trust between helper and helpee which is essential for subsequent teaching and interventions. Natural helpers or advisors who have special skills and talents should be sought and utilized within the community at all possible times. These individuals are the natural care givers who are the already known helpers or family members. They must be taught the advocacy role and reinforced for all successful endeavors. A system whereby residents become natural helpers for each other is one of the goals of the Kent model, which teaches self-help measures. If a neighborhood can be mobilized into a power position so that participation in the dominant social order of the community occurs, then responsible citizenship is learned and confidence gained in becoming a part of the democratic system that has influence upon local government. Nursing students can initiate the Kent model in neighborhoods showing potential for learning. They must first get well acquainted and be accepted in

[41] James A. Kent, C. Harvey Smith, and Sam Burns, *An Urban Strategy for Action against Poverty,* Foundation for Urban and Neighborhood Development, Denver, Colo., 1967, p. 1.
[42] Mary Bayer, "Community Diagnosis—Through Sense, Sight, and Sound," *Nursing Outlook,* 21(11):712-713, Nov. 1973.

the neighborhood before natural problems will be uncovered and natural assets discovered. They must know and understand the subgroups in the neighborhood and utilize the natural internal care-giver system before any effective action can be anticipated.[43] To enter a neighborhood utilizing the Kent model is an excellent learning experience that broadens the student's perspective of community organization and the problems of lower socioeconomic and disadvantaged populations.

WARREN'S MODEL FOR ASSESSING NEIGHBORHOODS

A typology of neighborhoods was developed by Warren[44] as a means for understanding and describing the variety of highly specialized roles that neighborhoods play in the lives of their residents. The typology is based on three dimensions of organization—interaction, identity, and connections. By examining a neighborhood in terms of the three dimensions, structural characteristics and differences in neighborhood organization are disclosed. The presence of social class, income, and ethnic factors do not change the basic elements of each neighborhood. Questions to ask in terms of the three dimensions are:

1 *Interaction* During the year do people in the neighborhood get together quite often?
2 *Identity* Do people in the neighborhood feel that they have a great deal in common?
3 *Connections* Do many people in the neighborhood keep active in political parties and other forces outside the neighborhood?

According to Warren, neighborhoods can be classified into six types, depending upon how each question in the typology is answered. A brief description of the six types of neighborhoods is summarized as follows:

1 *Integral* This neighborhood stands alone and is proud of its uniqueness and its ability to organize and function as an integral unit within the larger community. Prominent citizens live here and provide linkage between outside organizations and neighborhood groups.
2 *Parochial* Much activity and social interactions are observed in this neighborhood. People are friendly, and a sense of belonging is evident. However, the residents isolate themselves from the outside community with the attitude, "we take care of our own."
3 *Diffuse* This neighborhood has a sameness of homes, children, and attitudes. People are friendly yet place a premium on privacy. Neighbors have a good deal in common but share little. If they need help, they prefer to seek aid from their families rather than neighbors. They identify with their neighborhood but have little interaction with each other and feel little connection with the outside community.

---

[43] Kent, op. cit., pp. 3–19.
[44] Donald I. Warren and Rachelle B. Warren, "Six Kinds of Neighborhoods," *Psychology Today*, 9(1):74–80, June 1975.

4 *Stepping-stone* This neighborhood is open friendly, and marked with a transient characteristic. Moving vans are frequently seen in this neighborhood. Even though residents live here temporarily, there is close interaction between the people and their ties to the larger community. However, the sense of connection is not strong in this neighborhood.

5 *Transitory* There is a sameness of homes and structures in this neighborhood, but there is neither interaction nor community identification. The widespread distrust within the neighborhood communicates a feeling of "no one cares."

6 *Anomic* These neighborhoods lack all the predominant characteristics. There is little interaction between residents, a sense of isolation and disinterest, and little evidence of individuals engaged in activities outside the neighborhood. The prevailing attitude is, "we don't like people nosing into our business."

For nurses assessing neighborhoods with the intent to organize, it is important to examine the process of influence that goes on. Every neighborhood is an information-processing center—either keeping information out, absorbing it uncritically, or filtering its content so that interpretation of meaning is controlled via the individualistic "neighborhood perspective." Nurses should look for residents who are influential in the neighborhood information process. They represent three types: (1) residents who are officers in various kinds of voluntary organizations, such as PTAs or block clubs; (2) less visible residents who belong to no formal organizations but have the reputation for getting things done; (3) residents who are "opinion leaders," and who are approached frequently by neighbors for advice on a problem or for information about where to get help. With knowledge about the three types of residents to be on the lookout for, nurses must also understand how information is disseminated through the six types of neighborhoods.

1 *Integral* This neighborhood picks up resources and information from many outside points. Residents have influential jobs and links with many kinds of community groups. At the same time, they are active within their neighborhood. They bring new information and techniques into the neighborhood and let outside institutions know what people in the neighborhood are thinking. These "linking persons" have a real power base. They carry messages from local residents to outside organizations and back again.

2 *Parochial* People interact often and have a network of neighborhood groups. But unlike the integral neighborhood, it faces inward. Information seldom passes directly into the neighborhood; it is filtered and modified by key opinion leaders. These leaders have strong commitments to their neighborhood but are less likely than integral leaders to transmit to their neighborhood the concerns of the larger community.

3 *Diffuse* Residents identify with this neighborhood because they find it a pleasant place to live; but they seldom get together and do not depend on the neighborhood as a basis for shaping or protecting their lifestyle. Information flows slowly, and the neighborhood is often relatively slow in taking action, even though there is a great deal of organizational potential. Only under conditions of crisis does this neighborhood become organizationally active.

4 *Stepping-stone* This neighborhood has a high degree of internal organization as well as a large number of residents with outside connections. But the residents have no strong commitment to the neighborhood. There are usually formal mechanisms to

Table 4-2 Guide for Neighborhood Action*

Assessing the neighborhood characteristics	Taking action						
	Publish news-letter	Conduct door-to-door campaign	Adver-tise in mass media	Contact key neigh-bors	Use organi-zation lists	Form grass-roots group	Set up pipeline to city hall
1 *Interaction* Q During the year, do people in the neighborhood get together quite often? A Yes.	√	No	No	+	√	√	√
2 *Heterogeneity* Q Are there many people of differ-ent backgrounds, lifestyles, or social levels who live in the neighborhood? A Yes.	√	+	No	√	√	No	No
3 *Identify* Q Do people in the neighborhood feel they have a great deal in common? A Yes.	+	√	√	No	√	√	√
4 *Mutual aid* Q When someone has a problem, are neighbors willing to help? A Yes.	√	√	√	No	No	No	+
5 *Privatism* Q Do people in the neighborhood place more value on their family privacy than on being in touch with neighbors? A Yes.	No	No	+	√	√	No	No
6 *Insulation* Q If a bill collector came around ask-ing about a neigh-bor, would people in your neighbor-hood refuse to give out any informa-tion? A Yes.	√	+	No	√	No	√	No

Table 4-2   Guide for Neighborhood Action* (*Continued*)

Assessing the neighborhood characteristics	Taking action						
	Publish news-letter	Conduct door-to-door campaign	Adver-tise in mass media	Contact key neigh-bors	Use organi-zation lists	Form grass-roots group	Set up pipeline to city hall
7 *Connections* **Q** Do many people in the neighborhood keep active in groups outside the neigh-borhood? **A** Yes.	√	No	√	√	+	√	√
8 *Turnover* **Q** Are there many people who move in and out of your neighborhood? **A** Yes.	+	√	√	No	No	√	√

*For each "yes" answer, look across the list of strategies to find which action would be the best first step (+), which ones would be good follow-up actions (√), and which ones should be avoided (No).

Source: Donald I. Warren and Rachelle B. Warren, "Six Kinds of Neighborhoods," *Psychology Today,* **9**(1): 74–80, June 1975.

integrate new residents quickly and to tell them about neighborhood groups. However, residents usually continue to be more active in outside groups rather than local ones.

5 *Transitory*   The population turnover is so great and the institutional fabric so restricted that there is little action in this neighborhood. It often breaks down into cliques of longtime residents who belong to the same groups and never allow newcomers in. Neighbors feel they have little in common and usually avoid local entanglements. There may be pockets of intense activity, but there is no cohesion.

6 *Anomic*   This neighborhood has virtually no leadership structure. A few residents may have connections to outside groups but remain inactive on their home turf. Individuals and families are on their own, confronting outside institutions without any kind of support from their neighbors. Usually they are distrustful of outside groups, but almost never can they get help or guidance from anyone in their neighborhood. The residents are large consumers of the mass media, and the messages come through unfiltered.

Warren's examination of neighborhood structure and process provides a useful systematic description of neighborhood life in America. The typology shown in Table 4-2 provides useful guidelines for nurses wanting to organize a neighborhood for action.[45]

[45] Ibid., p. 76.

ROLE OF THE NURSE IN THE COMMUNITY

After assessing a neighborhood or local community, selecting a health problem, and becoming acquainted with community organization practices, the nurse is faced with deciding what role to play in terms of the diagnosis of the health issue requiring action. The role options available are: enabler, coordinator, catalyst, teacher, data gatherer, facilitator, activist, advocate, or negotiator. To perform intelligently in any of these roles, the nurse must be completely knowledgeable about the community and the risks involved in participating in any one of the selected community organization methods. Community life is plastic, and for the most part consumers seek positive betterment of their environment, living conditions, and way of life. Membership in a community derives from a conscious sense of "belonging." People are friends and neighbors and interrelate according to mutual interests, common problems, common values, and common hopes. Frequently, people are aware of and dissatisfied with negative aspects of their community yet give little thought to the improvement of things. Ideas for improved health conditions or focusing on situations revealing recognized health deficiencies can be a starting point for the nurse who wishes to be an enabler, a facilitator, or a catalyst in the community. Among members of every community can be found individuals with many capabilities, ideas, and skills. All that needs to be done is finding them and giving them some direction and positive reinforcement. It is in community effort that the personal meaning of a helping hand is discovered.

The teacher role requires knowledge of the selected subject. Delving into reference books or acquiring information that will catch the attention and interest of citizens is the challenge. Oftentimes, creativity is required in bringing out health issues previously taken for granted. For the most part, citizens do not get excited about health education until a personal health habit has affected their lives undesirably. One method for the teacher to choose is that of a lecturer. If this method is selected, visual aids and dramatizations which attract attention and lend charisma to the instructor-lecturer frequently are ingredients for success. The teaching role also can be accomplished by behaving as a consultant and/or facilitator. Citizens who are drawn to work actively on a health issue can be encouraged and reinforced to problem-solve, implement solutions, and evaluate outcomes in a teaching-learning situation that leads them to function autonomously, independently, and confidently.

If the coordinator or negotiator role is to be assumed, knowledge of the existing community services and acquaintance with key individuals of every discipline are desirable. The role of coordinator is valuable and time-consuming, as multiple telephone calls, negotiations about optimal meeting times and places, familiarity with particular interests of clientele, recognition of the input of members of each discipline, assignment of acceptable tasks, and delegation of responsibility for the completion of assignments are undertaken.

The activist or advocate role requires willingness to risk. In many instances, the nurse advocate must be assertive, oftentimes aggressive, and willing to take the consequences of actions as they occur. A knowledge of the legislative process, bargaining and/or making compromises, political maneuvers or strategies, power as exercised by influential persons, and counterstrategies are all essential. To become an effective advocate takes time, patience, perseverance, and practice. Learning to bargain and compromise or deliberately planning a strategy aimed toward winning a desired goal are skills that nursing students are not well-prepared to do. The word "manipulation" frequently has a negative connotation; yet, manipulation is part of politics and strategy.

It is in practice and experience that the nurse learns the essence and nuances of the role undertaken. Community organization work exposes the nurse to many facets of the community arena and prepares the nurse to deal realistically with life-and-death issues affecting the life and health of consumer populations.

PLANNING THE HEALTH CARE ACTION

Planning is a process considered essential for engineering actions which will produce desired outcomes. For the nurse, the diagnosis regarding a selected community health issue contains the implication that a nursing action is appropriate and feasible as a means for attaining desired outcomes and for which planning must be done. Consequently, objectives must be written which will provide direction for the accomplishment of desired ends. Objectives which are clearly stated, explicitly descriptive of desired outcomes, realistic, measurable, and attainable give purpose and consistency to the nurse and all other individuals involved with planning. Objectives must be congruent with the desires and wants of the consumers of the community. For more information about the writing of objectives, see Chap. 3.

Health care cannot be planned without considering how economic, political, social, religious, geographic, and other factors influence its utilization. In each community the visibility of health problems differs. Also, change occurs constantly in our dynamic society regardless of whether communities plan for it or not. Identification of a health problem for which planning is necessary does not ensure resolution of the problem. Often, a plan which culminates in an outcome desired by citizens produces a new situation in which new needs are created. In other words, planning is never completed because the process produces changes which require additional planning. Because planning is a continuous process in our changing society, short-term goals that depict tangible action and specify attainable realistic outcomes are best. A short-term goal can be attached to a long-term goal; however, the long-term goal should provide mechanisms for flexibility and adaptability in reaching the ends desired.

In addition to defining objectives, the well-prepared nurse must be cognizant of the factors that shape the community organization model deemed appropriate. The rationale for selecting the theoretical model of community organization should be appropriate for the population with which the nurse proposes to work. All variables of the community organization model must be examined, and strategies and role behaviors most likely to succeed must be consciously planned. When other individuals are teammates in the planning endeavor, a knowledge of group process and group behavior is facilitative. By keeping lines of communication with the multidisciplinary team of workers open, considerate of others, active, purposeful, and supportive, a plan generally satisfactory to all members will emerge.

When the environment in which the action will take place is comprised of social institutions or agencies, a knowledge of the structure of the institution or agency is imperative. All institutions or agencies have formal and informal organizational structures that can be shown on paper. The formal organization depicts a structure or picture by which the efforts or functions of the people fit together logically to accomplish some purpose. The organizational structure shows how the functions of members are interrelated and integrated. The informal structure or picture reveals the efforts or functions of people that have not been formally planned but have spontaneously evolved from the needs of the members within the organization. Informal work arrangements always exist, have rules or norms for guiding the behavior of its members, have leaders and followers, and are perpetuated as a means of social life within the organization.[46] When studying the structure of a particular social institution or agency, a formal structure or organizational outline can always be elicited from the person in charge. As the investigator becomes familiar with the activities and membership of the institution, the informal structure will emerge. Pictures of formal and informal structures are graphic visual aids that are descriptive of functions, membership, and interactions characteristic of the specified institution.

Health-planning agencies within communities, such as official health-planning councils, are informative, educational, and up-to-date on health issues and health legislation that are of concern nationally and locally. Involvement in some aspect of planning in such an agency is an excellent learning experience for nursing students. Opportunity to observe group dynamics, uses of power and authority, leadership strategies, bargaining, and decision making by community experts is provided at close proximity. The purposes, benefits, priorities, and communication styles of health-planning agencies acquaint students with business as it is actually conducted.

IMPLEMENTING THE PLAN OF ACTION

Implementing a plan is where the nursing process "goes into action." For some nurses, this is the "fun" part of the entire process. It is during the implementation phase that the nurse realizes if (1) all essential data was assessed and accumulated according to the need; (2) the diagnosis was accurate; (3) the plan was well thought out; (4) she or he possesses the attributes and skills necessary for the assumed role; (5) she or he is flexible; and (6) an oversight, an error in judgment, or a need for supervision and/or consultation can be admitted. Implementing a plan for action in the community often involves other persons who may behave as allies, show active resistance, require constant current reports of the ongoing situation, or interfere with unexpected, restricting rules or policies. It is during these times that the nurse becomes aware of personal capacity to be flexible, adaptable, frustrated, creative, persuasive, persistent, or firm.

When problems arise, it is well for the nurse and the members of the citizens' committee to review their activities up to the moment of intervention—their assessment of the problem, the selection of the community organization approach, the accuracy and completeness of their plan, the possibility that they overlooked a key individual or community resource, a breakdown in communication lines. Consideration should be given to what seems to be the issue of the opposition. Do opposing individuals understand the purpose of the planned action? Is clarification needed? Has language been of

[46]Joseph A. Litterer, *Organizations: Structure & Behavior,* John Wiley & Sons, Inc., New York, 1963, pp. 10-11.

a superior-subordinate nature? Does the opposition have an issue that must be taken into consideration? Perhaps the selected strategy for action needs to be redirected or modified. It is possible that the gathering of more supportive groups or influential individuals may be needed. Seeking consultation from experienced experts in the community inevitably brings forth useful ideas or alternatives for consideration. It is during the implementation phase of community organization practice that individuals come face-to-face with authority, power, politics, overt or covert resistance, and obstacles, particularly if the assessing and planning processes were hasty, incomplete, inadequate, or inaccurate. The implementation phase is the time for learning, accepting and readjusting mistakes or errors in judgment, examining effective leadership styles, studying the uses of power and authority, reassessing strategies, and determining stamina and commitment regarding accomplishment of original objectives. If a project is unsuccessful the first time it is implemented, this does not mean that it is a failure. If the purpose for the project is sound, persistence and commitment in working toward the attainment of desired objectives is essential, and eventually a way is found.

EVALUATING THE ACTION TAKEN

Reassessment or evaluation should be ongoing during every phase of the nursing process. If evaluation is done continuously and objectively, the attainment of goals or the success of the project is more likely to be assured. The input of new information, changes, or lack of progress requires examination of the objectives and methodology and may dictate new or revised approaches for the project. If changes or modifications are required in the plan of action, objectives can be rewritten and revised. The criteria inherent in the written objectives should help to determine the success or failure of goal attainment.

The focus of evaluation can be directed toward health services given, quality of care, processes, access, satisfaction, and outcomes.[47] In evaluating the provision of health services to a consumer population, accessibility of the services for the target group must be studied. Did the intended consumers make use of the services? If not, why not? Were the services relevant to the needs of the consumer group from their perspective? Did the health of the target group show measurable improvement?

Was any form of peer review utilized? How would the findings of the project compare with practices offered by other community resources? Were statistical norms changed for persons of a particular age or with a specified diagnosis? Were the results of the project as anticipated? Would case histories be descriptive of successful outcomes?

Was health behavior of consumers changed? Did the target group feel satisfied with the services as given? Were the individuals who did not utilize the services asked to contribute their views as another aspect of the evaluation study? Were results of the project interpreted accurately, objectively, realistically, and without bias? Were new, unanticipated needs created as a result of the project?

Evaluation of a project can be interpreted from a variety of perspectives—attainment of measurable objectives, change in health behavior of consumers, consumer

[47]Milio, op. cit., p. 260.

satisfaction, use of statistical formulas showing significance of data, visual graphs, comparison of findings with projects or studies done formerly, quantitative frequency distributions, and correlation studies. Whatever the means utilized for interpreting the results of a project for selected subjects or populations, data must be clear, accurate, complete, understandable, and accountable.

SUMMARY

In becoming oriented to any given community, the community health nurse must study its characteristics purposefully. The composition of each community has its own structure and personality, which is not duplicated by any other community. Information is gained about a community by synthesizing the community health nursing process with the community organization process. The nurse is able to identify a health care system in every community and the existence of several social classes of citizens. Getting involved in community action requires qualities of initiative, curiosity, and persuasiveness. Several community organization models are described, including Ross, Rothman, Kent, and Warren models. The role of the nurse in community action depends on the community organization model selected.

SUGGESTED READING

Adams, Richard: *Watership Down*, The Macmillan Company, New York, 1972.
Anderson, Ralph E., and Irl Carter: *Human Behavior in the Social Environment*, Aldine Publishing Company, New York, 1978.
Cox, Fred M., et al. (eds.): *Strategies of Community Organization*, F. E. Peacock Publishers, Inc., Itasca, Ill., 1974.
Delbecq, Andre L., Andrew H. Van deVan, and David H. Gustafson: *Group Techniques for Program Planning*, Scott, Foresman and Company, Glenview, Ill., 1975.
Gentry, John T. et al.: "Attitudes and Perceptions of Health Service Providers," *American Journal of Public Health*, **64**(12):1123–1131, December 1974.
Gilmore, Gary D.: "Needs Assessment Processes for Community Health Education," *International Journal of Health Education*, **20**:164–173, 1977.
Kent, James A.: *A Descriptive Approach to a Community*, Foundation for Urban and Neighborhood Development, Denver, Colo., 1972.
Kent, James A., C. Harvey Smith, and Sam Burns: *An Urban Strategy for Action against Poverty*, Foundation for Urban and Neighborhood Development, Denver, Colo., 1967.
Kent, James A., and C. Harvey Smith: *Involving the Urban Poor in Health Services through Accommodation: The Employment of Neighborhood Representatives*, Foundation for Urban and Neighborhood Development, Denver, Colo., 1966.
Klein, Donald C.: *Community Dynamics and Mental Health*, John Wiley & Sons, Inc., New York, 1968.
Milio, Nancy: *9226 Kercheval: The Storefront That Did Not Burn*, Ann Arbor Paperbacks, The University of Michigan Press, Ann Arbor, 1970.
Milio, Nancy: *The Care of Health in Communities*, The Macmillan Company, New York, 1975.
Murphy, Michael J., "The Development of a Community Health Orientation Scale," *American Journal of Public Health*, **65**(12):1293–1297, December 1975.

O. M. Collective: *The Organizer's Manual,* Bantam Books, Inc., New York, 1971.

Ross, Murray G.: *Community Organization,* Harper & Row, Publishers, Inc., New York, 1955.

Scutchfield, F. Douglas: "Alternate Methods for Health Priority Assessment," *Journal of Community Health,* 1(1):29–38, Fall 1975.

Suttles, Gerald D.: *The Social Order of the Slum,* The University of Chicago Press, Chicago Press, Chicago, 1968.

Terkel, Studs: *Working,* Avon Books, New York, 1972.

Warheit, George J., Roger A. Bell, and John J. Schwab: *Needs Assessment Approaches: Concepts and Methods,* U.S. Department of Health, Education, and Welfare Publication ADM-79-472, 1977.

Warren, Rachelle B., and Donald I. Warren: *The Neighborhood Organizer's Handbook,* University of Notre Dame Press, Notre Dame, Ind., 1977.

Warren, Donald I., and Rachelle B. Warren: "Six Kinds of Neighborhoods," *Psychology Today,* 9(1):74–80, June 1975.

Warren, Roland L.: *Studying Your Community,* The Free Press, New York, 1965.

Examining Families

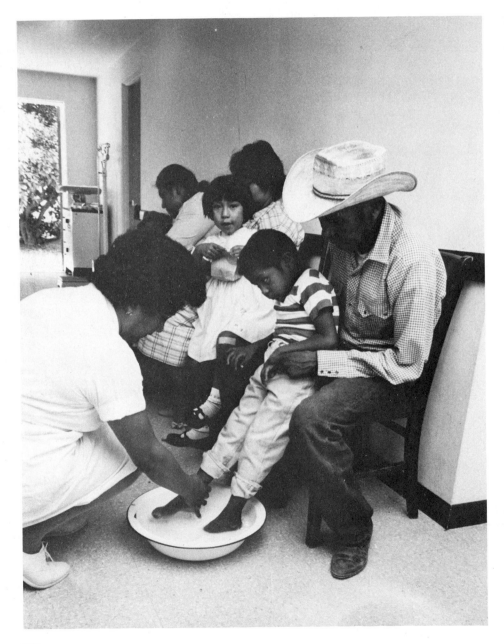

Traditionally the family has been the unit of service for the community health nurse. The orientation and practice of individual nurses, however, have varied for years on a continuum from client-centered to family-centered, dependent upon the nature of the family system and the illness of the identified client. Unfortunately, it is too easy to *speak* words like "family-centered," "caring," and "continuity of care" yet behave in *actions* differently from what the descriptive words suggest. Sometimes the nurse may consider that the family-centered approach is being used when she or he draws all the family members together for the goal of understanding and assisting the identified client of the family to make a more satisfactory recovery. A *truly family-centered approach* is one in which the nurse meets and continually assesses *all* the family members, either individually or as a group, is cognizant of the developmental role, power, and influence position of each family member, identifies the interactional patterns used by the family, and works with all members of the family to achieve a higher level of coping ability or health. The methods used for the family-centered approach are discussed in Chap. 6.

THE FAMILY

The common meaning of the word "family" is generalized to be the nuclear family, a structural unit composed of a man and woman who are married and have children. However, in view of the living patterns and kinship systems of people of different cultures and the emerging pattern of communal living among the youth of America, the family can also be considered a primary group possessing certain generic characteristics in common with all small groups.[1] These characteristics are mainly relationships with a high degree of intimacy, extensive communication, and common goals. When viewed in this manner, the family can be seen as a miniature society, with a culture all its own.[2] The concept of family tends to be a fluid one because of the accelerating changes occurring within Western Hemisphere societies. One-parent families, communal families, extended families living in a single residence, and other groups residing together in single dwellings must all be viewed in a common context, the nature of which supplies the nurse with a frame of reference, the family-centered nursing approach. For the purpose of this book, the family is the nuclear family or the primary group living and interacting together intimately in a common residence.

The Systems Approach

When the family is viewed from a systems approach, its role as a basic component of society is seen as a complex, many-faceted one. A system is an organized or complex whole—an assemblage or combination of things or parts forming a complex or unitary whole.[3] The world is made up of many systems, including social, biological, physical, and environmental systems. Parsons identified a social system as a plurality of persons

---

[1] F. Ivan Nye and Felix M. Berardo, *Emerging Conceptual Frameworks in Family Analysis,* The Macmillan Company, New York, 1966, p. 63.
[2] Ibid., p. 140.
[3] Fremont E. Kast and James E. Rosenzweig, *Organization and Management,* McGraw-Hill Book Company, New York, 1970, p. 110.

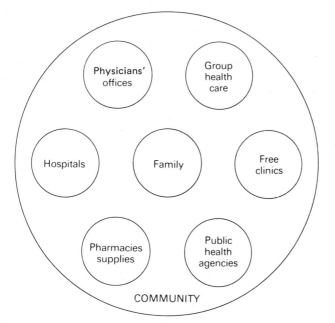

Figure 5-1 Health-care systems in the community.

or social roles bound together in a pattern of mutual interaction and interdependence. It has boundaries that enable us to distinguish the internal from the external environment, and it is typically imbedded in a network of social units both larger and smaller than itself.[4] The family is an open system which sustains relationships with other systems in the total transactional field and is interdependent and independent at the same time. When using the systems approach, the family's position in society can be identified in simple or complex terms. It is helpful to visualize a system by drawing a large circle and placing elements, parts, and variables inside the circle as components.[5] Circles representing components can be separate, touching, or overlapping depending on the strength of the attracting forces in operation among the components. For purposes of simplicity, the position of the family in relation to the health care system in the community can be illustrated as shown in Fig. 5-1. Each circle represents a subsystem that has boundaries but will admit individuals from other subsystems as necessary. It is possible for the community health nurse to act as a representative for any of the health subsystems, serve as a liaison agent with the family, and coordinate the health care delivery system in the community so that it has meaning and purpose to the family.

From another perspective, which includes a multidisciplinary approach, the family may be drawn as one of many social systems within the community with the possibility of having transactions with other systems on a frequent or infrequent basis. The

[4] Talcott Parsons and Robert F. Bales, *Family, Socialization and Interaction Process,* The Free Press, New York, 1955, pp. 401–408.
[5] Warren G. Bennis, Kenneth D. Benne, and Robert Chin, *The Planning of Change,* Holt, Rinehart and Winston, Inc., New York, 1961, p. 203.

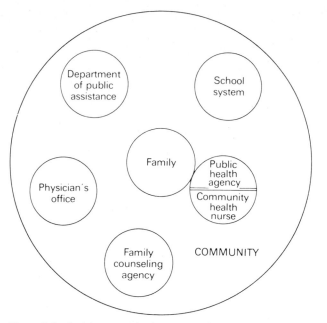

Figure 5-2 Social systems in the community.

community health nurse can act as the liaison agent for a dysfunctioning family and coordinate or integrate transactions with other participating social systems so that the family's equilibrium and coping abilities are eased. The illustration of social systems from a multidisciplinary approach may be drawn as shown in Fig. 5-2. The particular role of the community health nurse as a coordinator of services as shown in the figure can be elaborated from the following hypothetical example. The community health nurse was referred to the family initially through the department of public assistance because the mother was pregnant and was not seeking prenatal care. Following an appraisal of the family on a home visit, the nurse assessed the family as a dysfunctional one because of the evidences of marital strife, the lack of health care of older children, the lack of prenatal care for the mother, and the complaints regarding insufficient clothing and poor transportation facilities. After the nurse determined short- and long-term goals to be attained, immediate plans to talk with or make referral to personnel in each of the pictured social systems were instituted. For example, the nurse wanted to speak to the caseworker of the department of public assistance to share observations and assessment of the family with the worker. The community health nurse wanted to know if the data gathered were complete and if a cooperative effort by the caseworker and nurse would reap better results than working separately or discretely in predetermined subject areas. By conferring with the school nurse and teachers in the school system, the nurse wanted to learn if the school had been alerted to the health condition of the children of the family. Again, by a unified effort of all professionals concerned with family members, a change would be effected more easily if the family received concerted special attention. A first priority of the nurse was to refer the mother of the family to a private physician for prenatal care. The nurse planned to call the physician chosen by the mother to advise her or him of the current health status of the mother and the fact that continued supervisory visits would be planned during the antepartum and postpartum periods. When the mother and father of the family indicated a readiness to seek marital counseling, it was the plan of the nurse to call the family counseling agency to alert them to the nature of family problems and the fact that a professional has been guiding the family to seek additional assistance. Eventually, as the designated social systems within the community became acquainted with the family, a multidisciplinary conference of all representatives of the social systems would be arranged by the nurse to integrate and implement the health care needed by the family. By picturing the social systems involved with the family, the nurse clarified the coordination aspect of the nursing role.

Structure of the Family

The family structure is made up of individual members and the roles they play in interacting with each other. A *role* is defined as a goal-directed pattern or sequence of acts tailored by the cultural process for the transactions a person may carry out in a social group or situation.[6] No role exists in isolation but is always patterned to adjust in a complementary or reciprocal manner with the role partner. Traditionally, the assumption is made that a nuclear family consists of a male who enacts an instrumental role and a female who fulfills the expressive role. The instrumental role is one which emphasizes the performance of tasks and decision making and communicates power by the thinking, logical, perceptive approach. The expressive role emphasizes support of the instrumental leader and conveys power through the ability to mediate and influence feelings and emotions of others. In every small group there are persons who demonstrate either instrumental or expressive roles. Depending upon the nature of the group, an individual may interchange these two roles. The structural relationships in a family vary according to the particular mode of family organization, feminist awareness, social class, or culture. Thus, various manifestations of family structure are seen in terms of role behavior. The structure and role behavior of members of a given family must be determined by the nurse before an intelligent decision can be made on the best method for initiating a health activity. It is often clarifying for the nurse to illustrate the perceived family structure by means of a map, particularly if a family case study is being presented for group discussion. The map shows the number of family members in terms of their power, alignments, and boundaries. For the family that has closed boundaries, they are depicted within a closed circle, with the member demonstrating the greatest power in the center. Other family members are arranged within the circle as they relate to the person with the greatest power and their alignments with other family members. The family with closed boundaries is frequently a troubled family. They communicate defensively, are judgmental and dogmatic, maintain rigid roles and rules, have secrets, try to control others, and resist change.[7] The map of a troubled family of four with a dominant father, an alignment between

---

[6] John P. Spiegel, "The Resolution of Role Conflict within the Family," in Norman W. Bell and Ezra F. Vogel (eds.), *The Family,* The Free Press, New York, 1960, p. 363.
[7] Satir, V., *Peoplemaking,* Science and Behavior Books, Palo Alto, Calif., 1972, pp. 114–116.

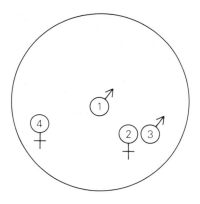

Figure 5-3 (1) Father, age 40. (2) Mother, age 38. (3) Son, age 12. (4) Daughter, age 14.

mother and son, and an independent daughter can look like Fig. 5-3. The space between the circles represents the psychological distance between family members.

For the family with open boundaries, the map is a broken circle, allowing for outside persons to enter as necessary. These families are considered healthy because they communicate supportively, help each other solve problems spontaneously, show understanding, share hurts with each other, have roles and rules that are flexible, give clear leveling messages, and consider changes to be normal and desirable.[8] Figure 5-4 is a diagram of a healthy family of four, in which all members work well together. The favored family cat is also included. It must be remembered that healthy families have disagreements, alignments, and variable distribution of power, depending upon day-by-day circumstances. They are considered healthy because family members are encouraged to grow and flourish in a supportive, flexible environment.

Any number of ingenious pictures of family structures can be devised by the nurse as evidence is gathered regarding the role behaviors, power, and alignments of family members. The pictures may change as the nurse's assessment of the family structure deepens. Sometimes families themselves will respond to the idea of picturing their placement in the family system when given the assignment.

Another way for presenting family structures before study groups is to do a

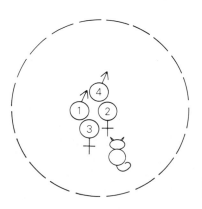

Figure 5-4 (1) Father, age 27. (2) Mother, age 26. (3) Daughter, age 4. (4) Son, age 3.

[8] Ibid., pp. 114–117.

family sculpture. Four volunteers from the study group can be requested to perform as models of the family. An assignment of a family role can be given to each volunteer, including a brief description of each one's appearance, life theme, and stance. Then, the nurse can arrange the volunteer-father, volunteer-mother, volunteer-son, and volunteer-daughter as a family unit with closeness and distance between members as she or he perceives it. Family members can be facing each other or standing back to back. When they assume the postures and facial expressions as described by the nurse, the visual scene of the family unit is graphic and communicates a situation with much greater impact than mere words.

Functions of the Family

In view of controversial opinions about the continuing existence of families as familiarly known in society, the function of the family assumes major importance.[9] It may be that the traditional concept of families should not be the focus of attention as much as the change or diversity of family functioning and structuring. Parsons stated that the functions of the family in a highly differentiated society are performed for the benefit of the personality rather than on behalf of the society. Families are necessary because the human personality is not "born" but must be "made" through the socialization process.[10] When babies are born and raised in their own distinct family environment, they learn to cope with the world by identifying with or in opposition to models with whom they have been intimate all their early years. Each child picks up individual characteristics from the adult models, mother and father. It is fascinating to observe small children at play and witness the behavior that is unconsciously mimicked from either the mother or the father. Children learn to perceive the world through the adult models in their environment, and they remember best the *actions* which gained their attention rather than adult words. Therefore, when adults rely on words to create an impression, they are often producing an inconsistency that is not understandable to a child. For example, when a mother cautions her child never to run across the street without first looking to the right and left for the presence of vehicles, and later runs across the street herself without following her own directives, the child takes note of this. The performed act has a much greater impact on the child's memory than the words. When the child is disciplined for running across the street without looking to the right or left, he or she tends to regard the punishment as unjust.

Hill outlined basic requirements for family survival, continuity, and growth. These included seven tasks:

1 Reproduction: planning and controlling family size
2 Physical maintenance of family members: providing food, clothing, shelter, and medical care
3 Socialization of offspring into functioning adults, capable of assuming adult family roles of husband-father, wife-mother
   a Organization of explicit expectations for children and adults
   b Organization of family objectives to which members are subordinate

[9]See Alvin Toffler, *Future Shock,* Random House, Inc., New York, 1970.
[10]Parsons and Bales, op cit., p. 16.

4 Allocation of resources and division of duties and responsibilities
   a Allocation of authority, including prestige, and designation of accountability
   b Allocation of economic income and output
   c Division of labor: specialization of roles to secure performance of essential family jobs
   d Division of time: scheduling of tasks and services
5 Maintenance of order within the family and between the family and outsiders
   a Within the family: meeting the emotional needs of members and determining types and intensity of emotional-affectional ties among members; channeling of sex drives; providing means of communication among members
   b Between family and outsiders: developing methods of articulating with other groups and the larger social structure
6 Maintenance of family morale and motivation to carry out family tasks: providing a system of rewards and punishments to keep members at family tasks; development of equilibrating and inspiring mechanisms for upset or discouraged members
7 Development of methods for orderly recruiting and releasing of group members; incorporating of adopted children, stepparents, kin, guests, and servants into family group; releasing members at adulthood to jobs and marriage[11]

The mastery of these seven tasks by families varies widely. The nurse can be of greatest assistance to families when she or he can identify the tasks which need strengthening, enlist the interest of family members in clarifying their own resources and methods of coping, and teach methods of problem solving and interaction skills adapted to the family and facilitative of family recuperative strengths.

Developmental Tasks

Families and individuals change and develop in different ways, according to the nature of their individual living processes, family interaction, and stimulation by the social milieu. Each family member and each family is unique in its complex of age-role expectations in reciprocity.[12] The family as a small-group system is interrelated in such a manner that change does not occur in one part without a series of resultant changes in other parts.[13] As stated by Lederer and Jackson, the family is a unit in which all individuals have an important influence—whether they like it or not and whether they know it or not. The family is an interacting communications network in which every member influences the nature of the entire system and in turn is influenced by it.[14]

The family role pattern constantly changes as each member grows, develops, and matures according to age and cultural role expectation. The developmental task concept takes into consideration the human needs of and the cultural demands made upon the individual. It is defined as a task that arises at or about a certain period in

---

[11] Reuben Hill, "Challenges and Resources for Family Development," in *Family Mobility in Our Dynamic Society,* The Iowa State University Press, Ames, Iowa, 1965, p. 255. Reprinted by permission of the Iowa State University Press.
[12] Nye and Berardo, op. cit., p. 210.
[13] Ibid., p. 203.
[14] William J. Lederer and Don D. Jackson, *The Mirages of Marriage,* W. W. Norton & Company, Inc., New York, 1968, p. 14.

the life of an individual, successful achievement of which leads to happiness and success with later tasks, while failure leads to unhappiness, disapproval by society, and difficulty with later tasks.[15] For example, one developmental task of the preschool child is to learn to develop physical skills appropriate to his or her stage of motor development.[16] The child who learns to button coats or tie shoes before going to school gains mother's approval, feels pleased, and is challenged to try new skills. A developmental task of the teenager is to achieve a satisfying and socially accepted masculine or feminine role.[17] When a teenage girl does not perceive herself as sexually attractive or lovable and has few girlfriends and no boyfriends, she is unhappy; all of her behavior reflects her dissatisfaction with herself. Her adaptation to all subsequent events in her life is affected and often dysfunctional if the developmental task is not satisfactorily resolved. Duvall lists in detail the developmental tasks of individuals for each age level in the life cycle in her book, *Family Development*. She states there are ten ever-changing developmental tasks which are faced by every individual. They are:

1 Achieving an appropriate dependence-independence pattern
2 Achieving an appropriate giving-receiving pattern of affection
3 Relating to changing social groups
4 Developing a conscience
5 Learning one's psychosocial and biological sex role
6 Accepting and adjusting to a changing body
7 Managing a changing body and learning new motor patterns
8 Learning to understand and control the physical world
9 Developing an appropriate symbol system and developing conceptual abilities
10 Relating one's self to the cosmos[18]

In addition to individual developmental tasks, there are family developmental tasks, which are the responsibility of the family as a whole if they are going to grow and develop in a healthy, satisfying manner. The family developmental tasks keep changing as the family grows, adjusts, and matures from a beginning family, which starts with the marriage, becomes a small group when children are born, allows outsiders to enter the family system when children marry, and becomes an aging family nearing the end of the family life cycle. Duvall lists nine ever-changing family developmental tasks that span the family life cycle. They are to establish and maintain:

1 An independent home
2 Satisfactory ways of getting and spending money
3 Mutually acceptable patterns in the division of labor
4 Continuity of mutually satisfying sex relationships
5 Open system of intellectual and emotional communication

---

[15] Evelyn Millis Duvall, *Family Development,* 2nd ed., J. B. Lippincott Company, Philadelphia, 1962, pp. 31–32.
[16] Ibid., p. 230.
[17] Ibid., p. 294
[18] Ibid., pp. 40–41.

6 Workable relationships with relatives
7 Ways of interacting with associates and community organizations
8 Competency in bearing and rearing children
9 A workable philosophy of life[19]

The defined developmental task concepts for individuals and families according to their stage of human growth are extremely helpful for the community health nurse to use as guidelines when working with individuals and families. The nurse who can assist or encourage an individual or family to achieve a difficult developmental task has facilitated growth, happiness, and movement toward maturity or self-actualization. It must be remembered that the individual must master the developmental tasks being faced, but it cannot be done in isolation.[20] The alert community health nurse who identifies the juncture at which developmental task progression may be stalemated can serve as an essential, facilitating change agent when it is most needed.

FAMILIES REPRESENTING SOCIOECONOMIC GROUPS

It has been said that the community health nurse works with *all* families in need at whatever stage of development or period of adjustment they are undergoing in their family life cycle. The nurse is a helpful assistant when the family has special problems for which they are not adequately prepared, such as illnesses, accidents, birth of handicapped children, emergence of undesirable health or social conditions, and personality disorders. As a generalist, the nurse views the family objectively from the perspective of wholeness. A key nursing function is to identify the coping patterns of the given family, the degree of discomfort they are experiencing, and to direct them, when they are ready, to community resources and facilities which most closely meet their requirements. The nurse's own energies are also directed to those professional consultants within the community from whom special instruction and guidance is needed to assist the family to cope better with explicit problems. Families representing socioeconomic groups are described in subsequent paragraphs to alert the nurse to her or his style of interaction and implementation.

Low-Income Families

Community health nurses have visited low-income multiproblem families for many years, have seen little discernable changes in the behavior of these families, have felt frustrated and sometimes angry with the apathy or lack of responsiveness of members of the family. In managing these families, some nurses regard them as a challenge, some view them as an unpleasant duty contained within their case load, and some see them as hopeless, worthless, and to be avoided, particularly if the family is resistant to any health measures offered. Obviously, these families have great need for health

[19] Ibid., pp. 478–505.
[20] Ibid., p. 42.

assistance. Being aware of one's values and sanctions is not easy but is essential in providing individualized, accountable nursing care.

The community health nurse visits all socioeconomic groups, but the low-income groups receive a proportionately larger concentration of time and services because of their high incidence of chronic diseases, multiple environmental hazards, high birth rates, high infant mortality rates, poor health standards, multiple social problems, and often inadequate delivery of health care services. These groups are generally identified as either poverty, multiproblem, hard-core, disorganized, or disadvantaged families. They are often families plagued by many serious problems, which they are unable to handle by themselves or through the services made available in the community, and they come repeatedly to the attention of community agencies in a negative connotation.[21] These families realize that health is an important reality for them but they often do not avail themselves of preventive health programs. Because community health nurses are very familiar health workers to the families, it is essential for the nurses to understand their lifestyles and implement methods of approach that will be successful in changing their health practices. Much research has been done in recent years from which nurses can profit as they experiment with new ways of developing self-esteem in these families and changing destructive health patterns to more acceptable, amenable practices.

Families of poverty are found in every community. Many of them reflect a design for living which Lewis has characterized as the culture of poverty. Regardless of their race, creed, color, culture, or setting, they have a lifestyle which shows remarkable similarity in the structure of their families, in interpersonal relations, in spending habits, in their value systems, and in their orientation in time. To demonstrate the culture of poverty, the social order of a population in general must be one in which members prize the value of thrift and work toward the accumulation of wealth and property and the advancement of upward mobility. In such a society, the individuals of a low economic status tend to be seen as personally inadequate and inferior.[22]

Once the culture of poverty has come into existence in a society, it tends to perpetuate itself. The family does not cherish childhood as a specially prolonged and protected stage in the life cycle. Initiation into sexual activity comes early. With the instability of consensual marriage, the family tends to be mother-centered and tied more closely to the mother's extended family. The female head of the house is given to authoritarian rule. In spite of much verbal emphasis on family solidarity, sibling rivalry for the limited supply of goods and maternal affection is intense. There is little privacy.[23]

Irelan described four distinctive life themes which are manifested in lower-class behavior. These include (1) fatalism, (2) orientation to the present, (3) authoritarianism, and (4) concreteness. When individuals have persistent fatalistic beliefs regarding unavoidable or uncontrollable external forces in their lives, a sense of powerlessness and resignation emanates, which acts as a definite deterrent to any efforts to break a

---

[21] L. L. Geismar and Michael A. La Sorte, *Understanding the Multi-Problem Family,* Association Press, New York, 1964, p. 33.

[22] Oscar Lewis, *La Vide,* Random House, Inc., New York 1966.

[23] Ibid.

chain of unfortunate circumstances. They receive their "hard luck" as their fate. Because of their basic need for survival (physiological and safety needs), they are oriented to the present rather than the future. They spontaneously take their pleasures and discomforts immediately or in the here and now rather than defer gratifications to a future time. They believe in the rightness of existing systems and in strength as the source of authority. By simplifying life experiences, they classify people as either weak or strong and will use authority, rather than reason, as the basis for decision making. The theme of concreteness deals with an emphasis on material rather than intellectual things. Because these individuals are preoccupied with tangible, day-to-day problems, they understand best any activity or emotion which is concrete and visible. They value action that has results or gives tangible rewards.[24]

In looking at their goals in life, they want the same things that any other citizen in America wants. They want to improve their life by acquiring security, material comforts and luxuries, and social values which appeal to all individuals. Their drive toward better occupations and more income is often based on escaping the discomforts of life in poverty. They want better housing, living conditions, and education. They value the opportunity to escape routines and pressures of day-to-day existence. Their desires are similar to the desires of any other social class; however, their life experiences have been such that their expectations for reaching toward their goals have been limited drastically. It is at this juncture that the community health nurse can play an active role in eliciting the feelings and desires of family members, encouraging the development of a plan of action which is conceivable to the family, and supporting and enabling the implementation of a plan so that success is achieved. To do this, the nurse must identify with the family minute goals that are achievable and have the strong possibility for culminating in a positive direction. Success breeds success, and families in poverty must begin at a level that they can see, understand, and trust. Oftentimes this means that the nurse must spend considerable time in developing the self-esteem and self-confidence of the clients before they are ready to move toward a projected desired goal, even though it may be a minute one.

It must be emphasized that not all poor families exhibit characteristics of the culture of poverty. There are stable lower-class families who are cohesive and function as integral parts of the society. The fathers are employed in steady positions as semi-skilled or unskilled workers, and have an elementary school level of education. In these homes the intellectual stimulation for the children is rather low. These families profit from the attention of the nurse but must not be managed or categorized in the same classification as the families who demonstrate the poverty culture.

It cannot be overemphasized that each family with whom the nurse comes in contact must be assessed *individually.* Successful interventions can come about only through joint setting of goals and mutual efforts. Textbook profiles and research studies point out important, significant data with which the nurse should be familiar to aid in understanding and implementing purposeful nursing actions. For example, the levels of social functioning are spelled out in detail for families classified as inade-

[24]Lola M. Irelan, *Low-Income Life Styles,* U.S. Department of Health, Education, and Welfare, Government Printing Office, Washington, D.C., 1966, pp. 7–9.

quate, marginal, and adequate by Geismar and La Sorte,[25] and descriptive characteristics which will help the nurse to work with disorganized and disadvantaged families
are elaborated upon by Minuchin et al.[26] The ultimate success of the nurse's work
depends on the synthesis of facts and data about families, an ability to relate, and the
individuation of the nursing effort with each family situation.

Health Perceptions of the Poor

Poverty is a health hazard because of crowded or deteriorated housing, inadequate
nutrition, and insufficient medical care. Consequently, low-income families are more
vulnerable to ill health and less able to cope with it. They are often ignorant about
causes, treatment, and outcomes of various diseases. They are not informed or particularly concerned about preventive measures. They accept poor health conditions as
inevitable, such as dental decay with ultimate loss of teeth. Physical discomfort is a
way of life, and only when one becomes incapacitated and unable to fulfill daily
responsibilities does one regard oneself as "sick." Therefore, treatment is sought at a
late stage of development, in contrast to early detection of disease symptoms. Many
low-income families do not participate in health activities or programs available in
the community, including the preventive type of programs. They do not conceive of
themselves as having a voice in community concerns since they lack contact with
community organizations and among themselves. They tend to practice self-medication,
and when they need medical advice, they ask friends, neighbors, or the druggist. They
feel a distrust of physicians and clinics, particularly if they sense that they are evaluated as being inadequate or uncooperative or are treated as impersonal objects. They
tend to set higher value on concrete physical improvements such as better housing,
better transportation, or improved household equipment than they do on health.[27]

Working with the Poor

The nurse will be better able to relate with the poor by understanding some of their
behavior patterns and attitudes. The community health nurse must be willing to
experiment with new ways of implementing nursing activities and health teaching,
since nursing actions in the past few years have not always ended in success when
applied to low-income families. When knowledgeable about characteristic patterns
of behavior as described by studies dealing with the poor, the nurse is better armed
to adapt the approach to the specific needs of any particular family. The nurse who
realizes that low-income families value material things will readily accept the fact that
they are more action-oriented than verbally oriented. When talking with an individual
who uses speech as a means of direct, specific communication rather than an elaboration of thoughts or intellect, the nurse will realize that a mutual understanding must
be created which does not rely on words alone. This forces the nurse to use ingenuity
and creativity in selecting an approach which will have meaning for the family. The use
of tangible rewards, demonstrations, active participation with tasks, role playing, or

[25] Geismar and La Sorte, op. cit., pp. 205-222.
[26] Minuchin et al., op. cit., pp. 192-242.
[27] Irelan, op. cit., pp. 51-62.

acting out behaviors or games are some approaches that may be more effective than words for the patient.

By being observant of the communication patterns of low-income families who are disadvantaged, the nurse can learn essential data which will have bearing on subsequent activities. She or he will become aware that family members do not expect be heard. No one really listens. If someone responds to a statement, it is not necessarily along the lines of the preceding communication. A high tolerance of interruptions and changing of subject material is demonstrated; therefore, a subject is rarely carried to any conclusion. Noise and motor activities often take precedence over the continuation of a subject being discussed. The mother is the central pathway for most transactions among family members when they are all together. Spouses rarely talk to each other but engage in a "parallel" type of conversation that is directed to a third party or to the children. The mother's messages to the children are mostly in terms of "don'ts." She rarely gives a message which emphasizes any positives to the children. Children learn to pay attention to the person rather than to the content of the message received.[28] Consequently, the children do not talk in long sentences or express their desires by words alone.

Because the intellectual stimulation at home is limited, the concepts of time, size, and shape have to be dealt with in terms of familiar objects and words. For example, children may have to be taught that a ball is a "circle," or a clock is a "square." It is not unusual that parental control is at times confusing, because of inconsistency in being at one moment completely authoritarian or at the next moment powerless. The ambivalence with which discipline and punishment of children are exercised in the home can be witnessed frequently. Often there is little evidence of commercial toys in the home, and the means by which children improvise playthings or give their attention in play can be instructive to the nurse. If no regular mealtime routine is practiced in the home, conversation at the dinner table or a parental focus on table manners is unknown.[29]

As the behavior and communication patterns of a given family are assessed, and data gained from an appropriate textbook or research study are synthesized, the nurse will be prepared to try new methods of implementation which will be stimulating to the family. For example, a goal can be set to encourage spouses to talk directly to each other or alert the mother regarding her predominantly negative messages to the children. The method for drawing the attention of family members to the goal may be through role playing, psychodrama, or role-reversal games. By bringing observed patterns of behavior to the attention of family members, the nurse has a starting point from which to determine if they want to do anything about it, and if so, to plan with the family regarding the best way of implementation.

It sometimes happens that family members express a desired goal which is too global, so the task of the nurse requires restricting the goal specification to a dimension possible for the family to attain. For example, a mother might express a desire for her 8-year-old son to stop wetting the bed, since this behavior causes her to be continu-

[28] Minuchin et al., op cit., pp. 201-206.
[29] Sol Adler, *The Health and Education of the Economically Deprived Child,* Warren H. Green, Inc., St. Louis, Mo., 1968, pp. 17-20.

ously annoyed and irritable with him. In order to implement successful activities with this goal, the nurse must elicit detailed information from both the mother and the son. There must be assurance of the desire of both to attain the stated goal. By requesting all the data related to the problem, gaining the individual perceptions of both mother and son regarding the causes of the problem, and discussing the activities each will feel able to carry out, a plan for eliminating the enuresis for one night only out of the week can be the stated beginning goal. Gathering baseline data before implementing a plan of action is always desirable. (See Chap. 6 for an elaboration of the behavior-modification method.)

Nurses must remember that the poor are distrustful of outsiders and have been exploited often, so considerable time and attention has to be given early to developing trust and a relationship in which communication has meaning for both the family and the nurse.

Middle- and High-Income Families

Many professional workers, including nurses, come from a middle-class orientation and are familiar with attitudes, values, and behavior patterns of middle-income families. Some of the characteristics descriptive of middle-class values are the desirability of the accumulation of material wealth, a belief in work and thrift as necessary attributes, an acceptance of upward mobility as indicative of success and progress, a future orientation for gratification of desires, and the importance of education. Children raised in a middle- or high-income family learn to express themselves with language which communicates observations, thoughts, and feelings. Curiosity is cultivated and questions are answered by parents. Children are raised in an environment which includes the stimuli of books, magazines, newspapers, and toys of all sizes and shapes. Meal-times are regular and attention is given to table conversation and proper use of eating utensils.[30]

In essence, the delivery of health care in any community is structured for and utilized mainly by middle- and high-income groups because they are the people who are alert and responsive to early disease symptoms, are able to pay for services, and expend much more energy in participating as planners and organizers of beneficial community services.

Working with Middle- and High-Income Families For nurses working with middle- and high-income families, the task of encouraging preventive health services is often made easy because of the acceptance and responsiveness of the consumer. The basis for a relationship may differ from that in low-income groups because the consumer is frequently well educated and has a cognitive understanding and natural desire to learn about any captivating phenomenon under study. For the consumer who prizes intellectualism, the nurse must prepare differently than for the customer who wants the concrete, pertinent facts and no more. Many middle-income family members have as great a need for strengthening their self-esteem as low-income families. However, some seem to have a high propensity for utilizing defense mechanisms, which

[30] Ibid., pp. 17–20.

makes the development of a therapeutic relationship difficult and time-consuming, yet essential. Defensive people respond to openness and honesty and can be convinced about an idea if it is presented in a logical manner which gives recognition to all the arguments or barriers opposing the idea. The necessity for the nurse to assess the consumer in terms of interests, personality, background, and education is vital as the nurse *plans* the teaching content and methods of approach on subsequent visits. Often it is not difficult for the nurse to recognize the need for a relationship with the middle-income family member if the consumer is friendly, receptive, and responsive—and most middle-class families are amicable. However, occasionally a family member is encountered who is hostile, openly questioning, highly educated, or unmistakably defensive, and the nurse tends to want to withdraw rather than pursue the difficult course of developing a relationship. The nurse must be encouraged to plan carefully the strategy with the challenging patient in a way that is convincing to the consumer. This requires extensive educational and psychological preparation on the part of the nurse, but the reward is a broadened educational and experiential background and a strengthened belief in oneself. If an open, honest style and refusal to react emotionally to any intentionally provocative statement by the consumer are maintained, nine times out of ten, the nurse can "win" the patient.

FAMILIES REPRESENTING CULTURAL GROUPS

To gain an understanding of families representing cultural groups, the meaning of culture is described, followed by a discussion of selected families representing cultures upon whom the focus of attention has been centered in recent years. The overview of families of other cultures as contained in this chapter represents only a "taste" of the vast amount of information that is currently available in a cross section of popular and professional books and periodicals.

Meaning of Culture

The concept of *culture* refers to those specific ways of thinking, feeling, and acting which differentiate one group from another. Culture varies in its patterns and meanings as represented by different groups who have been studied. Each group has developed its own way of life based on modifications and adaptations occurring through the course of history in the particular setting in which the group lived. The design for living of any particular group is transmitted to the children of the group directly and indirectly as they grow, develop, and learn to adapt to their physical environment and the people who act as their models and teachers. Culture serves as a subtle and systematic device for perceiving the world.[31] It stands for the way of life of a people, for the sum of their learned behavior patterns, attitudes, and material things.[32]

Every culture is of paramount importance to its possessor. It is a universal ten-

[31] Benjamin D. Paul, *Health, Culture and Community,* Russell Sage Foundation, New York, 1955, p. 467.
[32] Edward T. Hall, *The Silent Language,* Doubleday & Company, Inc., Garden City, N. Y. 1956. Copyright 1956 Edward T. Hall. Reprinted by permission of Doubleday & Company, Inc.

dency for human beings to accept that their way of thinking, acting, and believing is the right way and to rate one's own culture as generally superior to others. Each individual has no choice but to function in the culture of which he or she is part. It exercises a strong influence in the way individuals perceive themselves and others. As stated by Hall, culture is a mold in which we are all cast, and it controls our daily lives and behavior in many unsuspected ways. Culture hides much more than it reveals, and it hides most effectively from its own participants.[33] It is not because of any difference in the basic nature of humankind that the cultures of different ethnic groups differ so much from one another, but because of the differences in the history of experiences which each group has undergone.[34] Because people rely on learned behavior or culture for survival, it is this acquired guidance that enables them to adapt to change.[35]

The community health nurse talks and works with a wide variety of cultural groups and therefore must be constantly alert, consciously observant, sensitive, accepting of all differences, and curious about the behavior patterns and lifestyles that are revealed. There is much to be learned about other cultural groups, and according to Hall, much about our own culture.

Cultural Shock

The individual visiting a new country for an extended period of time or returning from another country after a long absence is apt to feel a "culture shock." This is a removal or distortion of many of the familiar cues one encounters at home and the substitution for them of other cues that are strange.[36] The person experiences great differences that seem to exist between oneself and the people with whom she or he is working. All things are regarded as strange and incomprehensible and communication is perceived as difficult because of the inconsistent response of the listener. In order to adapt to the new dimension in life to which the individual has been exposed, it helps to be ready to develop esteem in others who are different and at the same time maintain a personal sense of integrity and worth. The process of developing esteem for others who are different begins with getting to know them, by being willing to talk their language, using their particular jargon or phrases appropriately when their meaning is understood, and finding out their interests. It sometimes takes effort and involves periods of frustrations, but the outcome is satisfying and broadening to one's experience when dealt with successfully.

Frequently, selected groups of student nurses undergo culture shock when they are exposed to completely new patterns of family living, an experience which often occurs in community health nursing. They see and talk with families whose culture is greatly different from their own. For many nursing students, the actual experience of entering a dirty, insect-ridden, poverty-stricken home is a highly charged one. The student may have intellectualized these conditions for some time and feel "wise to

[33] Ibid., pp. 38–39.
[34] Ashley Montagu, *The Biosocial Nature of Man*, Grove Press, Inc., New York, 1956, p. 81.
[35] Benjamin A. Kogan, *Health, Man in a Changing Environment*, Harcourt Brace Jovanovich, Inc., New York, 1970, p. 34.
[36] Hall, op cit., p. 156.

the world and its ways," but coming upon the actual situations can be shattering.[37]
The nurses must be allowed to talk freely in discussion groups about their initial
impressions, followed by encouragement to look for factors in the strange home
environment that will reveal the family's strengths. As the nurses adjust to the reality
of accepting differences in family living patterns, they facilitate their productiveness in
implementing effective nursing services.

The Cultural Gap

The success of any health teaching is dependent upon the way in which it is understood, accepted, and implemented by the learner. The fact that there may be a gap or
difference between the culture of the family and that of the nurse must always be
remembered. Until the health worker or teacher understands the sociocultural patterns
of families, what purposes they serve, why they persist, and how they change, health
information believed to be desperately needed by the family will not be transmitted.
If the health teaching or activity is incompatible with the family's idea of illness and
curing, the obstacle and challenge of changing their beliefs and practices must be
attended to first. This necessitates many contacts with the family during which an
understanding of their beliefs as the basis for their reluctance to change is gained. Trust
is developed as the family members accept the health worker, and the subsequent
relationship of family members and health worker eases the willingness to change.
Cultural values give meaning and direction to life, and it is doubtful if anyone ever
really changes culture. What happens is that small, informal adaptations are continually
being made in the day-to-day process of living.[38] Until there is a hint of the cultural
value which seems to be impeding progress toward a desired goal with a family, the
nurse is working as though blindfolded. It is essential for the nurse to elicit the family's
perception of their health problems and needs, to *avoid* making assumptions based on
her or his *own* values, and to implement further actions based on an accurate understanding of the family's physical, mental, and emotional resources and the value they
place on health. This takes effort, patience, and ingenuity. Health practices and
adaptations may sometimes be initiated by appealing to pride or suggesting a gain in
prestige. Long-term goals have a better chance of being implemented if they are
combined with tangible measures to meet immediate health needs. For example, if the
nurse has a goal for convincing the mother of a family of the necessity of immunizations for her children, achievement of this long-term goal will be hastened by attending
to immediate illnesses, dental, clothing, or nutritional needs of the children. Early,
tangible proof of concern for the children will aid in convincing the mother that the
nurse genuinely cares about improving the overall health status of the family. Consequently, in due time the mother may be motivated to seek immunizations or practice
health measures as advised by the nurse.

Sometimes the values of both the health professional and the family can be met
by making use of means of adaptation and compromise. For example, for the adamant
elderly Scandinavian male who stubbornly insists on the use of kerosene dressings for

---

[37] Elaine C. Gowell, "Helping Student Nurses to Become Involved," *Internation Journal of Nursing Studies*, 7:225–234, Pergamon Press, London, New York, Nov. 1970.
[38] Hall, op. cit., p. 90.

his leg ulcers, the nurse can agree that kerosene is useful for superficial skin burns because of the property of being oil-based. For present purposes, however, the nurse can indicate firmly that the kerosene will be used only around the healthy skin edges. Only the prescribed medication as orderd by the doctor will be used on the leg ulcers.

It is good to remember that an individual, regardless of cultural background, wants to be recognized as an entity, a being who serves a purpose of some kind. When one is seen, heard, and made to feel that an impact of some kind has been made on the other person, then the individual feels a sense of satisfaction and fulfillment. If the nurse communicates a genuine desire to get to know the other person by learning the meaning of words, customs, foods, and dress specific to the person's culture and interests, an enduring rapport is often initiated. Universal inquiries that are responded to with warmth after two participants have established a mutual feeling of trust are, "What was your early childhood like?"; "How did you meet your husband or wife?"; "Tell me about the country where you were born"; "What are your favorite foods"; "Tell me about the holidays or celebrations that you particularly love." By eliciting descriptions of events that the client has experienced, the nurse becomes involved in a mutual exchange which is informative of the client's culture, habits, attitudes, and values and serves as a basis for future conversations about health practices. The nurse's scope of knowledge about learned behavior is broadened. Perhaps the nurse's curiosity will someday prompt a desire to visit the country or locale about which the client is speaking.

Ethnic Minority Families in the United States

Ethnic minority groups form a substantial portion of the American population. All have serious deficiencies in the area of health, education, and welfare which are due to impoverishment, cultural differences, or combinations of both. Even though each ethnic group is unique, has a different language, lifestyle, and world view, this does not mean that each group is monolithic in its views. A range of characteristics, lifestyles, and views exist within each ethnic group and stereotyping cannot be done based on exposure to one or two families.

A characteristic of all ethnic minority groups is the retention of their sociocultural-psychological identity existing either in harmony with or as complementary to the majority American culture. When discrimination is practiced by a majority group, minorities are forced to form their own social groups or enclaves where they find belongingness and solace.[39]

Black Families

Many books have been written recently that are informative and descriptive of the black people in America. A major factor which causes the black culture to be different from that of other cultural groups who have migrated to America involves the severance of traditional ties with the native land. Black people were brought to America forcibly and were completely cut off from their past. They were robbed of language

---

[39] Kanaur V. Chandra, *Racial Discrimination in Canada; Asian Minorities,* R. & E. Research Associates, San Francisco, 1973, p. 61.

and culture. They were forbidden to be Africans and never allowed to be Americans. While other cultural groups passed on proud traditions to their children, black people were denied a sense of worth about the values and rituals which they shared. The culture that was born during the days of slavery was passed on to later generations, with the result that the constricting adaptations which developed during that experience of bondage continue as contemporary cultural traits.[40] The traits and patterns of behavior that appear more often in black Americans than in nonblacks can all be traced to various aspects of life in America.

Grier and Cobbs describe the black family as weak and relatively ineffective because it has not been allowed the rights and privileges of protecting its members.[41] The black male is expected to maintain a family, educate his children, and provide the normal conveniences of modern living, even though he is more likely than his white counterpart to be unemployed, earn less money, and pay more for housing. Constant failures in his attempts to be a successful provider are great blows to his manhood. Often his wife is forced to work to add to the family income.[42] As parents, the husband and wife teach their children what the world is like, how it functions, and how *they* must function if they are to survive. All too often the children have the hope and desire to succeed in the world but because of futile and dangerous competition, they are unable to fulfill their ambitions. Despite these problems, the black family is first of all an extended family. Relatives share the responsibilities of child rearing and members of the family often come to the aid of a troubled member.[43]

Billingsley described in detail the three social-class groupings of black families. About 10 percent of black families may be considered upper-class because the working members are highly educated, are in high-income brackets, have secure careers and adequate comfortable housing. About 40 percent of all black families are middle-class as distinguished by educational, income, and occupational achievement and styles of family life. Half of all black families are in the lower classes. Of these, there are the "working nonpoor," the "working poor," and the "nonworking poor." The "working nonpoor" are the families with the males working as semiskilled, unionized laborers in industries. The "working poor" represent families whose working members work in unskilled and service occupations with marginal incomes. The "nonworking poor" are those families who receive the most publicity and who comprise 15 to 20 percent of black families. These are people who are unemployed or intermittently employed, supported by relatives and friends or by public welfare.[44] The majority of *poor blacks,* as classified by Billingsley, live in nuclear families headed by men and are self-supporting rather than supported by public welfare.[45]

Among the 15 to 20 percent of black families classified as *nonworking poor,* how-

[40] William H. Grier and Price M. Cobbs, *Black Rage,* Basic Books, Inc., Publishers, New York, 1968, pp. 22–24.
[41] Ibid., p. 71.
[42] A. Ludlow Kramer, *Race and Violence in Washington State,* Report of the Commission on the Causes and Prevention of Civil Disorder, 1969, p. 24.
[43] Grier and Cobbs, op. cit., p. 87.
[44] Andrew Billingsley, *Black Families in White America,* Prentice-Hall, Inc., Englewood Cliffs, N.J., 1968, pp. 8–9.
[45] Ibid., p. 139.

ever, a matriarchal pattern is frequently found. Many black families are headed by women because opportunities for welfare payments are better for the female-headed household. The woman is often overburdened by many children and substandard living conditions. The children may have a great deal of freedom outside the home and form important peer-group contacts early in life. The influence of the peer group is often more significant than that of the parents because of the sense of importance and identity conferred by "gang" membership.[46]

Grier and Cobbs describe a black norm of behavior which, when developed, involves a profound distrust of white citizens and of the nation. Many black people have learned self-preservation from physical hurt, cheating, slander, humiliation, and outright mistreatment by the official representatives of society. For survival, some black individuals view any white person as a potential enemy until proved friendly and any social system as oppressive to blacks unless their personal experience can prove otherwise.[47] This explains in part the many pent-up resentments and frustrations felt by blacks and expressed by them in many overt and covert ways.[48]

For the white nurse visiting the black family, verbal and nonverbal evidences of the resentments and frustrations are easily detected if the nurse is sensitive and alert to cues. Many of the traditional nursing behaviors in home visits, which had a logical basis for existence initially, are being interpreted in a different way by blacks. Standeven cited the example of the community health nurse's routine in placing a newspaper under the nursing bag. Blacks often saw this action as indicating their home was particularly repelling and dirty, and the nurse was avoiding contamination of herself and the bag.[49] Members of the black family are particularly sensitive to cues of behavior. As described by Pegues, the attitude of the interviewer (particularly if the nurse is white) is very important, and nonverbal behavior is watched closely. Blacks are sensitive to tone inflections, discreet pauses, subtle hesitations, the careful pattern of hidden meaning, facial expressions, bodily gestures and muscular tension of taut touch or "slimy" handshakes.[50] They are sometimes likely to "test" the sincerity and attitude of the nurse. When this factor is recognized as a possible behavior with which one must contend, the nurse has a better opportunity to initiate an empathic, client-centered relationship. It is also important for the nurse to focus on the particular family being serviced so as not to prejudge it in terms of the generalizations applied to a particular ethnic group. The interviewer's anticipation of ethnic commonalities can force the family members to respond in ways that are not characteristic of their particular style of behavior.

For many black groups the health status is complicated by environmental conditions, unemployment, and lack of money to obtain medical treatment. Residents of

---

[46] Martin Deutsch, Irwin Katz, and Arthur R. Jensen, *Social Class, Race, and Psychological Development,* Holt, Rinehart and Winston, Inc., New York, 1968, p. 204.

[47] Grier and Cobbs, op. cit., p. 149.

[48] Judson R. Landis, *Current Perspectives on Social Problems,* Wadsworth Publishing Company, Inc., Belmont, Calif., 1969, p. 108.

[49] Muriel Standeven, "What the Poor Dislike about Community Health Nurses," *Nursing Outlook,* 17:72–73, September 1969.

[50] Thelma Pegues, "Physical and Psychological Assessment of the Black Patient," *Washington State Journal of Nursing,* special supplement, 1979, pp. 4–8.

racial ghettos have a high incidence of major diseases. Health and illness tend to be dealt with on a crisis basis. Motivation to seek aid is only acted upon when there is impairment of function. As pointed out by Pegues, even though many blacks may have good medical care, they tend to favor foods which are identified as high risk because of fat and salt content. Examples of such foods are salt pork (fatback), fried foods (chicken, fish, pork), barbecued foods, potato salads, butter cakes, ham hocks and black-eyed peas with crackling cornbread, and the like.

One of the skills which the nurse must develop is that of doing a skin assessment of a black person to determine the general state of health. Skin assessments when done accurately and skillfully alert the health professional to changes in skin color, suggesting pathology and/or deviations from normal. Skin assessment for people of color has been described in articles by Roach, Paxton, and Roberts (see Suggested Reading). Each points out the value of astute skills in observation, the importance of adequate lighting, the effects of proper positioning and controlled environments to accurately assess the skin changes in black patients.[51] Practice in doing skin assessments reinforces skills.

Other tasks for which the nurse must be prepared include the raising of consciousness in disadvantaged families about available health care facilities such as medical and dental services, hospitals, and clinics dealing with family planning, abortion counseling, immunizations, child health, drug abuse, nutrition, health promotion, and other health-related matters. The nurse also must be prepared to cope with the problems of insufficient income, transportation, baby-sitting, and erratic hours. These obstacles often stand in the way of attendance to health care needs for blacks and their families. Black consumers have become active in exercising their right for health care and are playing a major role in the design and management of health care programs for blacks. According to Milio, blacks want to learn to be self-sufficient in meeting their health needs and appreciate efforts from white persons only when the goal is directed toward independent self-care for blacks. In striving for the "black is beautiful" concept, they are building their self-respect and gaining confidence in their own abilities to successfully determine and cope with the intricacies of modern living.[52]

American Indian Families

Increasing attention is being given to American Indian culture and the role of the Indian in our current society. Since different tribes live in various locations of the United States, information about local Indian families must be obtained from literature specifically describing the local tribe and from the Indian people themselves. There are a great variety of Indian tribes who have their own histories, languages, customs, religions, and traditions. In addition, strong Indian leaders and war chiefs of the past hold a revered place in the memories of their people and symbolize the great tradition of the Indian people. As described by Deloria, individual tribes show incredible differences. The single aspect of major importance is tribal solidarity. Tribes that can handle their reservation conflicts in traditional Indian fashion generally make more progress

[51] Ibid., p. 6.
[52] Milio, op. cit., pp. 191–195.

and have better programs than do tribes that continually make adaptations to the white value system.[53]

There are many differences between the white culture and the Indian culture, and also among widely scattered Indian groups. A ritual or value of one tribe may not necessarily be accepted as essential by another tribe. The different geographical settings and cultural characteristics of various tribes complicate the work of health workers because transference of knowledge about one Indian tribe will not necessarily be valuable when working with a different tribe. This fact is frustrating because the health worker must start anew with each new tribe. Consequently, the health worker when working with Indian families in a local community must become acquainted with the values and beliefs of that specific Indian community. This takes time and patience. One example of a difference between two distinct tribes in terms of their responses to the implementation of health care by professionals is cited to demonstrate that the values of each tribe must be understood and dealt with as individual to that particular tribe. In a Pueblo reservation it was found that when parents were expected to transport their own children with health problems to clinics and hospitals outside the reservation, they gained a clearer understanding of the health services provided to the children and followed through with the recommended health care much more dependably.[54] On a Tulalip reservation, however, the community health nurse was seen as more helpful if concrete health services were brought to the Indian child on the reservation or if the nurse personally transported the child outside the reservation to the clinics and hospitals providing the health services.[55]

Indian people place absolute dependence on their leaders and expect them to produce. Because leadership is physically and emotionally taxing, the usefulness of the leader is sustained only as long as he is able to withstand the pressures of leadership over a dependent people.[56] Indians welcome the future but don't worry about it. They like to meet other tribes, have a good time, and learn to trust one another. However, they reserve the right to change their minds about an issue whenever it serves their own purposes. Indians know the human mind intimately. They savor innuendo and inference and can dwell for hours on slight nuances that others completely miss. Because of this, Indians know the Indian mind best of all.[57]

The health status of Indians in some aspects is more appalling than that of blacks. The infant mortality rate is the highest in the nation, with infants dying of influenza, pneumonia, respiratory conditions, gastroenteric and parasitic diseases. The life expectancy of the Indian is less than that of all other races, and the suicide rate is triple the national rate. Suicide alone among Indian youth has caused great concern in recent years and for one tribe in western Washington led to the development of a progressive youth program in an attempt to forestall an epidemic of suicides among teenagers.

---

[53] Vine Deloria, Jr., *Custer Died for Your Sins,* The Macmillan Company, New York, 1969, p. 28.

[54] Lucille J. Marsh, "Health Services for Indian Mothers and Children," Children's Bureau, Division of Indian Health, Public Health Service, *Children,* November–December 1957.

[55] Rita Hoeschen Aichlmayr, "Cultural Understanding: A Key to Acceptance," *Nursing Outlook,* 17(7):23, July 1969.

[56] Deloria, op. cit., p. 214.

[57] Ibid., pp. 215–220.

Leading diseases among the Indians are otitis media, tuberculosis, trachoma, anemia, and dental caries. A high incidence of lethal accidents, cirrhosis of the liver, and alcoholism also occurs with Indian populations.[58] Because of crowded housing, unsafe water, unsatisfactory waste disposal facilities, lack of nutritious food, and adherence to practices hazardous to health, the nurse has much health teaching to do *after* overcoming the initial barrier of coming into the midst of the Indian people as a helping person and going through the long procedure of becoming acceptable.

As explained by Backup,[59] the extended family is a very important factor in the lifestyle of American Indians. The two most important groups in the family are the children and grandparents. Children are seen as assets to the family. The form of child care practiced by Indian parents puts very little emphasis on physical controls or overt punishment. Children are encouraged to be independent very early in life. They do not ask permission to do ordinary things of normal daily living. They eat when hungry and sleep when tired—there are no rigid schedules. Patience is expected of all children. If a child cries or whines, a parent or grandparent will hold, feed, or in some way help the child to gain control of the emotion. Children learn very early to behave in a quiet, unobtrusive, and most of all unassuming manner.

The aged are highly respected, loved, and looked to for wisdom and counsel. Indian grandmothers are important to the children and in some tribes they have as much authority as the mother in rearing practices and disciplines. In most tribes a child will have several sets of grandparents, all instrumental in the child's growth and development. This custom of adopting grandparents is important because it assures family unity and strength. To be really poor in the Indian world is to be without relatives.

Within the Indian family, individual freedom and independence are highly valued. This respect for individual rights is clearly seen in what is referred to as the principle of noninterference. No interference or meddling of any kind is allowed or tolerated, even when it is to keep the other person from doing something foolish or dangerous. No person has the right to speak for or to direct the actions of another.

American Indians have a profound spiritual relationship with nature and mother earth. They have a holistic view of life and believe that God (Great Spirit) is the primary giver and cause of life. The medicine man is an important and respected member of a tribe who believes the health of an individual includes body, mind, and the ecologic sphere. The treatment process, which could include religious rituals of chanting and dancing, is guided toward treating the whole person and bringing the person back into balance with the surroundings. When the services of the medicine man are needed, he comes to the home of the ill. The family is always involved in the healing process and assists with the ceremonies and rituals as directed by the medicine man.[60] When community health nurses recognize behaviors and beliefs of American Indian families, their interactions and services are greatly facilitated.

---

[58] Hilda Bryant, "Bad Health Adds to Indians' Woes," *The Red Man in America.* Reproduced by the information and editorial offices of the State Superintendent of Public Instruction, Olympia, Washington, by permission of the Seattle *Post-Intelligencer,* January 1970, pp. 15–17.

[59] Ruth Wallis Backup, "Implementing Quality Health Care for the American Indian Patient," *Washington State Journal of Nursing,* special supplement, 1979, pp. 20–24.

[60] Ibid.

For nursing students working with Indian families on a western reservation, Aichlmayr brought out the importance of starting a health program based purely upon the Indians' statement of need and desire and of being accepted as equals in a mutual endeavor. The concepts of social prestige, age, anonymity, time, patience, and generosity as perceived by Indians were gradually learned by the nurses over a period of 15 months. Indian people value sincerity, honesty, and absolute trustworthiness.[61] Similarly, as all people on the face of the earth, Indians are human beings who respond positively to treatment by helping persons when they are dealt with as having dignity, honor, and value. Regardless of race, color, culture, or creed, human beings have the universal need to be recognized and interacted with as worthy individuals.

Families of Spanish Origin

Persons of Spanish origin are the second largest minority group in the United States and live mainly in urban areas. About one-third of the total population is under 18 years of age. Only 4 percent of all Mexican-Americans are 65 years or older. Families of Spanish origin tend to be larger and include more children. Almost one-half of all persons 16 years old and over have not had more than an elementary education. The rate of Puerto Rican youth who have dropped out of school is particularly high. A great disadvantage of a large proportion of Spanish origin populations is their inability to use English. This is a factor that affects the amount of education that is available in schools, and the job opportunities which have been restricted mainly to low-skilled menial occupations. Spanish-speaking people are hard-working, with over three-quarters of the males in the labor force. A quarter of all persons of Spanish origin live in poverty and struggle with the basic problems of day-to-day survival. The lack of education seems to be a critical factor but not the sole one which prevents Spanish-speaking persons from advancing into secure and well-paying employment.[62]

Mexican-Americans represent a substantial portion of persons of Spanish origin. These individuals or their parents have come from Mexico and have brought with them many customs and traditions. They speak Spanish and have a noticeable accent.[63] Chicanos are also individuals whose ancestry is from Mexico; consequently, they have similar customs and traditions. Chicanos are the activists of the Mexican-American population and are working toward attainment of the qualities of self-determination and realization of inherent worth and value. Chicanos are a part of a cultural revolution, linking the past with the future in the bicultural world in which they presently live.[64]

Problems descriptive of families of Spanish origin include (1) bilingual, bicultural

---

[61] Aichlmayr, op. cit., pp. 20–23.

[62] *A Study of Selected Socio-Economic Characteristics of Ethnic Minorities Based on the 1970 Census,* vol. 1, *Americans of Spanish Origin,* Department of Health, Education, and Welfare, Washington, D.C., July 1974, pp. 1–118.

[63] Edward Casavantes, "Pride and Prejudice: A Mexican-American Dilemma," in Nathaniel N. Wagner and Marsha J. Haug (eds.), *Chicanos, Social and Psychological Perspectives,* The C. V. Mosby Company, St. Louis, 1971, p. 49.

[64] Eliu Carranza, "The Mexican-American and the Chicano," in Antonia Castaneda Shular, Tomas ybarra-frausto, and Joseph Sommers (eds.), *Literatura Chicana,* Prentice-Hall, Inc., Englewood Cliffs, N.J., 1972, p. 39.

conflicts with the Anglo society, (2) displacement of parents from the home environment, and (3) lack of adequate education.[65] Even though these families may have been residents of the United States for years, many have resisted acculturation into the Anglo culture and have remained apart from the mainstream of American citizens. They retain their own language and distinctive cultural beliefs and values.

The family is likely to be the single most important social unit in life because of the emotional and material security provided. The concept of family includes members of the extended family with whom there is much communication, sharing, and closeness of relationships. According to Murillo, in Mexican-American families interpersonal patterns within the family are organized around two dimensions—that of respect and obedience to elders and that of male dominance of females.[66]

Many minority families of Spanish origin are low-income, maintain cohesive connections with the extended family socially and in times of need, have a close social network system with members of the same culture, employ common channels of communication, and attend special events of common interest. They are a strong subculture with definite health-seeking behavior. For the most part, they believe in folk medicine and treatment as practiced by their ancestors and frequently combine the best of two belief systems—their own home remedies with the health care practices of American professionals.

Many Spanish-speaking people classify food, illnesses, and medicines according to an etiological and therapeutic system which goes back to ancient times and is now commonly called the *hot-cold theory* of diseases and treatment. As explained by Murillo-Rohde,[67] the cultural belief of Hispanics about the hot-cold theory of etiology of disease is one that should not and cannot be ignored by nurses and health professionals. They must become familiar with the theory as well as the hot-cold classification of diseases, foods, and medications. The hot-cold theory views health as a balance among the four humors of the body (blood, phlegm, choler, and melancholy). Each one of these varies in temperature and moisture. Blood is hot and wet; choler (yellow bile) is hot and dry; phlegm is cold and wet; and melancholy (black bile) is cold and dry. When a state of imbalance occurs between the humors, disease manifests itself. To restore the body back to a balanced state (a state of health), cold foods and medicines are used to treat "hot" diseases and hot foods and medicines are used to treat "cold" diseases. It is important for nurses to know the foods and medicines considered hot and cold, so that treatment regimens will be utilized which are in compliance with the hot-cold theory. Nurses can modify therapeutic regimes so that the patient's beliefs are respected and recommended treatments are followed as prescribed by physicians. Harwood and Currier (see Suggested Readings) are good reference sources for the hot-cold theory of disease.

[65] Robert Aranda, "Development Delivery and Evaluation of a Chicano Health Services Seminar," unpublished master's thesis, University of Washington School of Public Health 1974, p. 2.
[66] Nathan Murillo, "The Mexican-American Family," in Nathaniel N. Wagner and Marsha J. Haug (eds.), *Chicanos, Social and Psychological Perspectives*, The C. V. Mosby Company, St. Louis, 1971, pp. 97–108.
[67] Ildaura Murillo-Rohde, "Cultural Sensitivity in the Care of the Hispanic Patient," *Washington State Journal of Nursing*, special supplement, 1979, pp. 25–32.

Hispanics tend to distrust Anglos who do not speak Spanish or show respect for the existence and practice of cultural beliefs and folk treatment for specific illnesses. They do not reveal personal or family information to strangers (and/or nurses) if the information is not relevant to the situation.

For nurses who work with these families, fluency with the Spanish language is desirable. In addition, the nurse must be flexible in reconciling recommended health care practices with folk medicine and the use of herbs and rituals. The nurse's communication should provide clear explanations in response to family questions, suggestions for actions with positive consequences, and acceptance of positive values in ritual acts performed by the family. Understanding and respecting the ethnic culture is imperative; the nurse should not focus only on Anglo views of the nature and causation of illness. The needs of these families are many, and they accept help best from those people who allow them to retain their identity and encourage self-help measures.

Asian-American Families

Of the Asian-American population, the Japanese are the largest subgroup in the United States. Well over one-third of Asian-Americans live in the western states and 90 percent live in urban areas. The majority of Asian-American families consist of husband and wife; however, a trend toward dissolution of families with a female head of the household is on the increase. Among families of Asian-American populations, Japanese families are, on the average, the smallest. Of all Japanese males 16 years and above, 70 percent have finished high school, and 19 percent have completed college. One-quarter of the population of all Chinese males, 16 years or older, have obtained college degrees, which is double the United States average. Asian-American men and women have a high rate of participation in the labor force, and a high proportion of the Asian-American males are employed as professionals and managers. There are great contrasts in levels of income of Asian-American populations; however, family incomes tend to be better than or on a level with incomes of United States families in general. Despite a greater tendency among Asian families to look after surviving elders, the rate of poverty among Asian elderly is as serious as it is for the elderly in the country as a whole.[68]

Asian-American families combine two cultures which influence the magnitude of one's ethnic identity—meaning the extent of an individual's incorporation of "Japaneseness" or "Chineseness" into the total ego identity.[69] As expressed by Yoshida, "Mother was wise enough to know that American children could not be reared like Japanese children, that we were products of the new world and we required freedom." My father "always spoke to us in Japanese. I could understand him, but I couldn't express myself in Japanese, so I replied in English. . . . We did all the things white kids our age did for fun, but we never forgot we were Japanese Americans."[70]

[68] *A Study of Selected Socio-Economic Characteristics of Ethnic Minorities Based on the 1970 Census,* vol. II, *Asian Americans,* Department of Health, Education, and Welfare, Washington, D.C., July 1974, pp. 1-159.
[69] Gary M. Matsumoto, Gerald M. Meredith, and Minoru Masuda, "Ethnic Identity: Honolulu and Seattle Japanese-Americans" in Stanley Sue and Nathaniel N. Wagner (eds.), *Asian-Americans: Psychological Perspectives,* Science and Behavior Books, Inc., Ben Lomond, Calif., 1973, p. 65.
[70] Jim Yoshida with Bill Hosokawa, *The Two Worlds of Jim Yoshida,* William Morrow and Company, Inc., New York, 1972, pp. 17, 18, 20.

The structure and values of Asian-American families are changing. Traditional values, however, continue to influence the socialization of the offspring as parents interpret appropriate and inappropriate behavior. The families retaining traditional values are patriarchal, with communication and authority flowing vertically from top to bottom. The father's behavior is generally dignified, authoritative, remote, and aloof. Sons are highly valued over daughters. The primary allegiance of the son is to the family. The behavior of individual members of an Asian family is expected to reflect on the whole family.

The roles of family members are highly interdependent. Independent behavior which might upset the orderly functioning of the family is discouraged. If a person has feelings which might disrupt family peace and harmony, she or he is expected to hide them. Restraint of potentially disruptive emotions is strongly emphasized in the development of the Asian character. With the lack of outward signs of emotions, Asians have been stereotyped as reserved, passive, and/or inscrutable. Traditional Asian values also emphasize formality in interpersonal relations, obedience to authority, and achievement in academic and occupational life.[71]

In studying the interplay of the original ethnic culture with the American culture, an emergence of three personality types has evolved, which is described as follows: The *traditionalist Asian* has strongly internalized the basic ethnic values of her or his culture. Primary allegiance is to the family. Self-worth and esteem are defined by ability to succeed in terms of high educational achievement and occupational status. With success, this Asian feels respectable in American society and has brought honor to the family name.

The *marginal Asian* cannot give unquestioning obedience to traditional parental values. This Asian attempts to assimilate and acculturate into the majority society which causes personal suffering because of a marginal status between two cultures. The tendency to gauge self-worth as defined by Caucasians is accepted. The determination of acceptability is shown by the number of Caucasian friends she or he has and by fluency with the English language.

The *Asian-American* is in the process of formulating a new identity by integrating past experiences and heritage with present conditions. It is felt that complete obedience to traditional values limits self-growth. Parental emphasis on high achievement is too materialistic for the Asian-American who is trying to find meaning and self-identity. She or he believes in being assertive, questioning, and active in order to develop in the present environment. This Asian also faces conflicts and experiences a great deal of guilt and frustration in parental relationships. In individualistic ways this person is trying to help the Asian people; however, many do not understand the effort.[72]

The nurse's behavior when working with Asian families is similar to that described

---

[71] Derald Wing Sue, "Ethnic Identity: The Impact of Two Cultures on the Psychological Development of Asians in America," in Stanley Sue and Nathaniel N. Wagner (eds.), *Asian-Americans: Psychological Perspectives,* Science and Behavior Books, Inc., Ben Lomond, Calif., 1973, pp. 140–141.

[72] Stanley Sue and Derald Wing Sue, "Chinese American Personality & Mental Health," Tachiki, Amy et al. (eds.), *Roots: An Asian American Reader,* UCLA Asian American Studies Center, Los Angeles, 1971, pp. 72–77.

for working with middle-income families. These families are intelligent, educated, courteous, friendly—particularly when the purpose for the encounter is known, accepted, and a rapport has been established. A recognition and respect for the distinctive culture of the family can be acknowledged when eliciting a family health history which includes questions regarding values, beliefs, customs, treatments, and health practices. Incorporation of practices important to the family is essential, along with the health measures the nurse wishes to introduce. A curiosity about the family's particular beliefs, as shown by the nurse who actively listens, demonstrates his or her genuine desire to assist in the way most helpful for the family and contributes to their sense of worth and identity. At times the educational process may be reversed; the nurse may learn of remedies and health practices which have greater healing potential than the ones she or he came prepared to advocate.

Refugee Families

Refugee families from French Indochina started arriving in the United States approximately in 1975. The first families were mainly Vietnamese, followed in subsequent years by an influx of Thai, Cambodian, and Laotian families. Refugees are persons who remain closely allied to their culture and are away from home for political reasons. Refugees become immigrants when they assume permanent residence in a new country and as a consequence of the permanency, develop new cultural roots—not necessarily those of the new country but not those of the home country either.[73] Becoming an immigrant means coping with two worlds instead of one.[74]

In coming to America the Indochinese refugee families have had to adapt to a new way of life, the American way. They have had to accept opportunities and options made available to them by Americans, and adjust to expectations and situations which are not always congruent with their capabilities and/or skills. In a sense, many of these families have been cast in the position of "poor relatives" who are dependent initially on the willingness and generosity of sponsors to give, share, or instruct regarding the necessities of life in a new and unfamiliar country. In the process of learning to adapt to the American way of life and move toward the dignity of independence, these families have multiple needs for which assistance is required. First and foremost, they want to speak English with sufficient ease and clarity so that they are able to secure jobs which will make them self-supporting. Other needs with which they should have assistance include familiarity with the rate of exchange (dollars and cents), customs, and mores; access to appropriate clothing and housing (dependent upon the state in which they reside); knowledge of local clinics or medical facilities for health care and schools in which their children will be enrolled; opportunities to meet socially with similar refugee families to facilitate the initiation of support networks so vital to the mental and emotional health of people starting anew.

Indochinese immigrants who come to the United States tend to be young, part of a family group, and Catholic or Buddhist in religion. For the most part, the households consist of large extended families. When a household is incomplete (some family mem-

---

[73] Gail Paradise Kelly, *From Vietnam to America,* Westview Press, Boulder, Colo., 1977, p. 89.
[74] Ibid., p. 3.

bers have been separated or are missing), much effort is exerted toward finding the missing family members so that the goal of reunification of extended families is accomplished. Many of the immigrants are well educated, but are unable to find positions in the United States commensurate with their skills. For these individuals adjustment problems are primarily related toward accepting a lowered socioeconomic position and all that goes with it. Opportunities for advancement rarely exist in poorly paying jobs. In today's society, it is not uncommon to find successful ethnic restaurants run by well-educated Indochinese immigrants who opted to enter the restaurant business as opposed to attempting to meet the standards for legal qualifications in their given professions.

Nurses working with Indochinese refugee families should realize that Vietnamese, Cambodian, Thai, and Laotian families are not necessarily similar in behavior, characteristics, beliefs, religion, or customs. Ethnocentrism exists. To be most helpful when working with individual families, the nurse must be sensitive to the ethnic origin of the family; the roles of men and women in family units; the religion they practice; the foods they prefer; their beliefs regarding illness, the herbal remedies they utilize; the habits, customs, and rituals that are important to them; their likes and dislikes about their own country and about the United States, and their needs for recreation, socialization, and support systems. If families can be brought together and organization of self-help activities encouraged, the assimilation of refugee families into the American culture is facilitated and emergence of new ethnic groups diversifying the population of the United States is engendered.

Families of Other Cultural Groups

In each local community there are often families representing a given culture who can be found in residential pockets, neighborhoods, or cul-de-sacs. They may be groups of Scandinavians, Filipinos, Italians, Jews, and other groups representing a country, a particular section of the United States, or a religious creed. Each group has its own distinct culture in addition to some assimilation of United States culture. The task of the nurse is to become acquainted with each cultural group and attempt to understand the manifestations of behavior that arouse curiosity. Each family has characteristics and behaviors which need to be assessed before any effective action or teaching can take place. To learn more about a cultural group, the nurse can begin by inquiring about their foods, since people prefer to eat their own kind of food and often enjoy sharing their particular likes and individualized patterns of eating with others. The nurse can ask about the manner of dress and admire distinctive clothing, such as the sari of the women of India or the pina cloth of the Filipino. Historical tales can be requested about the early beginnings of the culture, such as the Puerto Rican history or the ancient civilization of the Aztecs. Descriptions of recreational festivities that have special meaning can be elicited, such as the bullfights of the Mexican and Spaniard, the Bon Odori of the Japanese, or folk dance festivals of the Scandinavian. Requests can be made for clarification of the roles of family members, such as the male dominance or machismo exercised in Mexican and Hindu homes. The meaning of religious procedures of Italians or Jews can be elicited in terms of the marriage ceremony or upbringing practices of the children. Clarification of beliefs about health practices that seem impractical, ritualistic, or incongruent to the nurse can be requested. Always, the nurse must remember that when asking additional information about a cultural group, genuine and sincere interest in the activities and practices of the family must be conveyed. If the nurse can promote a liaison with the family based on mutual understanding of existing behavior patterns, a solid base for teaching and counseling about practical and acceptable health practices is eased. Underlying the implementation of any desired health action is the implicit suggestion to both nurse and family that planned change is wanted. Consent to change is most easily acquiesced when a mutual understanding and agreement occurs between nurse and family. Preparing a family for change often takes time and patience and is most easily accomplished when a therapeutic relationship has been developed simultaneously with the strengthening of the family's readiness.

FAMILIES WITH DISTINCTIVE RELIGIOUS BELIEFS

Every nurse is obligated to develop a knowledge, understanding, and appreciation of the religious practices of the families under care, especially as they apply to birth, marriage, illness, and death. This is particularly true for the nurse working in the home, where patients can carry on their religious practices more freely than in a hospital. Such a knowledge and appreciation on the part of the nurse will help to overcome some of the barriers to communication. Priests, rabbis, and clergy are always willing to explain the meaning of the religious practices of their people and to be helpful to the community health nurse.

In general, the nurse should know and understand, to some degree, the main tenets or principles of the world's major religions as they affect family health practices, such as the status of women and children in the family, diet patterns, and acceptance of medical care. An understanding and appreciation of these points by the nurse will make it easier to communicate with families of various religious backgrounds.

Many times nursing students find it hard to accept what they perceive as proselytizing from their clients. All nursing students as well as all individuals have a right of choice. Listening and trying to understand another's beliefs, values, or religion does not necessitate a conversion. Listening and understanding broadens a person's perspective, gives clues as to the perception and emotional status of the speaker, and opens avenues for facilitative mutual discussions regarding beliefs and values that constitute the decisions each individual makes. Being open, curious, and respectful of another's religious beliefs is facilitating of a relationship. At the same time, the listener is not required to argue when beliefs differ or one's own beliefs are attacked. Nonjudgmental, nondefensive listening gives poise and the added knowledge gained about the client is valuable.

FAMILY MIXTURES

Families who are fragmented, mixed, or "mixed-up" present a special challenge to community health nurses. Flexibility and an ability to "roll with the punches" is required of nurses practicing in today's society. All kinds of family mixtures, combinations, and compositions are encountered in addition to nuclear and extended families.

The nurse must be nonjudgmental, curious, accepting, and see each family as unique and possessing potential for growth.

Single-Parent Families

Single-parent families become single-parent through death, divorce, or by choice. The number of single-parent families have mushroomed, due in part to the escalating divorce rate in the United States. Ninety-five percent of the heads of such families are women and their socioeconomic status is low-income. For example, in 1977 the average income for all families headed by a male with the wife present and at least one child was $17,600. The corresponding figure for father-only families was $17,500, but the income for mother-headed families was $7765. The poverty level in 1977 was identified as $6191.[75]

A major challenge for these families is creating a growth-producing environment for children when a significant adult is absent or the parenting role is assumed by transient-type role models. In our society, fathers and mothers are extremely influential in molding and structuring the environment of their children either positively or negatively. The early experiences of children are healthy and growth-producing, destructive and self-limiting, or a mixture of both. For the single parent who has major responsibility for parenting the children in the home, the task is tremendous because that individual must fulfill roles that are usually handled by two people, one male and one female. When the single parent is female, how does she talk to the children about their father, the departed male? How do the male children view maleness if they do not have a consistent model to observe? The same questions can be asked in reverse if the father is the single parent. How do children learn about common interactions and relationships between males and females unless they can observe a living demonstration on a daily basis? Is the single parent able to assume all the mothering and fathering capacities needed by the children? Does the single parent overprotect and create dependency? Are children of single parents confused about masculine and feminine sexuality?

A one-parent family is basically incomplete. If the single parent recognizes the incompleteness of the family, ways for providing a completeness can be managed, such as having the children live with a whole or nuclear family on periodic occasions or extending family relationships to include significant males and/or females who are warm and trustworthy role models.[76]

Single parents need a great deal of outside help and support for their roles. For example, when the parent works, acceptable day-care centers or baby-sitting facilities are needed. It is generally recognized that children do not have to be with their mothers or fathers all the time; however, they need a strong reciprocal attachment with loving adults. Efforts to provide children with constant, caring adults should be the aim of the single parent. Day-care experiences can be positive ones in encouraging children to learn cooperation, sharing, and new developmental skills.

---

[75] U.S. Department of Commerce, Bureau of the Census, *Statistical Abstract of the United States,* 1979, p. 451.

[76] Satir, op. cit., pp. 170–172.

Not all single parents are prepared initially to cope with the sole responsibility, the cost, the loss of freedom and privacy, and the loneliness of single parenthood. In many instances, they need a supportive person with whom they can share their concerns. This person can be a community health nurse who is able to assist in problem solving, suggest appropriate community facilities for particular concerns, bring in helping persons and resources representing a cross section of services available in the community, and strengthen the capabilities and confidence of the client.

In many single-parent families in which the woman is the head, there frequently is a boyfriend who lives with the family, is present only occasionally, or is a brief transient-type contact. For community health nurses it is important to know if a boyfriend exists because if so, he represents an influential position in the household for the time that he is connected with the family. It is desirable to meet the boyfriend and regard him as a substitute father for the period of time he is in the home, unless the mother definitely states otherwise. Besides being a sexual partner for the single parent female, the boyfriend is a male role model and often plays a role in disciplining the children. If he has successfully gained the acceptance of the mother's children, he contributes stability to the family system. If he is not accepted by the children or is present for a temporary time only, it is often helpful for the nurse to request and arrange family conferences with the goal of encouraging all members of the family to learn to communicate openly about their daily activities, concerns, routines, or questions. Whether a situation is seen as right, wrong, good, or bad is immaterial. What is important is for all members of a family unit to feel comfortable about talking openly and giving clear messages to one another so that self-worth grows.

Blended Families

Blended families, as described by Satir, put together parts of previously existing families. Individuals in these families consist of a wide range of possibilities, such as wife, wife's children, wife's ex-husband, husband, husband's children, husband's ex-wife, children of the current husband and wife, etc. Even though all of these individuals do not live under one roof, they are in each other's lives—whether acknowledged or not. All these individuals are significant to the growth and success of the blended family.

Some problems that can occur in blended families include: (1) differing directions children receive from the various "responsible" adults concerned about their development; (2) the "hurt" of a divorce which has been satisfactorily resolved or is still unfinished business; (3) the inclination of natural mothers or fathers to be protective of their "own" children and to resist new perspectives brought into the family by the new mate; (4) the expectation of mothers that the new male spouse will take over the role of disciplining before a relationship has been developed with the children; (5) the new mate's feeling of exclusion when the family enjoys a joke or memory that is reminiscent of the former marriage; (6) the sharing of the parenting role by natural parents with stepparents; (7) the fact that some parents may be in closer contact with their stepchildren than with their natural children; (8) the difficulty of knowing how to manage rituals, traditions, holidays, birthdates, visits with in-laws, and grandparents;

and (9) the uncertainty of children that they are free to love whomever they want to regardless of the shadows of the past.[77]

A major task of community health nurses is to encourage open communication in blended families, bring out the concerns or problems that are troubling family life, be supportive of problem-solving attempts, and strengthen the resources of all family members so that they are able to learn, accept, and grow. This is most easily done by means of family conferences or talking with both parents of the new marriage. The nurse performs the facilitative role of suggesting potential problem areas, eliciting feedback from each parent of the new marriage, and encouraging open, honest discussion of all implications, alternatives, and consequences of behavior. For guidelines about a family conference see Chap. 6.

Potentially Abusing Families

Child abuse is a family affair. Everyone in the family knows about it, but no one talks about it. When abuse is known to have occurred, it is not so important to find out which parent did the abusing, as it is to counsel both parents to assess the basis for trouble in the family and the precipitating factors that led to the abuse. When potential for abuse is suspected, a family history elicited by the nurse is helpful for determining early interventions before anything happens. If the nurse decides to ask for a family history, attempts must be made to help the parents relax and be comfortable with the history-taking process. The nurse must be person-centered and initiate the interview by indicating concern for each parent's feelings. For example, the nurse might say, "I sense that your life is pretty difficult at times. Do you see it that way?" Be honest at all times, and give concrete examples of what you want to communicate. For example, *do not say,* "I think you punish your child when she cries too long." (Too threatening.) *Do say,* "When your daughter cries for a long time, it must be frustrating and hard to know how to stop it."

For actual abuse to occur, there are three qualifications that must be met. There must be (1) potential for abuse, (2) a special kind of child (either obnoxious or passive), and (3) a crisis. In assessing the potential for abuse, the nurse must perceive how parents see themselves, their spouse, their parents, their child, and other people. Some questions that may be helpful in eliciting the information you want are as follows:

1 Feelings about self
   a How were you punished as a child when you did something wrong?
   b Would you say you had a happy or unhappy childhood?
   c Were you close to either parent as a child?
   d Did you feel your parents were pleased with you?

Many "abusing" parents feel isolated, have low self-esteem, and had a primarily negative childhood. These individuals were not "mothered" or nurtured lovingly and may not know how to nurture others.

[77]Ibid., pp. 173–195.

2 Feelings about parents
   a Do you think the way your parents punished you is the best way to get children to behave?
   b What kind of relationship did you have with your mother when you were a child?
   c How would you describe your relationship with your mother now?
   d Do your parents help you out in any way now when you need it?

Frequently, "abusing" parents communicate the feeling that they were not regarded as worthwhile by their parents, and they believe their parents were justified in that viewpoint. They strove to please their parents but never quite made it. Seldom were their needs as children understood by their parents.

3 Feelings about spouse
   a What happens when you and your spouse disagree on how to handle the children?
   b Does your spouse recognize when you are "uptight"?
   c Does she (or he) help you out at these times?
   d In what way is your spouse helpful with the children?
   e Is there anything in your marriage that could be better?

The relationship with the spouse is extremely important. Frequently, an individual will marry a person with similar feelings of low self-esteem. "Abusing" parents do not always know how to be supportive of each other, particularly when one is "uptight."

4 Feelings about other people
   a Do you ever feel helpless and want help from others when problems with the children occur, such as crying, disobedience, or misbehavior?
   b Whom do you turn to at times like this?
   c How do you reach this person?
   d Do you use a baby-sitter? How often? Who?
   e What do you do when you are concerned about your children?

"Abusing" parents rarely have coping mechanisms or solutions with which they are satisfied. If they do not turn to other persons for help, or do not know how to reach others, the following information assists in determining the risk for abuse:

5 Feelings about their child
   a Are you having any problems with your child's behavior?
   b What kind of things make you feel really nervous and upset?
   c How do you handle accidents when they happen to your child?
   d How do you feel inside when your child cries?
   e How well do your children understand your feelings?
   f Do your children know when you are upset, and do they help you then?
   g Do your children live up to your expectations?

Parents who abuse tend to have unrealistic expectations of their children. They anticipate the attainment of certain developmental tasks based on their own desires rather than on the readiness or ability of the child. A rigid, righteous attitude of the parent should be watched for, if present.

For abuse to occur, the child must be a special kind of child who is either the wrong sex, was born at a wrong time, looks or behaves like someone the parent dislikes. The fussy baby or ornery little kid is more vulnerable to abuse than the "good" baby or child. It is helpful for the nurse to watch the behavior of a child when a parent is in a period of stress. If a child comforts and meets the parent's need, this often suggests that the child doing the comforting may be the one at risk.

Finally, for abuse to occur, there must be a crisis or precipitating factor. Perhaps, the crisis was triggered in this particular family because the child did something that taxed the patience or tolerance of the parent at a time when the parent was feeling particularly "low" anyway. The parent wanted reassurance or nurturing, and instead, it was at this time that the child did something wrong—triggering an emotional reaction. In such families, it may be that stress and recurring crises are a normal way of life, and abuse is one way of releasing feelings of frustrations and incompetence.[78]

For the nurse suspecting abuse in a family, it is necessary to initiate a relationship of trust with the parents before eliciting a detailed family history. The nurse must focus attention on parents and demonstrate a genuine concern for their thoughts, feelings, and actions. If allowed to do tangible activities with the children, the nurse can interact sociably with them, read to them, have them draw pictures, and demonstrate caring concern based on each child's level of understanding and readiness. In all interactions with each parent, reinforcement must be given for positive behaviors or actions so that self-esteem starts to build. If a homemaker or baby-sitter is needed in the home, the nurse can assist in finding appropriate resources for these services. Parents Anonymous groups are excellent resources for families willing to go to such groups. At all times, members of other disciplines who are working with the "abusing" family must be called by the nurse and all activities coordinated in such a way that goals are similar, congruent, and attainable.

When the nurse suspects abuse and feels that interventions have made no difference in the activities of the family, it is advisable to discuss the observations and data regarding potential for abuse with the nursing instructor or supervisor. Dependent upon the policies and rules of the local agency, the correct procedures for reporting child abuse in that community will be explained.

Families with Suicidal Members

Often community health nurses inadvertently learn that persons to whom they are giving service have formerly threatened suicide or are giving it serious thought because of their feelings of despair and helplessness and a belief that nothing can be done about their lives. In order to be responsive to any "cry for help," the nurse must be cognizant of prevention or follow-up phases of suicide. Prevention of suicide involves the identification of high-risk groups and/or individuals; the ready availability of responsive services, such as crisis clinics; the dissemination of information, particularly about pro-

---

[78]C. Henry Kempe and Ray E. Helfer, *Helping the Battered Child and His Family*, J. B. Lippincott Company, Philadelphia, 1972, pp. 55–64.

dromal clues; the lowering of taboos so that citizens can more easily ask for help; and the sensitization of professionals and ordinary citizens to the recognition of potential suicide. Follow-up activities are those that occur after a suicidal event, such as (1) working with an individual after a suicide attempt or (2) working with survivor victims of a committed suicide to help them with their sense of anguish, guilt, anger, shame, and perplexity.[79] Life has two aspects, its duration (length or shortness) and its scope (richness or aridity).[80] Community health nurses have frequent opportunity to enable others to see life as having meaning and richness, provided they recognize early behavioral clues of ambivalence regarding the value of life in their clients.

McLean defined a suicidal crisis as a period of time during which a person experiences an extremely strong wish to die, which conflicts with the wish to live. The crucial element that makes suicide prevention possible is the ambivalence. The nurse must utilize all knowledge and relationship skills to keep a potentially suicidal client focusing on the desire to live. Crisis intervention in suicide prevention is outlined in detail by McLean, consisting essentially of the following elements:

1 Establishing a relationship, maintaining contact, and obtaining information
2 Identifying and clarifying the focal problem or problems
3 Evaluating the suicidal potential
4 Assessing strengths and resources of the client
5 Formulating a therapeutic plan and mobilizing the resources of the client and others.[81]

When the nurse tells the client contemplating suicide, "Don't do it," a sense of caring is communicated. If a promise which is purposely designed to be fulfilled at a later time is extracted from the client, the nurse has probably assisted the client in overcoming the existing ambivalence of the moment. Few persons contemplating suicide renege on a promise. By being aware of the nature of suicide, in either the prevention or follow-up phase, another dimension is added to the intervention skills.

When working with the family following the suicide of a family member, it is necessary that the nurse initiate a relationship of trust and concern. Each family member must be allowed to ventilate their feelings. The nurse assesses all family members individually and as a group to identify interactional patterns, coping mechanisms, and health status, and assists each to identify mechanisms for achieving a higher level of coping ability.

SUMMARY

The family has traditionally been the unit of service for the community health nurse as a means for focusing on all members of the family toward achieving higher levels of health or wholeness. The family was defined as a nuclear family or primary group living

---

[79] Edwin S. Shneidman, *On the Nature of Suicide,* Jossey-Bass, Inc., Publishers, San Francisco, 1969, pp. 20–21.

[80] Ibid., p. 29.

[81] Lenora J. McLean, "Action and Reaction in Suicidal Crisis," *Nursing Forum,* 8(1):28–41, 1969.

and interacting together intimately in a common residence. From the perspective of a systems approach, one of the roles of the community health nurse was described as that of coordinating the health care systems and social systems within the community with the health needs of the family. The nurse also assesses the structure of families, the functions, and developmental task levels of families and individuals within the family. Interacting with families representing different socioeconomic positions requires careful preparation by the nurse, as implementation of successful activities is planned with each family according to its values, beliefs, and culture. Low-income families frequently cope with multiple health problems and health hazards of a different nature than middle- and high-income families. The existing health behavior and health needs of families representing cultures unfamiliar to the nurse are studied in order to facilitate changes of health practices which will be desirable, acceptable, and beneficial to the family.

SUGGESTED READING

Ackerman, Nathan W.: *The Psychodynamics of Family Life,* Basic Books, Inc., Publishers, New York, 1958.

Angelou, Maya: *I Know Why the Caged Bird Sings,* Bantam Books, Inc., Publishers, New York, 1970.

Bell, Norman W., and Ezra F. Vogel: *The Family,* The Free Press, New York, 1960.

Billingsley, Andrew: *Black Families in White America,* Prentice-Hall, Inc., Englewood Cliffs, N.J., 1968.

Blackwell, James E.: *The Black Community Diversity and Unity,* Dodd, Mead & Company, Inc., New York, 1975.

Branch, Marie, and Phyllis Paxton: *Providing Safe Nursing Care for Ethnic People of Color,* Appleton-Century-Crofts, New York, 1976.

Clark, Margaret: *Health in the Mexican-American Community,* University of California Press, Berkeley, Calif., 1959.

Craven, Margaret: *I Heard the Owl Call My Name,* Doubleday & Company, Inc., Garden City, N.Y., 1973.

Currier, Richard L.: "The Hot-Cold Syndrome and Symbolic Balance in Mexican and Spanish American Folk Medicine," in Ricardo Arguijo Martinez (ed.), *Hispanic Culture and Health Care: Fact, Fiction, Folklore,* The C. V. Mosby Company, St. Louis, 1978.

Deloria, Vine, Jr.: *Custer Died for Your Sins,* The Macmillan Company, New York, 1969.

Duvall, Evelyn Millis: *Family Development,* J. B. Lippincott Company, Philadelphia, 1962.

Farris, C. E., and L. S. Farris: "Indian Children: The Struggle for Survival," *Social Work,* 21(5):386–389, September 1976.

Geismar, L. L., and Michael A. La Sorte: *Understanding the Multi-Problem Family,* Association Press, New York, 1964.

Ginott, Haim G.: *Between Parent and Child,* The Macmillan Company, New York, 1965.

Good Tracks, Jimm G.: "Native American Non-Interference," *Social Work,* 18(6):30–34, November 1973.

Grebler, L., J. W. Moore, and R. C. Guzman: *The Mexican American People,* The Free Press, New York, 1970.

Grier, William H., and Price M. Cobbs: *Black Rage,* Basic Books, Inc., Publishers, New York, 1968.

Hall, Edward T.: *The Silent Language,* Doubleday & Company Inc., Garden City, N.Y., 1959.

Harwood, Alan: "The Hot-Cold Theory of Disease: Implications for Treatment of Puerto Rican Patients," *Journal of the American Medical Association,* **216**(7) May 17, 1971. pp. 1153–1160.

Henry, Jules: *Pathways to Madness,* Random House, Inc., New York, 1971.

Herzog, Elizabeth: *About the Poor: Some Facts and Some Fictions,* U.S. Department of Health, Education, and Welfare, Children's Bureau, 1967.

Hoyt, Edwin P.: *Asians in the West,* Thomas Nelson Inc., New York, 1974.

Hymovich, Debra P., and Martha Underwood Barnard: *Family Health Care,* McGraw-Hill Book Company, New York, 1973.

Irelan, Lola M.: *Low-Income Life Styles,* U.S. Department of Health, Education, and Welfare, Government Printing Office, Washington, D.C., 1966.

Kane, Robert L., Josephine M. Kasteler, and Robert M. Gray (eds.): *The Health Gap: Medical Services and the Poor,* Springer Publishing Company, New York, 1976.

Kelly, Gail Paradise: *From Vietnam to America,* Westview Press, Boulder, Colo., 1977.

Kempe, C. Henry, and Ray E. Helfer: *Helping the Battered Child and His Family,* J. B. Lippincott Company, Philadelphia, 1972.

Keyes, Charles F.: *The Golden Peninsula: Culture and Adaptation in Mainland Southeast Asia,* The Macmillan Company, New York, 1977.

Kerr, Lorin E.: "The Poverty of Affluence," *American Journal of Public Health,* **65**(1): 17–20, January 1975.

Kitano, Harry, H.: *Japanese Americans–The Evolution of a Subculture,* 2d ed., Prentice-Hall Inc., Englewood Cliffs, N.J., 1976.

Langsley, Donald G., and David M. Kaplan: *The Treatment of Families in Crisis,* Grune & Stratton, Inc., New York, 1968.

Leininger, Madeleine M.: *Nursing and Anthropology: Two Worlds to Blend,* John Wiley & Sons, New York, 1970.

Lewis, Oscar: *Five Families,* Basic Books, Inc., Publishers, New York, 1959.

Lewis, R. G., and Man Keung Ho: "Social Work with Native Americans," *Social Work,* **20**(5):379–382, September 1975.

Lyman, Stanford M.: *Chinese Americans,* Random House, New York, 1974.

MacVicar, Mary G., and Pat Archbold: "A Framework for Family Assessment in Chronic Illness," *Nursing Forum,* **15**(2):181–194, 1976.

Messner, Gerald: *Another View: To Be Black in America,* Harcourt Brace Jovanovich, Inc., New York, 1970.

Minuchin, Salvado et al.: *Families of the Slums,* Basic Books, Inc., Publishers, New York, 1967.

Nye, F. Ivan, and Felix M. Berardo: *Emerging Conceptual Frameworks in Family Analysis,* The Macmillan Company, New York, 1966.

Patterson, Gerald: *Families: Applications of Social Learning to Family Life,* Research Press Company, Champaign, Ill., 1971.

Pratt, Lois: *Family Structure and Effective Health Behavior: The Energized Family,* Houghton Mifflin Company, Boston, 1976.

Primeaux, Martha: "Caring for the American Indian Patient," *American Journal of Nursing,* **77**(1):91–94, January 1977.

Roach, Lora: "Assessment Color Changes in Dark Skin," *Nursing '77,* **7**(1):48–51, January 1977.

Roberts, Sharon: "Skin Assessment for Color and Temperature," *American Journal of Nursing,* **75**(4):610–613, April 1975.

Rogers, Carl R.: *Becoming Partners: Marriage and Its Alternatives,* Dell Publishing Co., Inc., New York, 1972.

Satir, Virginia: *Peoplemaking,* Science and Behavior Books, Inc., Palo Alto, Calif., 1972.

Shneidman, Edwin S.: *On the Nature of Suicide,* Jossey-Bass Inc., Publishers, San Francisco, 1969.

Sheehan, Susan: *A Welfare Mother,* New American Library, New York, 1976.

Shepard, Katherine F.: "Family Focus," *American Journal of Public Health,* **65**(1): 63–65, January 1975.

Spector, Rachel E.: *Cultural Diversity in Health and Illness,* Appleton-Century-Crofts, New York, 1979.

"The Sick Poor," *American Journal of Nursing,* **69**(11):2423–2454, November 1969.

Tachiki, Amy et al. (eds.): *Roots: An Asian American Reader,* UCLA Asian American Studies Center, Los Angeles, 1971.

Tapia, Jayne Anttila: "The Nursing Process in Family Health," *Nursing Outlook,* **20**(4):267–270, April 1972.

Toffler, Alvin: *Future Shock,* Random House, Inc., New York, 1970.

Wagner, Nathaniel N., and Marsha J. Haug: *Chicanos: Social and Psychological Perspectives,* The C. V. Mosby Company, St. Louis, 1971.

Personalizing Health Services for Families

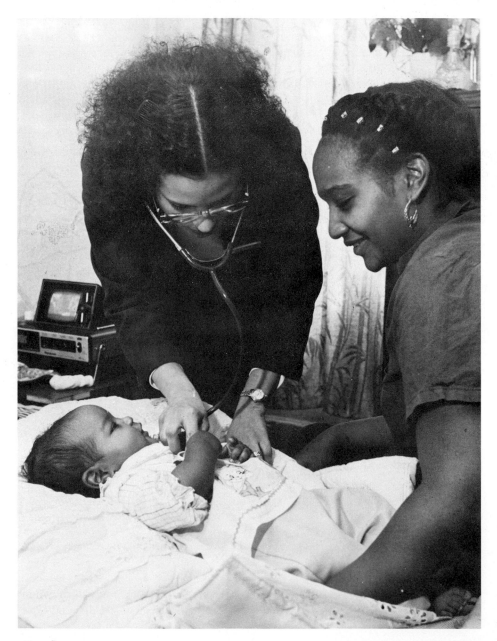

For years the home visit has been the principal means by which community health nurses interacted with families. Recently, however, the uncertainty about the efficacy of outcomes and costs of home visits have been critically questioned. As a result, many agencies have required a severe reduction of visits to homes. It must be realized that families can be worked with in a variety of settings, including the home, office, school, industry, job, clinic, neighborhood center, and any other location that is acceptable to the family and the nurse. Careful consideration of the environmental aspects of the selected setting must be taken into account by the nurse. The nurse wants the family to be relaxed and comfortable and must therefore check the setting for noise, distractions, privacy, lighting, warmth, arrangement of furniture, facilities for refreshments, if wanted, and availability of site for family, transportation, and parking requirements.

For nursing students, the home continues to be a desirable setting for working with families because of the learning opportunities existing in the home for observing family interactions, patterns of coping, and lifestyles. Families are the most natural in their own familiar territory. Nursing students learn that the implementation of the nursing process seems different in territory away from institutions. To become comfortable in a community environment, the nurse must be familiar with the great variety of health facilities; the differences in settings, atmospheres, and helpfulness of personnel; and the feeling of practicing as an independent agent for health promotion.

Community health nurses increasingly are making use of telephones and group meetings in place of home visits on a one-to-one basis. Group meetings are advantageous for reaching and educating numbers of people and providing stimulating health teaching in a practical manner. (For more discussion about groups, see Chap. 7.) The nurse must be prepared to do both individual and group work and sometimes may wish to diversify the methods of working with the family by talking with individual members occasionally, on a one-to-one basis, and meeting with the entire family at other appointed times.

COMMUNITY HEALTH NURSING PROCESS

The community health nursing process consists of five steps. They are

1 *Assessing* Identifying the need for the act
2 *Planning* Arranging for the methods and techniques necessary to meet the assessed need
3 *Implementing* Taking the action required to carry out the plan to meet the need
4 *Evaluating* Testing the outcome of the actions against previously determined criteria
5 *Studying and researching* Searching for knowledge in a systematic way

A model which summarizes the meaning of the first four steps of the nursing process as applied to families in community settings and discussed in this chapter is shown in Fig. 6-1. The nurse and family are mutual participants in moving toward therapeutic outcomes. The nurse initiates the nursing process and works with the family as they

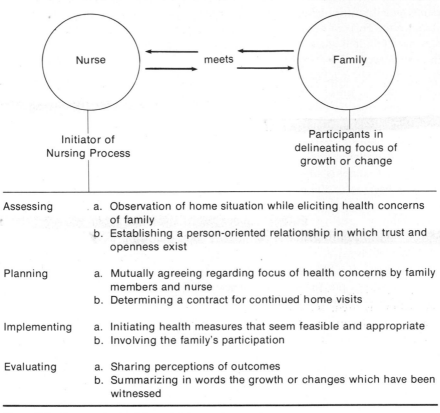

Figure 6-1 Community health model for nursing process.

are ready to grow, learn, and become responsible for attainment of desired goals. For more discussion about study and research, see Chap. 10.

COMPONENTS OF A VISIT

When making a visit, the community health nurse is faced with many functions, immediate or latent, which include preparation for the visit, introduction to the family, contract with the family, assessment, plan, implementation, evaluation, and written summary. These functions occur on every visit, but the depth of purpose and emphasis changes as movement toward an agreed-upon goal by family and nurse becomes more resolute. The ultimate objective of the nurse is to assist the family's advancement toward wellness or an acceptance of their present reality as exemplified by their improved coping skills, increased self-confidence, and attainment of better levels of health. *Wellness,* as defined by Dunn, is an integrated method of functioning that is oriented toward maximizing the potential of which the individual and family are capable, within the environment where they are functioning.[1] When the family and nurse

[1] Halbert L. Dunn, *High Level Wellness,* R. W. Beatty Co., Arlington, Va., 1961, pp. 4–5.

agree that essential and desired goals have been reached satisfactorily, then the nurse has accomplished the purpose of a helping change agent.

PREPARATION FOR A VISIT

There are two acceptable methods used by nurses when preparing for a visit. The first method consists of thorough preparation and assimilation of all data before making the first visit, and the second method postpones the gathering of related data until the first visit has been made and initial impressions have been received by the nurse. The first method requires a careful reading of the family folder in order to become familiar with the family constellation and the unique considerations of cultural, ethnic, religious, and social conditions. By reading all the nursing notes thoroughly, an impression is gained about the past events and successful and unsuccessful maneuvers which have occurred between the family and former nurses. Talking with other nurses or personnel from related fields who know the family also helps the nurse to form a mental image of the anticipated situation. The second method consists of a brief perusal of the family folder to make note of the family constellation and reason for the referral or continued visits. A conscious effort is made to avoid reading nursing notes or talking with personnel who are acquainted with the family before making the first visit. When the second method is used, the nurse is dependent upon individual skills of on-the-spot observation, assessment, and the family's feedback of events that have occurred in the past as seen from their perception. After gaining a picture of the situation from the family's point of view and her or his own appraisal of cues which occurred on the first visit, the nurse consequently reads the family folder and nursing notes thoroughly and talks to all individuals who are acquainted with the family to ascertain if all viewpoints coincide. It is a matter of individual preference and knowledge of one's own style of proceeding which determines the method selected by the nurse. The nurse who prefers to make her or his own assessment believes that the first method gives an unconscious predetermined bias, which may be deceiving and difficult to overcome. The nurse who relies on the first method feels more thoroughly prepared for any occurrence which may arise and will respond more successfully with tactics that may be attempted by the family.

When the family has a telephone, the nurse has the opportunity to call and arrange for a visit at an appointed time. One introduces oneself and gives the reason why one wants to meet the family. By making an appointment in advance, the nurse and family member become psychologically prepared for the visit. Also, the nurse is assured that someone will be available when the visit is made, and the family has been allowed the courtesy of arranging a time interval most suitable for them.

Once the visit is planned, the nurse should take several safety measures to assure safe passage into the community. Before walking out of the agency, the nurse should leave a list of expected visits for the day. The list should include names, addresses, and telephone numbers and the expected order in which the families will be visited. The nurse should be familiar with the area and map out the travel route. Never use short-cuts such as alleys or infrequently traveled streets. Purses should not be taken into homes; spare change can be carried in the nursing bag for necessary phone calls. When driving, cars should be locked and parked as close to the home to be visited as possible.

As the nurse enters the neighborhood, say "hello" to residents and be relaxed and open in manner while walking through the area. Conversing with the people in the area conveys a warm, caring attitude and demonstrates to them that the nurse has a genuine interest in the neighborhood. Common sense dictates that the nurse be aware of surroundings, not walk through large congregated groups, and use elevators rather than stairways when available. The uniform and nursing bag provide identification about the nurse in the community. Dress should be conservative and shoes should be comfortable. The nurse's image should reflect the public's expectation of the nurse.

INTRODUCTION TO THE FAMILY

When the time comes to knock on the door or ring the doorbell, it always is a moment of uncertainty for the nurse. One knows *why* one is making the visit but never is certain what tableau will be revealed when the door is opened. Feelings vary as the nurse waits for the door to open. One student nurse described her thoughts as follows:

> (knock, knock) As I stood outside the door, I could hear the radio playing within, and various images of stubborn, suspicious, frightened, or confused countenances flashed across my mind; I hoped to meet any or none of them as best I could.

Unless the nurse is well known to the family, the first step in the visit is the introduction, stating clearly one's name and that of the agency. The nurse explains the reason for the visit and the source of the referral for the visit if that is necessary, e.g., "Good morning, Mrs. Brown, I am Mr. Jones. I am the community health nurse from the Ocean County Health Department. Your physician, Dr. Smith, asked that we call on you about your pregnancy." Or, "Good morning, Mrs. Brown, I am Mr. Jones, the community health nurse from the Ocean County Health Department and Ocean City Visiting Nurse Service. I came in response to your telephone request this morning to visit your little boy who has a cold." The introduction or social phase will vary with the situation, but warmth, friendliness, and expressed interest on the part of the nurse will help establish rapport with the family and to develop a relationship on which to base effective teaching later.

The social phase of the visit cannot be overemphasized, because it is during this time that the family member becomes acquainted with the nurse as having the potential for being a warm human being and not another official professional entity who must be treated with awe, respect, and compliance. When anxiety is moderately high for the nurse and the family member, recall of all the words that were spoken during the home visit is limited. When comfort and relaxation occur, facilitated during the social phase of the visit, then the professional content of the visit has more possibility of being remembered and the family member and nurse are better able to absorb the implications of subsequent interactions.

On early contact the nurse must become acquainted with all the members in the household. Their ages and interactional patterns between family members must be learned and observed whenever feasible. It is extremely important to meet the father or head of the household, since he often holds an influential role in the family. In the past, many nurses have not made a practice of meeting the man in the family because they do not know how to cope with him for one reason or another.[2] However, when the organizational makeup of any family is studied, the conclusion reached is that the man holds an important position of influence and power and therefore must be involved. Sometimes, in order to meet the man in the family, special arrangements have to be made, such as a visit in the evening or an appointment visit near the father's place of employment. Generally when the nurse expresses a desire to meet the man of the family, the response of family members is favorable. Until all members of the household are met and actively involved, a truly accurate assessment of a complex family health situation cannot be accomplished.

When entering a home, the nurse must consciously greet all the family members present. If all members of the household are recognized by verbal or nonverbal means, the nurse is making her or his presence known and is in a position of catching their attention even though the initial response of individual family members may be one of indifference or withdrawal. Even the family's pets should be acknowledged, particularly if they seem to hold a position of esteem. For example, a staff nurse who was visiting a young couple with a new baby recognized early that the friendly Dalmatian held an important position in the affections of the new mother. It was not until several visits had been made that the nurse came to the realization that the dog was treated as a firstborn and the new baby was regarded in attitude very similarly to that of a second-born child. By making this assessment of the dynamics of family life, the nurse was able to give more appropriate, cogent assistance to the young mother.

If the household contains a sick member who is unable to respond verbally or tangibly, the nurse should make a point of speaking directly to the client, in a manner which indicates the belief that the client understands. By recognizing the existence of the client, the nurse communicates a respect for the client's dignity and serves as a model to family members regarding the appropriate attitude to assume toward the sick person.

Beginning Relationship with a Family

By recognizing all the members of the household and being cognizant of the interrelationships and family dynamics, the nurse is in an excellent position of soliciting and gaining cooperation from family members and eliciting health goals that will be beneficial to all. When a meeting with the whole family is desired, the nurse must purposefully make an appointment with the family, specifically stating the goal of the meeting and that all family members are to be present. When the appointed time arrives, the nurse should take the initiative for starting the conversation by introducing the reasons for wanting to talk with the family. The nurse should consciously create a climate that is relaxed and aimed to put family members at ease. Each individual should be encouraged to state a particular view of the health issue by means of direct and nonthreatening questions. Being present in the family group as an outsider or a third-party consultant, the nurse should realize that this role can facilitate conversation that is not usually

---

[2] Rosemary Pittman, "The Man in the Family," *Nursing Outlook,* 16:62–64, April 1968.

openly expressed between family members. Feedback about their verbalizations should be given to individuals within the family as perceived by the nurse. The nurse should be accepting of positive and negative information and, by listening carefully, should request further clarifying and factual information. The nurse should be cognizant of assets and express recognition of individual and family strengths as they become apparent. By engaging the family as a whole, the nurse is able to assess the family situation, enable the family to focus on the issue of the moment, and provide the impetus to help them to move toward stated, desired, unified goals. Because all family members have been brought together and encouraged to discuss a health situation openly, and decisions regarding goals to be achieved have been elicited and perhaps decided upon, the predictability of a favorable outcome for future events is much more assured.

To cite an example, a student nurse who was visiting on a regular basis a family with multiple problems frequently discussed with the mother the current problems of the father's unemployment, finances, transportation, school adjustment of the four children, and discipline in the home. There was no noticeable progress in the family's ability to cope with their daily problems as reported by the mother until the nurse conceived the idea to meet the father and arrange a family conference. An appointment was made to meet the entire family and an open discussion of their situation was aired. No issues were resolved as a consequence of the meeting other than a complete reassessment of the family by the nurse. This initial meeting did provide the family the opportunity to identify and review problems that they felt they were confronted with at the time. After three more meetings, during which several health issues were discussed, the family demonstrated much more unity, a happier and more secure attitude, a better insight into some of their behaviors, and an improved ability to cope with daily events. Because of the positive change in the family's functioning, the nurse felt that she benefited most because she learned that all families are a dynamic whole, made up of individuals who must be met and involved as participating members, and resolution of health needs is facilitated with the least amount of nurse energy.

CONTRACT WITH THE FAMILY

When working with a family, it is essential that the family members and the nurse know the purpose of the nurse's visits, that there is a mutual agreement to work toward a desired end or goal, and that both family members and nurse will direct their activities or abilities toward the achievement of the mutually determined goal. In essence, a *contract* is made in which the family and the nurse are involved. It can be written and signed by both parties or verbally agreed upon. As a consequence of the contract, both know the goal or goals toward which they are striving, both realize what is expected of them as participants, and both will know when the contract has been completed.

If the word "contract" seems too officious, the word "agreement" can be substituted. What is important is that the family and nurse have a contract or an agreement which has been mutually determined. As pointed out by Sheridan and Smith, students frequently feel a discomfort in developing a contractual approach to care because of their basic uncertainties and perception of self in the responsible role of nurse working with family X.[3] A contract must be a sharing process, a partnership in which both parties openly express their opinions and thoughts regarding changes that seem advisable, benefits and barriers that may occur concurrently, and the likelihood of successful and/or desirable outcomes. The nurse has a great deal of knowledge and many skills and services which, when shared with families, facilitate their progress toward improved states of health. The first agreement or contract can be a "small" or nonthreatening one such as, "The nurse will visit weekly to take vital signs and do a health assessment of the identified patient in the family." Very often, the nurse must "sell" services she or he is prepared to offer, such as doing Denver Developmental Assessments on children; explaining and interpreting birth control measures that are contained in kits; bringing explanatory and appropriate audiovisual aids, books, and pamphlets; checking blood pressure and temperatures; looking into throats.

There are four patterns of responses from family members when faced with making a decision regarding a contract: (1) They know what they want help with and say so; (2) they know their own needs and priorities but are reluctant to say anything for fear the nurse might not indicate approval; (3) they are uncertain of their own needs and priorities and want others to tell them what to do;[4] (4) they cannot think of any needs or priorities at the moment of the inquiry but if given a time span in which to reflect (1 week) will be able to state their desires at the appointed time.

One must be aware that there are also three states of mind when it comes to an agreement or contract. A client may state "I want to know how to stop my 6-year-old boy from wetting the bed." This client may be stating (1) an intention—"I want to," (2) a decision—"I will," or (3) a commitment—"I will do it." If the nurse can determine the state of mind of the client accurately, it will help in setting up a workable contract.

If the family needs suggestions about suitable and desirable contracts, it may be helpful for the nurse to explore their perceptions of their current lifestyle. Is there anything that they would like different? Perhaps one child is annoying the mother, but she is not thinking of it as a health need. With some suggestions from the nurse about possible ways to change the behavior of the child, an agreement or contract may evolve.

The contract can be renegotiated every week, if necessary. Perhaps the first agreement was too easily attained, was not really what the client wanted, was not specific enough, was not realistic, or was not focused on the client's greatest need.

When a satisfactory agreement has been negotiated verbally between family and nurse, it is desirable for the goals and/or contract to be written in understandable language. It can be written by the client or by the nurse. Both the nurse and client should read the contract and sign their consent. A contract can be written as follows:

1   John will say one word clearly (other than Daddy and Momma) by the end of 2 months.

[3] Ann Sheridan and Ruth A. Smith, "Student-Family Contracts," *Nursing Outlook,* **23**:114–117, February 1975.
[4] Nena O'Neill and George O'Neill, *Shifting Gears,* M. Evans & Company, Inc., New York, 1974, p. 149.

2 Children will brush their teeth properly at bedtime for five consecutive evenings without protest.

3 Mrs. M. will prepare balanced low-budget lunches for the children for 1 week.

Initially it helps if the contract is small, specific, attainable, and reasonable. For a goal to be reachable, small "steps" must be taken which show the family that movement and progress toward the desired goal is possible and within their capabilities. The nurse must be patient, persistent, and reinforcing of the family as they move slowly and sometimes hesitantly toward the desired goal.

The ability to implement a planned goal is facilitated for the nurse when the contract is written, has specific desired terminal behaviors, and has a time limit. A methodology or theoretical framework can be easily integrated into the learning situation when terminal goals are mutually agreed upon and accepted by both family and nurse. Psychological readiness is present. Designating a time limit for specific goals is particularly important for nursing students, since their time period for working with families is generally fixed. When families are forewarned that the nursing student will be working with them for 2 months, that a terminal behavior can realistically be achieved within the stated time period, and when discernable progress becomes apparent, excitement and hope are engendered. The nurse learns to be self-confident of the ability to be an influential change agent, and feels satisfied and rewarded.

For families who have had nursing visits in which contracts have not been made, there is often an uncertainty about the reason for nursing visits. Families many times relate, "Our nurse is coming to visit today," but when asked the purpose of the visit, they seldom are able to identify the planned focus of the visit. They find the nurse a pleasant person and attempt to meet her or his needs by telling about their past illnesses or reasons for failure to attend clinics. After the nursing visit, however, they resume their life patterns as always.

THE NURSING PROCESS: ASSESSING

Nurses are accustomed to assessing the client's needs based on a medical and nursing model and can often identify many more needs than can a client. However, unless a client also sees a need as one that exists and for which help is desired, there is little point in making the assessment.

Assessment is a continuous process which becomes more accurate as knowledge of the consumer deepens. As defined by Harpine, *nursing assessment* is the continuous, systematic, critical, orderly, and precise method of collecting, validating, analyzing, and interpreting information about the physical, psychological, and social needs of a patient, the nature of self-care deficits, and other factors influencing condition and care.[5] While determining client needs, the nurse will concentrate only on those needs which can be influenced or changed by nursing intervention. The nurse will seek to

[5] Frances H. Harpine, "Assessing the Needs of the Patient," in Helen Yura and Mary B. Walsh (eds.), *The Nursing Process: Assessing, Planning, Implementing, and Evaluating,* The Catholic University of America Press, Washington, D.C., 1967, p. 22.

know the client as a distinctive person so that the nurse's abilities as a therapeutic agent can be utilized as effectively as is possible.

All persons have needs, but which needs will the client confirm as indeed existing and for which will accept assistance from the nurse? For low-income families, the needs which have to be focused upon early are often the physiologic and safety needs, whereas with middle- and high-income families the needs for love, belonging, esteem, or self-actualization may be the ones that are most urgent and in need of attention. All persons, regardless of social class, periodically regress in their individual fashions toward seeking satisfaction for the more basic physical needs when they indulge in overeating or lose their appetite, seek additional sleep or have insomnia, or reveal similar manifestations of stress.[6] The ability to assess and observe the client's present reality makes use of the nurse's senses, knowledge of hierarchy of needs, and ability to relate to the client's verbal and nonverbal cues in a facilitative manner. Upon observing and noting the client's cues, the nurse must share and explore perceptions with the client to ascertain if they are both in agreement.[7] Sometimes, the client has difficulty expressing desires and must be helped by the nurse to articulate needs. A facilitative way to do this is to state, "You look worried. Are you concerned about something that I am unaware of?" Or the nurse may say, "Sometimes it is difficult to ask for help because we all like to think we can handle our own affairs. However, there are times when each one of us needs the help of another, and I sense that you may feel that way now. Is this true?" By admitting that we all are human beings and have moments of need, a relationship is facilitated in which each participant feels a greater freedom to exchange inner meanings with the other person involved.[8] When the nurse is authentic, she or he excludes the possibility of seeing the client as a problem and self as a person who can solve the problems. The nurse tries to be responsively aware so that the client, in turn, can be authentic and reveal true concerns.[9]

Obstacles which tend to blunt the perceptions of nurses and deter the attainment of accurate assessments of clients and families have been experienced by all nurses and must be watched for as undesirable behaviors. The first one is taking a partial view of the person, labeling or stereotyping that person with descriptive labels such as uncooperative, slow, immature, incompetent, and so on. Once the judgment has been made or the label attached to the client, the nurse tends to miss other positive or negative attributes which may change her or his mind about the person. All people have likable and dislikable characteristics, and an attempt should be made to view all persons as accurately as possible.

A second obstacle is that of viewing the client as a thing instead of a person. All too often in nursing and medicine, clients have been referred to as a room number, a bed number, or a diagnosis. In fact, sometimes the common practice of calling a person a client is discriminatory and not always beneficial for the person. When the person is viewed as an object, it is all too easy to deal with the individual purely as the receiver

[6] Sister Kathleen M. Black, "Assessing Patients' Needs," in Helen Yura and Mary B. Walsh (eds.), *The Nursing Process: Assessing, Planning, Implementing, and Evaluating,* The Catholic University of America Press, Washington, D.C., 1967, p. 8.
[7] Harpine, op. cit., p. 22.
[8] Black, op. cit., p. 17.
[9] Ibid., p. 18.

of nursing ministrations and to deny the individual the choice of accepting or refusing procedures that are designed as helpful whether the client agrees or not.

A third deterrent is viewing the client in terms of potential to meet the nurse's needs, rather than the nurse's potential to meet the client's needs. This obstacle has to do with the esteem needs of the nurse and the natural desire to be influential and successful with the person receiving the nursing assistance.[10] It is difficult for the nurse to know that the client can be helped yet have the client refuse nursing service or observe the client as demonstrating no improvement in spite of nursing ministrations. It is also sometimes difficult to accept the fact that the client no longer requires nursing services and is competent to make decisions. For example, a student nurse during a routine visit to a young mother with a new baby was shown the diaper rash of the baby, which was causing the mother considerable concern. The nurse instructed the mother carefully and thoroughly about the care of the buttocks, and in the event that no improvement was demonstrated, referral to a well-baby clinic was given. The nurse promised to return in a week. Three days later, the student nurse felt a compelling urge to visit the young mother and baby to see for himself if the diaper rash was better or not. After a vigorous conflict within himself, the nurse decided that his *own* need to see the mother and baby must take second priority to the knowledge that the mother had been carefully instructed, had understood, and was probably competent to manage the situation. On the home visit the following week, the nurse received the report from the mother that the diaper rash had cleared after the mother implemented the instructions she had received from the nurse.

Factors in Assessing the Family

On the initial visit to a family many early impressions are secured, which form the initial basis for the ongoing assessment. As data are gathered and assembled continuously during subsequent visits the nurse becomes better acquainted with the family and responds to the assessment process similarly to that of assembling a jigsaw puzzle. The early pieces of the jigsaw puzzle give one an early image of the completed picture, but while sorting and trying various pieces for size, there are frequent periods of puzzlement and frustration. Until all the pieces are in place, a complete understanding of the picture is not reached. Families are like jigsaw puzzles in that sometimes it takes several months before an understanding of the mechanisms operating within families is gained by the nurse. Early impressions are important but not always accurate. Therefore, the nurse must be flexible, patient, and willing to adjust the assessment as new data are revealed over the course of time.

To make a comprehensive assessment of the family is time-consuming and must involve all the following factors on a superficial or detailed basis. When specialized information is needed in addition, many nursing texts and professional periodicals are available that describe more specifically the data required for special diagnoses and conditions. These factors include: (1) the family's physical and environmental status, including the medical history and present health of each family member, with special consideration of housing, number of rooms in relation to size of family, ventilation, cleanliness, sanitation, source of water supply, sewage disposal, and general safety, e.g.,

---

[10] Ibid., pp. 14–15.

fire protection. (2) The family's cultural background, which is important to the nurse in understanding and appreciating the needs of the client and family. What are the family's attitudes and practices with regard to religion, medical care, nutrition, and eating habits? To what degree does the family participate in the life and activities of its neighborhood and wider community? (3) The economic factors, including the occupation of the family breadwinners and the family's approximate income. The latter is helpful to the nurse when assisting with budget problems and purchasing. It will help the nurse determine, also, the family's eligibility for medical and dental care in clinics if it is needed and there is no medical insurance. (4) The developmental levels of family members, including ages and levels of achievement, both physical and mental. (5) The psychological factors, including family relationships both within and without the home, the emotional tone of the family life, and patterns of family behavior and intra-family relationships, e.g., parent-child relationships and sibling relationships. (6) The educational, vocational, and recreational interests of its members. Knowledge of these interests is important in the nurse's appraisal of the family because teaching is planned according to the apparent knowledge, educational background, interests, and levels of understanding of the family members. An appreciation of the recreational needs and interests of the family and the facilities available in the neighborhood and community for meeting them is helpful to the nurse. Does the family plan its recreation together? Does their church meet some of these needs through church clubs and classes? What other community resources are available? a library? a playfield? a zoo? (7) The family's use of resources within the community. Is the family knowledgeable about resources available within the community? Are they willing to visit the resources? Are they ready to avail themselves of needed services or would they like the nurse to serve as a liaison agent initially?

In order to provide a family health service, the nurse must be alert to the health and welfare needs of all the members. For this reason the many facets of family life are explored in order to try to answer the questions, "What information do I need so that I can plan constructively with this family?" and "Which family need or needs should be given top priority immediately?"

At times nurses are confronted with numerous needs of a family. This can be most frustrating and overwhelming. The nurse must be aware of feelings of competency and should not solely identify need areas with which she or he feels most competent and comfortable when working with families. Multidisciplinary consultants as well as team members can assist with problems revealed by families. Care should be taken to deal with family needs in order of importance, so that the problem with greatest urgency is dealt with first. Other needs and/or problems can be recorded until such time that their resolution can be managed.

Interviewing

Purpose distinguishes an interview from a casual conversation. The following account reveals the purposefulness with which a nursing student interacted with a client:

> I initiated my interview with Lola by asking her, "How are things going?" This gave her the opportunity to take the lead in the conversation, and focus on the issue of most concern to her at the moment. By doing this first, I felt the client

would be better able to concentrate on subjects I had planned for teaching in relation to the problems which were mutually identified during our last visit. In addition, the client would feel you care about her as an individual with her own life and unique problems, not just as "another case."

I always greet the dog, Tramp, at the beginning of the visit, pet him, and ask how he has been feeling. To Lola, this is giving recognition to her personal possession and loved one. Tramp is the most worthwhile thing she feels that she has. She states that she could never leave him. She gives him medicine when he is ill, and shares her food with him. By accepting Tramp, I show that I accept Lola and her way of life.

In its simplest form, interviewing is a method of securing information, such as facts, opinions, or personal histories. When used on a professional level, interviewing, according to Abramovitz, involves "a process of interaction and communication between people. Through this process individuals can mutually clarify feelings, attitudes, and meaningful information. In this way professional people can gain increased understanding of the behavior and personal reactions of individuals they serve."[11] Abramovitz points out further that the interview process can help individuals come to recognize and understand their own problems.

Meanings are transferred from one person to another during an interview. For the individual transmitting a message to another, the meaning is what the transmitter believes it to be. For the person receiving the message, the meaning is as the receiver perceives the message. However, it cannot be assumed that the meaning to the second person is identical to that of the first person. Each person lives in an individual world of reality, and reality is *not what is,* but what each person *believes it to be.*[12] Consequently, communicating clear messages from one person to another is much more complex than the average individual assumes. People behave in terms of their personalized perceptions of discovered meanings, and they view the world from a perspective of attitudes and values which have been learned from experience and which provide a frame of reference for subsequent meanings. Because people have internalized attitudes and values which constitute their own world of reality, the helping person must attempt to understand meanings and behavior as individualized by the client.

An *attitude,* as defined by Rokeach, is a relatively enduring organization of beliefs around an object or situation predisposing one to respond in some preferential manner. A *value* is a type of belief, centrally located within one's total belief system, about how one ought or ought not to behave, or about some end-state of existence worth or not worth attaining. Values are abstract ideals, positive or negative, representing a person's beliefs about ideal modes of conduct and ideal terminal goals. Once a value is internalized it becomes, consciously or unconsciously, a standard or criterion for guiding action, for developing and maintaining attitudes toward relevant objects and situations, for justifying one's own and others' actions and attitudes, for morally judging self and

---

[11] Abraham B. Abramovitz (ed.), *Emotional Factors in Public Health Nursing,* University of Wisconsin Press, Madison, 1961, p. 72.
[12] Arthur W. Combs, Donald L. Avila, William W. Purkey, *Helping Relationships,* Allyn and Bacon, Inc., Boston, 1971, p. 82.

others, and for comparing self with others. Within each person is a value system which has a hierarchical organization or a rank ordering of ideals or values in terms of importance. To one person truth, beauty, and freedom may be at the top of the list, and thrift, order, and cleanliness at the bottom. To another person, the order may be reversed. Many individuals have inconsistent values within themselves and are not conscious of their contradictory beliefs. For example, a person may be asked to rank a set of values in order of importance and find that freedom ranked first and equality last, or salvation first and a comfortable life second, or making money first and health sixth. When the discrepancy of the ranking is pointed out to the respondent, awareness of the dissonance may lead to a cognitive reorganization of values and possibly a change of behavior. Values clarification is a method by which clients are helped to consider whether their stated beliefs and values match their behavior and actions.[13] If not, the individual must decide how to handle the apparent dissonance or contradictory behavior. Any decision made is a reflection of what we value.[14] Nurses who use the values clarification method concentrate on making responses which encourage clients to cogitate about their life and ideas. For example, for the client who rates making money first and health sixth, the nurse can point out, with realism and drama, how maintenance of health is essential and desirable while in the process of making money and enjoying its benefits. The purpose of values clarification is to stimulate the problem-solving capabilities, self-direction, and responsible behavior of clients.

Essentials for a successful interview of any type include a satisfactory environment, privacy, and the assurance of confidentiality. The home is a suitable place for the community health nurse's interview, especially if the interview is that nurse's first contact with the family. As the host, the client (or family) will feel more secure and relaxed in their own environment. For the nurse, the intrafamily relationships and the atmosphere of the home will be more apparent and will provide clues on which to base the interview. Furthermore, the photographs, framed certificates of birth, confirmation, and marriage seen in many homes, and also the books, musical instruments, and arrangements of household living will provide silent answers to some of the nurse's questions and cues for others.

Settings other than the home can be used for the interview, such as the office, a clinic, a health center, a place of business. When interviews take place in settings other than the home, the nurse is the host and the client or family are guests. In the role as host, the nurse must take this into consideration, recognizing that they may not be as comfortable as in their own home. During an interview the client and family need ample time to develop their point of view. It is as valuable for the nurse to listen as it is to talk, and knowing *when* to do each is a skill in itself. The nurse should determine what her or his own reaction is to the expectations of the interviewee.

In an eagerness to help, the nurse should be careful not to impose on others her or his own attitudes and standards in such matters as cleanliness, mode of dress, food, medical care, or social behavior. An understanding tolerance is important here. It has

[13] Milton Rokeach, *Beliefs, Attitudes, and Values,* Jossey-Bass Inc., Publishers, San Francisco, 1970, pp. 112-160.

[14] Nena O'Neill and George O'Neill, *Shifting Gears,* M. Evans and Company, Inc., New York, 1974, p. 157.

been said that the true meaning of tolerance is to be found in the Sioux Indians' definition: "If you wish for tolerance you must ask the Great Spirit to help you never to judge another until you have walked for 2 miles in his moccasins." This is especially true when client and family are trying to meet their problems not only in the light of their own traditions, culture, and religious customs but also within the general patterns of American culture. The nurse must try to recognize what the client and family really want, need, and are ready to accept from the professional services being offered. The nurse needs to look for and consider causative factors in the client's background that may be operating in her or his behavior. The nurse's expressed appreciation for what the client has accomplished and the difficulties that have been encountered will help to establish rapport. A judicious use of sympathy and empathy enters the relationship. There will be times when the client or interviewee needs help in differentiating between reality and confusion created by personal defenses. Setting limits to prevent the client from wandering too far from problems under discussion will help.

In planning for the interview, the nurse considers and selects those questions that will elicit the information needed, questions that are concise, clear, and pertinent to the situation. These questions need to be phrased carefully, with no evidence of disapproval or personal value judgments by the nurse. Weissman has listed some concerns that community health nurses and other public health workers have expressed in relation to their skills and techniques in the interviewing process. Following are some of these concerns:

1   How can the interviewer ask questions that will elicit meaningful responses?
2   How can the interviewer secure information and understanding about some of the underlying emotional aspects of problem situations?
3   How does the interviewer deal with personal anxieties and tensions during an interview?
4   How can the interviewer comfortably meet silences on the part of the interviewee?
5   Can a silence be constructive?
6   How can the interviewee be encouraged to break the silence?
7   How can the client's or the family's anger or unwillingness to talk be handled?
8   What does it mean to be supportive, and how is it done?[15]

Helpful Hints   Questions which have been found to be helpful in eliciting desired responses are:

When did it start?
How did it happen?
How often does it happen?
Where did it happen?
In what way do you let other people know how you feel?
What would you like different in this situation?
What have you done about this situation so far?

[15] Isabel G. Weissman, "Make Interviewing a Creative Process," *California's Health,* **22**(22): 201–203, May 15, 1965.

A question to avoid is "Why?" In most instances, a "why" question elicits a defensive response. As an experiment, the nurse can ask a series of "why" questions of a friend and observe the friend's progressive self-protective responses. Questions that may be answered with a "Yes" or "No," e.g., "Does May eat the right kind of breakfast?" are usually of little help to the nurse. Such a question elicits little information about May's eating patterns. A more specific question, such as, "What did May eat for her breakfast this morning?" would provide a more helpful answer.

It is advisable also to think twice before giving advice! Human behavior seems to dictate that each person will do as she or he wants to do or perceives what must be done. When asking advice this person often is weighing possible alternatives, is curious what the nurse will advise, is "playing an acceptable game," or is waiting to hear a solution she or he will *not* use. The clairvoyant nurse will avoid giving advice, and instead, will elicit the possible solutions the client has been considering in an effort to encourage self-direction and responsibility.

It is important to remember not to ask two questions during one verbalization. The client is forced to decide which question takes top priority for answering and, consequently, the direction of the discussion can be changed.

When a relationship of trust exists between nurse and client, direct appropriate questions can be asked which will elicit direct honest responses. Some nurses tend to seek information via the circuitous indirect route rather than being open, honest, and direct about the questions for which they want answers. When clients trust the nurse, they feel comfortable about responding honestly, directly, and without embarrassment.

"I" messages are an effective means of verbalizing language which states meanings the interviewer is thinking about. The client, upon hearing the "I" message of the interviewer, can affirm or deny the meaning of the statement and not feel overtly attacked. For example, the nurse interviewer can say, "I sense, at times, that your baby's crying is more than you can stand." Or, "I am uncertain if you are taking the medications as regularly as you say." In these instances, a message is being conveyed that the nurse wants the client to hear, and the client can accept or deny the implications of the message. The relationship between the nurse and client is not necessarily disrupted, and clarification of concerns may be facilitated. An "I" message can be initiated by the nurse when feeling uncomfortable during the interview. For example, the nurse can say, "I am uncomfortable with this silence. I am uncertain if it is because I cannot tolerate silences or if you are waiting for me to say something?" Again, if the client is perceived to be angry, the nurse can say, "I feel you are angry and am not certain if it is due to something I said or did?"

When the nurse engages in *active listening,* several techniques are being utilized which assist in clarifying the concerns of clients, including emotional aspects of problem situations. *Paraphrasing* is repeating a message back to the client, but putting the thought together with the client's words or with new words to convey what was heard. *Perception checking* is closely related to paraphrasing but deals more overtly with the meaning of the message as heard by the nurse. The content of the message is repeated to the client and concluded with, "Is this what you mean?" or, "Is this how you see it?" *Behavior description* is very effective in giving objective feedback to clients. It consists of reporting your observations of specific behaviors or actions without interpretation of a good or bad value. For example, the nurse can say, "You are telling me how troubled you are with all your problems, yet you are smiling." Or, "I notice you clench your fist every time you talk about your son." For beginning nurses, practice of these interviewing interventions is recommended so that utilization of them becomes natural and spontaneous. Frequently, important information is gained through the use of these techniques—information that was not anticipated but turns out to be valuable.

There are several components of the communication process which must be understood as underlying all messages and meanings which are transmitted from one person to another. They also contribute to the way in which the listener interprets the message. The *content* of the message is the cognitive level which most adults listen for and deal with. The *vocal process* of the speaker transmits meanings that the listener interprets according to perception of tone quality, style of speech, and method of delivery. *Body talk* reveals nonverbal behavior descriptive of the emotional status of the speaker. Use of the *metaphor* (a figure of speech in which one thing is likened to another) assumes the understanding of the listener according to the perspective meant by the speaker. The *life theme* or script of the speaker is apparent to all the senses of the listener as the message is received and interpreted from the listener's frame of reference. Upon examination of the components of the communication process, it must be realized that most adults deal mainly with the content of messages, and because they miss cues revealed by the remaining components, they misinterpret or misunderstand messages. The remaining components of the communication process are understood much more readily by children as they are attentive to the speaker, but not necessarily to the speaker's words.[16] The effective nurse must use all the senses in the most effective way possible when interacting with a client in a therapeutic relationship and interpreting meanings as intended by clients. Abramovitz points out that skillful interviewing is a medium in which "an integrated understanding of people is combined with the knowledge of one's own professional field in order to enable the patient to help himself.[17]

Assessment Tools

It is always sound nursing practice to make use of screening devices, tests, or measurements whenever possible to determine more accurately what the nurse suspects based on early observations or intuitive hunches. An essential tool for assessing the basic reflex patterns of newborns, infants, and preschool children up to 3 years is the reference *A Developmental Approach to Casefinding,* by Una Haynes.

This booklet describes the reflexes, how to elicit them, and how to appraise the baby during the bathing procedure. A wheel device for quick recall of developmental skills in conjunction with age in months is included with the booklet.[18]

A second excellent tool is the *Denver Developmental Screening Test,* which evaluates the gross motor, fine motor, adaptive, language, and personal-social areas of a child's functioning from birth to 6 years of age. It is easy to administer and utilizes

---

[16] Peter J. Hansen, *Family Counseling: A Workshop for Nurses,* Notes taken during workshop, October 1975.

[17] Abramovitz, loc. cit.

[18] Una Haynes, *A Developmental Approach to Casefinding,* U.S. Department of Health, Education, and Welfare, Social Rehabilitation Service, Children's Bureau, Publication HSA-79-5210, 1967.

participation of the parent during the testing procedure. Most parents respond with great interest to this screening device and are motivated subsequently to assist the child in practicing the skills that are in need of further development.[19]

Many more assessment tools are available for nurses to use for gaining more data about families, infants, children. The *Neonatal Behavioral Assessment Scale* as developed by Dr. T. Berry Brazelton is one example.[20] The *Developmental Profile* for children from birth to preadolescence by Alpern and Boll is another example.[21] Meister has developed a nursing tool to assess and record family status information and identify interventions.[22] A *Psychosocial Framework for Assessing Family Strengths* by Herbert Otto is valuable for the purpose of mobilizing family strengths.[23] Because new tools are constantly being developed, it is essential for community health nurses to maintain ongoing curiosity about research studies reported in professional journals. In this way the nurses remain up-to-date and knowledgeable about new screening devices and procedures which more accurately assess the health needs of clients and families.

HEALTH CARE ASSESSMENT

Nursing students are learning and practicing primary nursing care skills throughout their educational program. While working in community settings and with families, every opportunity must be utilized for screening the health status of each family member. When a systematic screening examination is done routinely and as needed by the nurse, family members tend to respond favorably. The examination in no way approximates the physical examination of a physician. It is mainly a health appraisal in which the nurse gains a general impression of the physical status of each family member. Checking the skin, vital signs, and blood pressure; listening to heart sounds and the lungs; looking into the throat; inspecting the condition of the teeth and gums; and inquiring about essential data for the compilation of a health history for each family member is advisable. Interpretation of normal ranges of findings and the rationale underlying the systematic health appraisal impresses and educates the family as to the nurse's competence as a professional.

When a family member complains of a specific ailment, examination of the designated body system or distressed body part is essential. Physical examination techniques which include inspection, palpation, percussion, and auscultation must be done as appropriate to gain objective data along with securing a history from the client regarding subjective data. Interpretation of the nurse's findings in language understandable to the family member is facilitative of future follow-through when advised by the nurse.

---

[19] Manual, form, and kit are available from *LADOCA,* Project and Publishing Foundation Inc., E. 51st Ave. and Lincoln, Denver, Colo. 80216.

[20] T. Berry Brazelton, *Neonatal Behavioral Assessment Scale,* J. B. Lippincott Company, Philadelphia, 1973, pp. 1–66.

[21] Gerald D. Alpern and Thomas J. Boll, *Developmental Profile,* Psychological Development Publications, Indianapolis, Ind., 1972, pp. 1–70.

[22] Susan Meister, "Charting a Family's Developmental Status—For Intervention and for the Record," *Maternal Child Nursing,* January–February, 1977, pp. 43–48.

[23] Herbert A. Otto, "A Framework for Assessing Family Strengths," in Adina Reinhardt and Mildred Quinn (eds.), *Family-Centered Community Nursing: A Sociocultural Framework,* The C. V. Mosby Company, St. Louis, 1973.

Referral to appropriate resources is eased when the nurse explains the reason for the referral and the probable corrective activity that will be performed by the designated professional. Making use of physical examination skills should be given top priority by every practicing community health nurse whose objective is to educate and promote optimal health of all individuals.

NURSING DIAGNOSIS

After gaining essential data about the family and determining a contract with the client and/or family about the immediate need, a nursing diagnosis must be made that will form the basis for the plan and implementation of nursing services. Implicit with the making of a diagnosis is the assumption that judgments are made based on what the nurse observes, hears, and consequently infers about the client and family. Organizing data involves collecting, clustering, weighing, and validating information in a family situation which is relevant for nursing services. Frequently this process is difficult in a home environment because of the multiplicity of complex and/or irrelevant factors occurring simultaneously. Making judgments pertinent to the health status of the client and/or family requires that the diagnosis is congruent with the data which document the need for nursing services.

Nursing diagnoses have been defined by many authors, and classification systems or taxonomies have been recommended for the purpose of standardizing phenomena relevant to the practice of nursing. Gordon states nursing diagnoses describe health problems in which the responsibility for therapeutic decisions can be assumed by a professional nurse. In general, these problems encompass potential or actual disturbances in life processes, patterns, functions, or development, including those occurring secondary to disease.[24] Roy is more succinct in specifying that a nursing diagnosis is the summary statement or judgment made by the nurse about the data gathered during the nursing assessment.[25] A compilation of summary statements commonly expressed by nurses can lead to development of diagnostic classifications.

Classification systems for nursing diagnoses require a systematic description of the domain of nursing, agreement by nurses of the nomenclature or terms used, grouping of identified diagnoses into classes or subclasses so that patterns and relationships among them can emerge.[26] Gordon elaborates about components essential for the development of diagnostic categories. These include the state of the client or health problem, the etiology of the problem, and the signs and symptoms. The state of the client requires a description about the client rather than a nursing activity, i.e., the client is anxious rather than "needs reassurance." The etiology of the problem represents the probable cause of the client's problem, i.e., noncompliance with drug treatment due to lack of knowledge regarding the benefits of the drug action. Signs and symptoms represent client behaviors used to make the diagnosis.[27]

---

[24] Marjory Gordon, "Nursing Diagnoses and the Diagnostic Process," *American Journal of Nursing,* 76:1298–1300, August 1976.

[25] Sister Callista Roy, "A Diagnostic Classification System for Nursing," *Nursing Outlook,* 23:90–94, February 1975.

[26] Kristine Gebbie and Mary Ann Lavin, "Classifying Nursing Diagnoses," *American Journal of Nursing,* 74:250–253, February 1974.

[27] Gordon, op. cit., p. 1298.

A tentative list of nursing diagnoses were published in 1974 by Gebbie and Lavin as a beginning step in the development of a standard nomenclature of nursing diagnoses.[28] Acceptance and utilization of a classification system universal with all nurses is yet to be achieved. In a study by Sutcliffe,[29] a small sample of community health nurses were asked to read a case study, list nursing diagnoses they identified in the case study, and state the cues in the case study which led them to determine each selected nursing diagnosis. It was found that the majority of nurses studied identified incorrect diagnoses or identified medical disease-oriented diagnoses. It was found also that the nurses who tended to identify many cues were more apt to identify a correct diagnosis. This study demonstrates the advisability for a standard diagnostic classification system for nurses. Once a system is ultimately accepted and universally utilized by all nurses, the probability is increased for accurate diagnoses within the domain of nursing.

Listed in Table 6-1 is the nursing diagnostic nomenclature accepted at the fourth national conference in 1980 as delineating the domain of nursing practice.[30] Nursing students are encouraged to make nursing diagnoses of their clients and families, utilizing the suggested nomenclature. Basing the diagnoses on state of the patient, etiology, and signs and symptoms also is encouraged for the purpose of identifying cues used in making the diagnoses. Testing of the diagnostic classifications will reveal the usefulness of the terms as stated and may provide important data which can be communicated to the National Group for Classification of Nursing Diagnoses, a group which meets every two years.

The following example very briefly illustrates an assessment of a family made by a student nurse and the subsequent nursing diagnosis:

It wasn't until after I made my initial visit that I realized that health encompassed more than just the physical and mental, but included the social, cultural, environmental, and socioeconomic factors. . . . Identifying the medical needs of the family was not difficult since this was one of the mother's major concerns for herself and the children. The mother was very open and willing to talk about her own ailments, which were many, and the medical care needs of the children. . . . The family's economic situation was precarious, which had an effect on the follow-through of medical needs. . . . Focusing on the mental health of the family made me acutely aware of how the manner of communication can deeply affect the mental attitudes of family members toward each other. I was able to make a home visit when the mother and father were home. Even in my presence, it was quite apparent that these two people annoyed each other. The father was very intolerant of the mother's naive concepts about the subject we were discussing at the time. The mother likewise voiced her anger toward the father on a separate occasion. The mother views the father as a very egocentric individual and feels rejected by him. The problem with both of these people is that they do not have the appro-

[28] Gebbie and Lavin, op. cit., p. 251.

[29] Kathleen Marnik Sutcliffe, "The Diagnostic Labels Identified by Community Health Nurses When Provided with a Specified Client Situation," unpublished thesis in Nursing, University of Washington, 1980.

[30] M. J. Kim and D.A. Moritz (eds.), *Classification of Nursing Diagnoses: Proceedings of the Fourth National Conference on Classification of Nursing Diagnoses,* McGraw-Hill Book Company, New York, 1981.

Table 6-1 List of Nursing Diagnoses Accepted at the Fourth National Conference

Airway clearance, ineffective
Bowel elimination, alterations in: Constipation
Bowel elimination, alterations in: Diarrhea
Bowel elimination, alterations in: Incontinence
Breathing patterns, ineffective
Cardiac output, alterations in: Decreased
Comfort, alterations in: Pain
Communication, impaired verbal
Coping, ineffective individual
Coping, ineffective family: Compromised
Coping, ineffective family: Disabling
Coping, family: Potential for growth
Diversional activity, deficit
Fear
Fluid volume deficit, actual
Fluid volume deficit, potential
Gas exchange, impaired
Grieving, anticipatory
Grieving, dysfunctional
Home maintenance management, impaired
Injury, potential for
Knowledge, deficit (specify)
Mobility, impaired physical
Noncompliance (specify)
Nutrition, alterations in: Less than body requirements
Nutrition, alterations in: More than body requirements
Nutrition, alterations in: Potential for more than body requirements
Parenting, alterations in: Actual
Parenting, alterations in: Potential
Rape-trauma syndrome
Self-care deficit (specify level: feeding, bathing/hygiene, dressing/grooming, toileting)
Self-concept, disturbance in
Sensory perceptual alterations
Sexual dysfunction
Skin integrity, impairment of: Actual
Skin integrity, impairment of: Potential
Sleep pattern disturbance
Spiritual distress (distress of the human spirit)
Thought processes, alterations in
Tissue perfusion, alteration in
Urinary elimination, alteration in patterns
Violence, potential for

Diagnoses "accepted" without defining characteristics*

Cognitive dissonance   TBD
Family dynamics, alterations in   TBD
Fluid volume, alterations in: Excess, potential for   TBD
Memory deficit   TBD
Rest-activity pattern, ineffective   TBD
Role disturbance   TBD
Social isolation   TBD

*Therefore unacceptable, but to be listed separately as diagnoses to be developed (TBD).
Source: M. J. Kim and D. A. Moritz (eds.), *Classification of Nursing Diagnoses: Proceedings of the Fourth National Conference on Classification of Nursing Diagnoses*, McGraw-Hill Book Company, New York, 1981.

priate outlets upon which to release their anger. They are unable to discuss their feelings on a rational, adult level; consequently, they use their children to release their anger on. It comes through in their communication to the children. I am sure they are unaware of how their communication is perceived by the children or anyone else. They sound intolerant, impatient, and very angry. . . . The nursing diagnosis for this family is ineffective family coping secondary to existing and constant economic, environmental, and psychosocial stressors. Cues leading to this diagnosis are the destructive communication patterns used by the mother and father, the economic situation of the family, occasional expressions of anger, and the apparent inability of mother and father to "level" openly with each other.

NURSING SERVICES AND FEES

The nurse describes the purpose and philosophy of the agency and explains that its services are available to all in the community according to their health needs. If, however, the agency is private or nonofficial, a combination agency, or an official agency that charges for some services, the nurse explains the fee schedule for services.

Although these services of the agency are available to all in the community according to their health needs, today's concept that clients and families pay for services as they are able has become fairly well established and accepted. Most people wish to pay what they can, and agencies have found that clients and families tend to value nursing services and teaching more when they pay at least something for them.

In discussing the fee schedule with the family or client, the nurse keeps the following points in mind:

1 The actual cost to the agency of the visit, including costs for travel, professional nursing services provided, equipment used, overhead expenses, i.e., rent, light, and telephone, and the necessary personnel in addition to the nurse, i.e., administrative, supervisory, and secretarial personnel.
2 The family's ability to pay for nursing service. This is based on a consideration of the family's overall income and fixed expenditures, e.g., food, rent, utilities, and financial commitments such as insurance. When the client is the wage earner, it is to be expected that the family income will be markedly reduced. In such situations, some families may be unable to pay the full fee but might find it possible to pay on a partial basis.
3 The type of illness and the nursing care needed. If the illness promises to be short, requiring two to three visits, a full fee might be indicated, but if it appears that the illness may be long, such as cancer or disability following a stroke, the nurse might consider the probable number of visits necessary and then evaluate with the family their ability to pay under the circumstances.
4 The fee schedule is flexible and may be adjusted easily to the family situation.
5 Many families today have certain types of medical insurance that provide for nursing services. Often they are not aware of the provisions in their policies.

When a family requests a nursing visit on an appointment basis in order to meet their convenience, the full "cost-of-visit" fee or more is charged by some agencies. On the other hand, if the family can adjust to the nurse's plan for the day, the full fee or less may be charged.

Most official agencies make no charge for visits for nursing service, demonstrations of nursing care, or teaching when the request was made because of a communicable disease; when the visit is for the purpose of supervising maternal and child health or handicapped children; when families are faced with problems of mental or emotional difficulties or mental retardation; or when the visit is a first one that has not been requested by the client or family.

If a fee is to be charged for a visit to a new family, and for later visits, the client, family, and nurse discuss the fee, but before making a final decision, the nurse may wish to discuss aspects of the situation with the supervisor. Sometimes a client or family, prompted by an appreciation of the nurse's help, will want to pay more for the services than their budget actually allows.

Generally speaking, nurses find it very difficult to discuss fees with clients and families. They recognize that their visits merit payment but are reluctant to evaluate their services in terms of monetary value. Establishing fees tends to be considered a cold, mercenary task, and talking about money conflicts with the nurses' view of themselves as warm, helping persons. For this reason, nurses have responded favorably when some official agencies have hired a person whose title is that of fee clerk. The fee clerk's primary task is to visit all new families who have been accepted for nursing services, interpret the agency's policies in regard to fees, and establish a fee for services that is satisfactory to the family. Whenever the nurse reports a change in the family's financial status after the initial encounter, the fee clerk visits again to adjust the fee according to the ability of families to pay. In many agencies a graduated fee schedule based on family income is used as a guide for determining a fair fee.

Every 3 to 5 years, community health nursing agencies conduct "cost-of-visit" studies. The findings will reflect the current cost of each visit made by the nursing agency. On the basis of this information, the fee is adjusted. Established fee schedules are helpful to the nurse as the agency services are discussed with the family.

MEDICARE

In 1978 over 13 percent of the nation's total health care bill was paid in medicare benefits. Medicare (Title XVIII) is a federally administered program providing hospital and medical insurance protection for eligible elderly people. The medicare program is under the overall direction of the Secretary of Health and Human Services. Within the department, the Bureau of Health Insurance of the Social Security Administration is responsible for policy and administrative control of the program with much of the day-to-day operational work of the program performed under contract by 100-plus commercial insurance companies and Blue Cross–Blue Shield plans. These organizations have the responsibility for reviewing claims for benefits and making payments.

In each state, health officials assist the federal government in determining whether facilities that wish to provide services to medicare beneficiaries meet the conditions for participation in the medicare program. These conditions relate to the quality of client care and various health and safety requirements.

The medicare program consists of two parts—the hospital insurance plan (part A) and the supplementary medical insurance plan (part B). Hospital insurance benefits include: (1) inpatient hospital services for up to 90 days in a benefit period, plus a lifetime reserve of 60 additional days of hospital care after the 90 days have been exhausted; (2) posthospital extended care in a skilled nursing facility for up to 100 days in a benefit period; (3) posthospital home health services for as many as 100 home health visits. A benefit period begins with the first day an individual is furnished inpatient hospital or skilled nursing facility services, and does not end until that individual has not been an inpatient in either a hospital or skilled nursing facility for 60 consecutive days.

Supplementary medicare insurance benefits (part B) include: (1) physicians' and surgeons' services, certain nonroutine services of podiatrists, limited services provided by chiropractors, and the services of independently practicing physical therapists; (2) certain other medical and health services such as diagnostic services, diagnostic x-ray tests, laboratory tests and other diagnostic services, x-ray, radium and radioactive isotope therapy, ambulance services, and additional medical supplies, appliances, equipment, and prostheses; (3) outpatient hospital services; (4) home health services (with no requirement of prior hospitalization) for 100 visits during a calendar year; and (5) outpatient physical and speech therapy services furnished by approved providers.

Both the hospital insurance and medical insurance plans contain limitations on program benefits in the form of deductible and coinsurance amounts for which the beneficiary is responsible. The most important of these are a variable deductible with respect to part A hospital services and a deductible and 20 percent coinsurance amount with respect to most part B services.

Hospital insurance (part A) coverage is available to (1) all people age 65 and over who are entitled to receive social security cash benefits or railroad retirement benefits; (2) social security beneficiaries under age 65 who have been entitled to social security or railroad retirement benefits for at least 24 consecutive months on the basis of a disability; (3) otherwise ineligible persons, age 65 and older, who elect to enroll in the hospital insurance program and to pay the full cost of their coverage; (4) almost all people under age 65 or nearly that age when the program was enacted in 1965 but who were not eligible for cash benefits.

Supplementary medical insurance is available to all hospital insurance beneficiaries and to all other people age 65 and over, except recent immigrants.

Payments of medical benefits is on the basis of (1) reasonable costs in the case of hospitals and other institutional providers and (2) reasonable charges in the case of physicians and other noninstitutional suppliers of services. Reasonable costs are determined on the basis of actual costs incurred by the individual provider in furnishing covered services to beneficiaries. The principles of reimbursement provide that all necessary and proper costs which maintain the operation of client-care facilities and activities will be included in the computation of medicare reimbursement. A provision in the Social Security Amendments of 1972 now permits establishment of upper limits of "reasonableness" of costs by hospital category or type of service.

The determination of the reasonableness of charges is made by carriers pursuant to policy guidelines issued by the Social Security Administration, which are established within the framework of general statutory instructions. In determining reasonable charges, the carrier must take into consideration the customary charges for similar services by the physician or other person furnishing the services, as well as the prevailing charges in the locality for similar services. The prevailing charge for a service is limited to the 75th percentile of the customary charges in an area. The 75th percentile amount is increased over time by a factor which takes into account increased costs of practice and increases in earnings levels in the area. Reimbursement for medicare supplies and equipment is based upon the lowest charges at which supplies of similar quality are widely and consistently available in a locality.

The hospital insurance part of the program is financed primarily through social security payroll contributions paid by employees, employers, and self-employed people covered under social security.

Of the 21-plus million people age 65 and older in the United States, almost 98 percent now have hospital insurance protection. Requests for medicare payment for covered services generally are submitted by the provider of services; they must be signed by the beneficiary (or someone designated, if she or he is unable to do so). The provider is reimbursed on the basis of reasonable costs of covered services and bills the beneficiary for deductible and coinsurance amounts as well as for services not covered by the program.

Claims for payment of supplementary medical insurance benefits may be submitted to the carrier either by the client or by the physician or other supplier of services. If the client submits a claim (an itemized bill) directly to the carrier, direct payment of benefits for covered services is received; the client remains responsible for the physician's bill. The client may assign the benefits to a physician or other supplier of services willing to accept assignment. In this case, the physician agrees that the allowed or reasonable charge determined by the carrer is the total charge. The physician submits the bill and is reimbursed. In this situation, the client remains responsible for the remaining 20 percent of the allowed charges for covered services and the deductible.[31]

MEDICAID

It was in 1950 that Congress first authorized "vendor" payments for medical care—payments from the welfare agency directly to physicians, health care institutions, and other providers of medical services. In 1960 a new category of assistance recipient was established by Congress for the "medically needy" aged, whose incomes were greater than that which would have qualified them for cash assistance payments, but who needed help in meeting the costs of medical care. In 1965 a new medical assistance (medicaid) program was enacted as part of the Social Security Amendments of 1965. The medicaid program had the following features:

1 It substituted a single program of medical assistance for the vendor payments under the categorical cash assistance and medical assistance for the aged programs, with a requirement that beginning in 1970 federal sharing in vendor payments would be provided only under the medicaid program.

[31] Committee on Ways and Means, *National Health Insurance Resource Book,* Government Printing Office, Washington, D.C., 1974, pp. 429-433.

2 It offered all states a higher rate of federal matching for vendor payments for medical care.

3 It required each state to cover all persons receiving cash assistance.

4 It permitted states to include medically needy aged, blind, disabled, and dependent children and their families at the option of the state.

5 It required that states include inpatient and outpatient hospital services, other laboratory and x-ray services, skilled nursing home services, and physicians' services, and permitted other forms of health care at state option.

In 1967 congressional concern over rapidly rising medical costs led to legislative action. The Congress chose as its basic method of cost control, limiting the definition of "medically needy" to persons whose income did not exceed 133½ percent of the maximum payments for similar size families under programs of aid to families with dependent children. The 1967 amendments also included an amendment designed to focus on the health needs of medicaid children. Specifically states were required by 1969 to implement early and periodic screening, diagnosis, and treatment programs for children under 21.

Increasing congressional concern with the rapidly escalating costs of the medicaid program as well as with the quality of care provided recipients led to an extensive review of the entire program. In 1972 legislation (P.L. 92-603) was enacted which contained a substantial number of amendments designed to control costs, strengthen program administration, and improve the delivery and review of services. Cost control amendments included provisions limiting federal participation for capital expenditures not approved by planning agencies, establishing limitations on prevailing charge levels, repealing the "maintenance of effort" and comprehensive goal requirements, and instituting mandatory and optional client cost-sharing requirements. Amendments designed to improve program administration included provisions increasing federal matching for installation and operation of management information systems, establishing penalties for fraudulent acts and false reporting, and assigning responsibility for the establishment and maintenance of health standards to the state health agency.

Congress also focused attention on improvements in existing utilization review programs. Incentives were established for states to establish effective utilization review activities under medicaid and required coordination of these activities with those required under medicare. Congress was particularly concerned that existing utilization controls had been ineffective and that rising costs were in part attributable to the provision of medically inappropriate services. It therefore included a provision providing for the establishment of professional standards review organizations (PSROs), formed by organizations representing substantial numbers of physicians in local areas, to undertake the comprehensive and ongoing review of services under medicaid and medicare. PSROs determine whether services are medically necessary and provided in accordance with professional standards.

P.L. 92-603 also established a supplemental security income program (SSI) which, effective 1974, replaced federal and state welfare programs for aged, blind, and disabled individuals. States were permitted to establish programs supplementing the basic federal payment. Medicaid eligibility determinations for these individuals could no longer be tied to eligibility under the old federal and state cash assistance programs.

Subsequent legislation specified the requirements for mandatory and optional coverage.

Increasing medicaid costs have had a particularly severe fiscal impact on the states. Welfare costs typically constitute one of the largest items in the state budget, and vendor payments have increased 583 percent in 10 years (from 1965 to 1974).[32]

Medicare and medicaid should not be considered as static programs. Their requirements have continued to develop and change, depending somewhat on the economic, social, and political climate in each state. New programs and practices have been devised to meet specific needs and new conditions and some old ones have been discarded, having proved to be ineffective. It is anticipated that legislation will be passed by Congress at some date for a national health insurance plan that will meet the medical, nursing, and health needs of the nation's entire population at a reasonable cost. This will demand a tremendous amount of comprehensive planning and thought on the part of all concerned. Nurses must utilize the opportunity to contribute their ideas because of their present experience in working with medicare, medicaid, and other federal medical programs.

In recent years, increasing numbers of nurses have been actively monitoring major health legislation for its effects on the health care delivery system and the quality of care available to clients. Sharing ideas with legislators facilitates development and implementation of health care bills that allow for comprehensive quality care for clients. At the same time, nurses become sophisticated in their dealings with the political process. For more discussion about the political process, see Organization is Key to Political Influence in Chap. 7.

THE NURSING PROCESS: PLANNING

When nursing diagnoses about the health needs of a client or family have been gained and a contract with the family established, the nurse is faced with the necessity for planning. A plan is the method of action or the blueprint for activity based on the resources available and the goals desired.[33] Of primary concern is the client with her or his knowledge, capabilities, customary patterns of coping, resources, needs, and desires. The nurse must also consider her or his own knowledge, capabilities, ways of coping, resources, needs, and desires, as well as limitations, which may have a bearing on the attainment of the client's desired goals.[34] The setting of the client must be viewed from a realistic and objective standpoint to ensure that desired goals have the potential for successful fulfillment.

While talking about realistic goals the client desires, the nurse can give valuable assistance by suggesting practical, short-term and long-term goals. The long-term goals exemplify the ultimate objectives desired by the client, whereas the short-term goals represent the graduated steps marking progression toward the desired long-term goals. When short-term goals are attained, they build confidence that the next

---

[32] Ibid., pp. 487–490.

[33] Joan Nettleton, "Planning to Meet Patient Needs," in Helen Yura and Mary B. Walsh (eds.), *The Nursing Process: Assessing, Planning, Implementing, and Evaluating,* The Catholic University of America Press, Washington, D.C., 1967, p. 44.

[34] Ibid., p. 47.

goal can likewise be achieved. For example, for the mother who wishes her son to be toilet trained, the long-term goal is independent self-care in toileting for the son. The short-term goals may be (1) determining the boy's physiologic and psychological readiness for toilet training; (2) ascertaining the boy's present toileting patterns; (3) setting up a toileting procedure which is feasible for the mother and son and includes rewards or positive attitudes for activities done successfully; and (4) determining a measuring method or chart for observing frequency of success. Early expectations should be minimal, then show progress as the boy develops skill in his toileting activities. Charts with gold stars can often be motivating stimuli for preschool children. When toileting accidents occur infrequently, then the mother realizes that the long-term goal has been achieved.

It is important that the family and nurse plan toward desired goals together because goals decided upon are a prelude to action for both family and nurse. Dependent upon the health care needs of the family, the goals may be directed toward care of sickness and handicaps or health teaching and counseling.

Care of Sickness and Handicaps

For those client's needing physical care, the nurse plans the administration of nursing procedures and treatments prescribed by the physician and also includes an inventory of all medications used by the client to ensure that the drugs are being taken properly as ordered and are having the desired effect. The nurse remains up-to-date on rehabilitation and exercise measures and plans for execution of activities for daily living for those clients who desire to acquire new self-help skills. For those clients on special diets, the nurse obtains a history of their nutritional practices and plans for implementation of ideas which seem practical and geared to the client's needs, desires, and limitations.

Frequently the nurse will need to adapt nursing equipment and procedures to the home situation. Family members can be encouraged to work with the nurse in improvising many articles to contribute to the client's safety and comfort, such as a back rest from a cardboard carton or a wheelchair made by attaching castors to the bottom of each leg of a sturdy chair. The use of disposable, self-help, and low-cost equipment is always an important consideration. Utilizing transfer procedures which ease the difficulty of moving a client from one object to another or from one room to another is sometimes a major feat to accomplish in the setting of some homes.

Many ideas for assisting the client with personal grooming and eating may be found in current nursing periodicals and pamphlets. On occasion, families work out helpful ideas for the comfort and safety of the client that will contribute to independence. They should be encouraged to do this, and appreciation should be shown for their efforts.

During bedside nursing activities, the nurse has the opportunity to observe the client and assess his or her condition. The nurse may note also the degree of understanding the family has for the situation. Whenever possible, certain responsibilities should be delegated to family members so that they may participate in the care of the client, such as assembling equipment for a bath or a treatment. One or more of the family members can be shown how they may care for the client in the nurse's absence and the nurse observes them in a return demonstration. Family members will watch closely the nurse's techniques, even when she or he is not consciously teaching. The care the nurse takes with the contents of the nursing bag, with handwashing, and with the use of equipment is of great interest to them.

Clients and families like to know what is causing the client's distress, so interpretations of the medical phenomena underlying the disease process are appreciated when explained in an understandable manner. Also, explanations of the treatment, its purpose, its length, and what can be expected as an end result are important in enlisting the intelligent cooperation of the client and family members.[35] The client faced with a choice of two acceptable treatment plans should be allowed to make the decision regarding the treatment plan desired after being made cognizant of the benefits and limitations of both plans. At all times in community health nursing, the resourceful nurse is prepared for situations requiring adaptability and flexibility. As reported in a study by Johnson, a limiting factor in the delivery of nursing care that was documented repeatedly was the variability of clients' reactions to services rendered by nurses.[36] To meet unexpected challenges successfully takes skill, planning, ingenuity, acceptance of risk, and the belief that all persons have potential talents just waiting to be tapped.

Health Teaching and Counseling

Much of the work of community health nurses consists of teaching and counseling clients and families about better ways of coping with health problems so that they are able to increase their competency in dealing with their health needs and desires. The utilization of client and family strengths and resources requires involvement of the client and family in the plan of care. Also, an effective relationship of the nurse with the family must be developed before success can be assured.

In health counseling the approach varies with the family. In one family, the nurse may feel the direct approach will serve the best purpose. In another family, one of.the members may be able to assume leadership and make plans and decisions with little assistance from the nurse other than encouragement and support.

Anticipatory guidance is an important part of health counseling. A guided discussion of probable happenings or events provides an opportunity for clarifying ideas, for lessening anxiety, and for constructive teaching. By anticipating the occurrence of an expected event, various ways of handling the event can be explored so that when it actually happens, few surprises transpire. For instance, the nurse can explain objectively to the expectant mother the mechanics of labor and delivery, using a birth atlas or similar teaching material. This also may provide the mother with emotional support, so that she may be better prepared to accept the experience of her delivery.

New methods for teaching and counseling families appear constantly in books and professional periodicals. Some of them are easily adapted for use in community health

---

[35] Letha Hickox, "Planning to Meet Patient Needs," in Helen Yura and Mary B. Walsh (eds.), *The Nursing Process: Assessing, Planning, Implementing, and Evaluating,* The Catholic University of America Press, Washington, D.C., 1967, p. 65.
[36] Walter L. Johnson, *Content and Dynamics of Home Visits of Public Health Nurses,* Part II. American Nurses' Foundation, Inc., New York, 1969, p. 124.

nursing. Methods which should be considered when planning for selected families, dependent upon the nurse's assessment of the situation and knowledge of the implementation of the method, are described briefly under the following subheadings.

Strengthening Approach During the period of formal nursing education, the student nurse is encouraged to look for deviations from the norm. The student is alerted to symptoms that are indicative of a pathology and patterns of behavior that are not accepted as healthy behavior. For example, symptoms can be identified that are descriptive or indicative of specific biologic diseases, emotional dysfunctions, or unacceptable social conditions. Because of the identifiable nature of the symptoms, the student learns to look for those signs which represent pathology and often anticipates manifestations of progressive disease. Concurrent with learning to identify and anticipate pathology, the nurse also experiences performance evaluations of work with ill patients. When nursing performance is evaluated, the nurse seems to be conditioned to expect critical statements rather than positive reinforcing statements regarding the skills exhibited. Otto stated that in our problem-centered culture most people's perception of their own personality strengths and resources is very limited. Research has shown that the average healthy, well-functioning person with 1 year or more of college training, on being asked to list personal strengths, writes down only five or six items. If asked to list weaknesses, the respondent can usually fill one or two pages.[37]

It is generally accepted that all persons have unrealized potential and frequently live a life within self-imposed boundaries or limitations inflicted by others. One way for assisting these persons (including clients and/or nurses) to recognize their strengths and disclose thoughts about potential is to do a personality inventory of strengths. This method is new to many persons, and the results of such an inventory can be strengthening to individuals as their self-image and self-confidence soar to a new level of acceptability. Sometimes a false idea of humbleness blocks their receptivity to the idea of personality strengths. Yet if these persons believe in themselves and their innate skills, they must recognize those strengths that exist and realize that a deepening and broadening of their positive capabilities can yield results beneficial to themselves and to those around them.

Nurses themselves and clients are enriched mentally and emotionally from a personality inventory of strengths. It is a procedure that a person can do alone, or two persons can share identification of strengths for each other. Herbert Otto prepared a list of headings under which strengths could be identified.

Sports and outdoor activities
Hobbies and crafts
Expressive arts
Health
Education, training, and related areas
Work, vocation, job, or position
Special aptitudes or resources

[37]Herbert A. Otto, *Guide to Developing Your Potential,* Charles Scribner's Sons, New York, 1967, pp. 171–172.

Strengths through family and others
Intellectual strengths
Aesthetic strengths
Organizational strengths
Imaginative and creative strengths
Relationship strengths
Spiritual strengths
Emotional strengths
Other strengths such as a sense of humor[38]

In the practice of writing down assets, additional related strengths often come to a person's mind and should be added to the list. When two people are using the inventory method, they inspire each other with many additional ideas. It must be remembered that the process of taking inventory of strengths is strengthening in itself to all participants.

Nurses who have used the strengthening approach with clients have received a variety of reactions, mainly positive. Clients are initially surprised to have strengths pointed out to them but respond with pleasure, and if the approach is a consistent one, they increasingly show pleasure of an improved self-image and confidence in decision making. One situation in which the strengthening approach was conducive in moving the client toward an increase in self-respect involved a nurse's weekly visits to a young mother for emotional and practical support; the nurse decided to try the method, explained the process to the client, and asked her to write down her own strengths in preparation for the next visit. The nurse assured the client that she too would write down the client's strengths as she had observed them. On the subsequent visit the client read her list of strengths first. They were mainly positive statements regarding her relationship with her husband and child. None made a direct reference to herself. When the nurse read the list of strengths that she had observed in the client's behavior and lifestyle, the young mother perceptibly straightened up in her chair, responded with a radiant glow, and exclaimed, "Do you really see that in me?" In this case, by accepting the positive opinion of the nurse, the young mother was started on the road toward development of greater self-respect, which involved the recognition and internalization of *her* strengths. This she needed, the nurse believed, in order to cope more effectively with her daily life.

Inquiry or Problem-Solving Approach The inquiry approach is based on the idea of encouraging the client or family member to think through to new understandings alone. The nurse serves as a facilitator in introducing this process and making use of questions that stimulate thought, expression, and divulgence of new insights. It is known that thoughts are often fuzzy when the mind is mulling all aspects of a given problem, and the act of verbalizing one's thoughts tends to clarify and crystallize ideas which have been previously vague and disjointed. Language influences thought and the putting together of an idea verbally helps to organize and clarify the problem. When attentively figuring out a personal problem with the assistance of a facilitator and

---

[38] Ibid., pp. 236–239.

considering possible methods for solution, an individual attains greater depth of understanding of the issues involved, is more apt to follow through with devised solutions, and feels satisfaction with the conclusions and self-directed learning.

The role of the nurse in facilitating an inquiry approach is to elicit those problems that are of concern to the client. As the concerns of the client unfold, by being responsive to the client, the nurse can pose questions that enable the client to delve investigatively and sometimes with discovery into all aspects of the problem. If there are omissions or patterns of information given, the nurse can assist in looking for the gaps. This can be done by asking the client pertinent questions or recognizing patterning by making comparative analogies or checking the nurse's perception of the information already heard from the client. The nurse's goal in the inquiry approach is to stimulate the client to think by creating an environment responsive to the client and enabling the client to verbalize concerns in a self-investigative, creative way. Rather than giving direct suggestions or advice, the nurse elicits the self-knowledge the client has about the problems, the possible solutions and resources with which the client is acquainted, and the possibility of implementing activities which the client believes to be feasible. Through this approach the client is an active participant in her or his own learning, is enabled to find answers to questions, discovers the joys of doing problem solving, and consequently feels a boost of self-esteem. The nurse may have known the best answer to the problem and given the needed advice early in the interview, but by engaging the client into doing her or his own problem solving, the probability that the client will carry through with the "discovered" solution is greatly enhanced. At the same time the sharing of information and wrestling with a problem between nurse and client produces a supportive relationship that is satisfying to both. There are times when the client is unaware of the role the nurse has played in facilitating inquiry, and the client thinks the problem solving has been unassisted. At these times the nurse may express pleasure that the client is so adept at problem solving or may recap the sequence of the interview as it progressed.

The following example illustrates the facilitating role of the nurse as she talked to a mother who was concerned about her 14-year-old boy, who had been known to steal but on the day of the interview was playing hooky from school. The nurse makes use of the inquiry approach and she also takes advantage of the teachable moment when it occurs.

Nurse: Now, why do you think Mike played hooky today? He hasn't been in any real trouble for quite a while, although he has been stealing by picking things up.

Mother: (then recounted his habit of "lifting things" and told about her husband's sister, who is married and has a habit of "lifting things") I don't intend to excuse myself, but really, there has been no stealing on my side of the family. I've thought about it very carefully. My husband and his sister and her twin brother do "lift things," but the sister does it more than any of the others.

Nurse: (getting back to Mike) You asked me why Mike stole and why I think he may have played hooky. Shall we look at this together?

Mother: Well, I sure would like to understand why he does things like this.

Nurse: There are several theories or ideas why children steal. We can look at these and think about it. One idea is that the child is looking for love and affection and he steals because he is trying to grab on to love. Another idea is that stealing is attention-getting. It is one way to be a "big man" around one's friends, to be important. Another idea is that stealing and behaving badly is a way of getting back at your parents or authority figures. It will get your parents in trouble. Because he has not stolen this time, but played hooky, and you and Mike have been fighting about the dishes this week, I would tend to subcribe to an underlying dynamic that he is hitting back at *you*. Here is one way that will really hurt you, and get you into trouble.

Mother: I hadn't thought about that. I really would like to understand him better. (Said with sincerity.)

Nurse: He knows you have been angry with him. Have you said any kind things to him at all this week?

Mother: (looked at the table for a while in thought. Then she raised her head and said) No, I don't think I have.

Nurse: Well, no matter how badly the children have behaved, they need praise. You may have to look hard sometimes to find something to praise them about that is real, but look, and look hard and give praise and appreciation to the children, especially those who misbehave the most. At the same time you need to stand firm—as you are doing—on your expectations for them.

Mother: I wonder what I should do to him.

Nurse: What do you plan to do?

Mother: I'm really going to lay into him when he comes home. I'm really going to tell him what I think about him and his friend (a pause). But I've done that before and it doesn't work.

Nurse: I offer this as a thought. Why not tell him you know he is angry with you about this past week and you realize he's trying to get back at you and hurt you. Tell him he has succeeded. Let him know he really has hurt you, and ask him how he feels now and if hurting you has done him any good.

Mother: I never thought of that. Do you suppose it would help?

Nurse: I really don't know, but it is an honest approach, isn't it?

Mother: Yes, it is. I've never approached him in that manner. I suppose I might as well try it. Nothing I have done has worked.

Nurse: There is one thing about discipline; you must fit it into the framework of *your* family and the values *you* hold. Consistency is the key, and teenagers in the rebellion of seeking the independence of adulthood still want the security of limit setting. This is how you tell them you love them, that you care what happens to them.

Goal-Oriented Approach   The goal-oriented approach makes use of the fact that any person will actively strive to attain a goal that is truly desired when it is believed to be within reach. The optimal time to set a goal or goals is when the individual feels dissatisfied with a specific condition or aspect of life. Upon reflection and considerable thought, a person can be encouraged to decide what is wanted, then set definite, desired goals. Goals must be known and desired, must be clearly stated and preferably written, must have a deadline for achievement, and in reality, must have the possibility for attainment.

Life is a continuous process of development and maturation from birth to death.

Developmental tasks are dealt with as the person progresses in age. Tasks such as learning to walk and talk, to relate effectively with others, preparing for marriage, adjusting to physical changes of middle age, and adjusting to retirement often are taken for granted and managed as the particular stage of development and age are reached. However, life at any stage also has periods of obstacles and challenges which each individual can view as opportunities if one wishes to realize potential for growth and make optimal use of any situation. One method of coping with life's problems is to set goals. Goals help to focus attention on coping mechanisms, facilitate movement or progression toward a desired end, help in motivation, give a sense of inner, compelling urge, and often expand the individual's view of existing opportunities. When goals are reached, the reward of achievement develops increased self-esteem and confidence.

The role of the nurse in utilizing the goal-oriented approach is to introduce it as a method for the client, explain the purpose and desired ends of goal setting, and offer encouragement and support as the client needs it when obstacles are encountered. When the nurse makes use of goal setting in her or his own life, she or he can serve as an excellent model and proponent of the efficacy of the method. Examples of benefits and pitfalls from the nurse's own experience can be offered. The nurse can stress the importance of *clearly stated goals, written goals,* and *time limits* for achievement. The difference between goals and wishes as a difference of commitment can be discussed. A wish is a desire that a person may dream about and truly want. It can be changed from a wish and become a goal when one is committed to achieving it by writing the culmination of the desire in clearly stated terms, setting a target date for achievement, and persisting in the belief that the goal can and will be attained, regardless of the obstacles that may appear.

The nurse can utilize the goal-oriented approach in planning her or his own work for and with the client. This is shown in the nursing care plan written specifically for the client. The nurse can also introduce the client to goals by advocating the use of the goal-oriented approach. The client can be helped in writing a clearly stated goal that is conceivably attainable within a specified time limit. Together they can work toward achieving the stated goal. By involving the client in goal setting and demonstrating success in achievement, the nurse serves as a teacher in opening up new avenues for the use of goal setting. For example, the client may be encouraged to write personal goals which will benefit her or his life. Personal goals do not necessarily need to be shared with others; sometimes a personal goal is best attained when the individual writes it privately and works toward it alone. At other times the individual needs the reinforcement of a helping person such as a husband, wife, friend, or nurse. This person's role is to give positive encouragement as it is needed to overcome motivational obstacles and periods of discouragement and to reinforce the individual's belief in his or her ability to attain desired goals.

An example of a goal-oriented approach utilized by one nurse with a client was demonstrated when the nurse visited a young woman who stated the desire to lose weight. A discussion ensued about the variety of crash diets which the client had utilized in the past, the successes and failures that had been experienced, and the pitfalls that often occurred. The nurse asked the client what weight she wished to attain and tried to determine if the client was truly earnest about wishing to lose weight. When the nurse sensed that the client's motivation was purposeful, she suggested the goal-oriented approach. Together the nurse and client wrote down the desired loss in weight and the target date for achievement. In this instance, the client weighed 135 lb and wished to lose 15 lb. A target date for achievement was set for 2 months hence. The weekly goal of weight loss was determined to be a minimum of 2 lb. A chart for notation of weekly weights and specified target dates was devised. The nurse advised the young woman to set up the chart where it would be seen constantly and remind the client of her resolve to lose weight. The nurse also encouraged the client to cut out pictures that would image her goal and put them where she would see them frequently. In this case the client chose a photograph of herself when she had weighed 120 lb. She put the chart with blank spaces for weekly weights and target dates and the photograph of herself on the door of her refrigerator. In addition, she pasted a statement in large lettering which read, "I weigh 120 pounds and it looks *good.*" Together the nurse and client worked out a low-calorie diet that the client felt she would be able to follow and that would enable her to lose the 2 lb needed per week. On every subsequent visit the nurse requested the client's account of how things were going. When success was achieved in losing the 2 lb weekly, the nurse gave praise and reinforced the client's self-discipline. When pitfalls were encountered, the nurse encouraged the client to recall the events preceding the period when the diet was forgotten. Together the nurse and client looked at the stresses which the client had experienced and talked about ways in which the client might respond differently if a similar event or temptation occurred. The nurse maintained a constant belief in the client's ability to lose and communicated this belief to the client verbally and nonverbally. When the client attained her goal of 15 lb weight loss ahead of her target date of 2 months, she felt elated and proud of her accomplishment and emanated a new sense of self-confidence in her demeanor.

Behavior Modification or Social Learning Approach   The behavior modification approach is used widely in schools, institutions, and homes for children and adults who have special learning needs, such as those persons with distinct handicaps or who are retarded. Social learning theory is similar to the behavior modification approach, but it focuses on concepts and methods aimed at facilitating positive behavior or attitude change. The approach differs from the behavior modification approach in its emphasis on the use of the individuals in the existing environment as the main sources for reinforcement. For the community health nurse assisting the mother in the home in helping the identified client to acquire necessary new skills or acting as a liaison agent between special schools and the home environment, an understanding and application of behavior modification and/or social learning methods is essential.

According to an operant point of view, an individual tends to behave in certain ways as a result of events which immediately follow particular behavior. One tends to repeat behaviors that have been rewarded. An operant response is simply a behavior which is governed by its consequences. For the nurse who is observing specific behaviors in a client, emphasis is placed on noting those events or occurrences which immediately precede and immediately follow a behavior of interest. To become completely knowledgeable about the occurring events requires *direct observation* of client interactions and behaviors by the nurse. The nurse is in a position to observe antecedent events, behaviors or responses of the client, and consequent events which give cues as to which conditions produce a positive or negative behavior in the client.[39] By recording observations and the frequency with which the observed behaviors occur, the nurse has a base of knowledge from which to plan for effective intervention. The basic premise of the operant method is that behaviors can be shaped by the consistent use of reinforcers. Reinforcers are rewards, behaviors, or events which increase the probability of the desired response. Reinforcers are used to strengthen, weaken, or shape behavior.

When visiting a family with a child who is in need of assistance with a growth and development pattern and may respond to the behavior modification method, the nurse must interpret the method and its purpose to the parents, enlist their interest and cooperation, assess the child's functional level of development, and plot on a chart the variability in the child's achievement of self-help skills in daily living—feeding, toileting dressing, play, discipline, sleep, and motor development.[40] When the data about the child and family has been assembled, it is advisable to consult with behavior modification experts. It must be decided whether to attempt to work with the family on a concentrated basis or refer the child and family to an appropriate community facility which will give a comprehensive and complete indoctrination of the method.

If the nurse has been encouraged to proceed alone with the family, the parents should be consulted regarding the one behavior which they would like strengthened or weakened first. By selecting one behavior, the nurse is then ready to make direct observations and write down precise baseline data about the behavior. By allowing for specific time intervals on several different days for data gathering, a base rate of the frequency of the selected behavior is gained, in addition to the antececent events which stimulated the behavior. Also, ideas are accumulated about which reinforcers of the behavior have positive or negative results. When sufficient data have been charted, the nurse is ready to work out a plan of action with the parents regarding the shaping of desired behavior. See Table 6-2 as an example for recording data. By showing the parents the frequency with which the behavior occurred in conjunction with the antecedent events, a plan of action can be devised where agreement will be reached whether to strengthen or weaken the specific behavior. A reinforcer will be selected which the parents and nurse will use consistently to shape the desired behavior. At selected time intervals, the nurse will observe and chart the behavior to measure if the plan of action is demonstrating progress. The successful use of the behavior-modification method requires frequent consultation with personnel who are skilled in using the method, a team approach with the parents, and patience of the nurse, since predictability of child response is variable.

The method can be modified for use with many families who desire to change specific behaviors in "normal" children. Since the use of positive reinforcers (rewards,

---

[39] Linda Whitney Peterson, "Operant Approach to Observation and Recording," *Nursing Outlook*, **15**(3):28–32, March 1967.
    [40] Ibid.

Table 6-2 How to Write Down the Observed Baseline Data of the Feeding Abilities of a 5-Year-Old Retarded Child during One Mealtime
Setting: Child Was Sitting at Luncheon Table. Soup, Crackers, and Applesauce Were in Small Dishes on the Table. The Time Was 12 Noon.

Antecedent event	Behavior	Consequent event
1. Mother gave graham cracker to child.	2. Child grasped cracker with left hand and ate entire cracker.	3. Mother smiled and said, "You liked that, didn't you?"
4. Mother offered a spoonful of soup of a thickened consistency to child.	5. Child opened mouth expectantly, took food, and swallowed all of it.	6. Child looked expectantly for next spoonful.
7. After several spoonfuls, mother offered spoonful of soup to child.	8. Child opened mouth, took food, and held it in mouth.	9. Mother said, "You've had enough of that, hmm?"
10. Mother was talking to nurse and not feeding child for several minutes.	11. Child spontaneously picked up spoon awkwardly, dipped it into applesauce dish, and successfully maneuvered the spoon to mouth and swallowed the applesauce.	12. Mother did not notice child's behavior until nurse said, "Good girl! You fed yourself some applesauce."
13. Mother offered spoon to child and said, "Here, take another spoonful of applesauce."	14. Child refused spoon, would not touch it, and cried.	15. Mother said, "OK, I'll feed you."

praise) is less common than the use of negative reinforcers (criticisms, punishment) in the average American home, the social learning method can be successfully implemented to shape desired behaviors in children by instructing parents to use effective positive reinforcers in a consistent pattern with the children. For example, to shape a desired behavior, the parents can be instructed to consistently notice and praise their son every time he hangs up his coat after school. On the days when he does not hang up his coat, the parents can be instructed to consistently give him a chore that he does not find attractive. In this way, the shaping of the desired behavior is secured as the boy realizes the consequences of the original act. An excellent self-help type of book for parents to use who want to teach their children desired behaviors is *Living with Children*, by Patterson and Guillon.[41] The ingenious community health nurse is able to adapt the use of the method to the capacities of a family by observing significant family behavior patterns and providing a method of implementation that catches the interest of parents.

The Family Therapy Approach Family therapy is a procedure that makes use of

---

[41] Gerald R. Patterson and M. Elizabeth Gullion, *Living with Children*, Research Press, Champaign, Ill. 61820, 1968.

a true group, a primary group. The sphere of intervention is not the isolated individual client but rather the family viewed as an organismic whole.

> Family psychotherapy . . . is a procedure that makes use of a true group, a primary group; the sphere of intervention is not the isolated individual patient, but rather the family viewed as an organismic whole. . . . It is developing a body of knowledge, ... illuminating those processes by which the family supports or damages individual development and also those by which the individual supports or damages family development. . . . It is evolving a specific system of therapeutic intervention, disclosing how the family member may be related to and combined with other means of supporting the goals of family life. . . . It merges the efforts of treatment with the goals of prevention of illness, maintenance of health, and education in the problems of family living.[42]

Community health nurses can make use of a modified form of family therapy when they accept the premise that an individual can change and adjust behavior in a healthy manner only when the family system allows it. In other words, for one person's behavior to change, the responses of family members must likewise change. The basic procedure in family therapy is to gather the family members together to talk about their relationship with each other.[43] By so doing, the nurse is able to view family interaction patterns and reactions of individual family members to each other. Until the entire family has been met and the family's interaction system assessed, the nurse cannot hope to change coping behaviors of any individual family member with any pronounced degree of success.

Virginia Satir makes use of a growth model for families based on the idea that people's behavior changes through process and that the process is represented by transactions with other people. Growth occurs when the system permits it. The therapist is intimately involved in the transactions, and anything he or she may offer the client or family to expedite learning and exchange is utilized to help them grow within the context of the relationship. This model requires willingness of the therapist to be experimental, spontaneous, and flexible. The goal of the growth model is to teach people to be congruent, to speak directly and clearly, and to communicate their feelings, thoughts, and desires accurately. The therapist serves as an example of an active, learning, fallible human being who is willing to cope honestly and responsibly with whatever is confronted, including her or his own vulnerabilities.[44] The implementation of a family therapy approach on a modified basis by the community health nurse can be an exciting learning experience for both the family and the nurse. One thing to be remembered by the nurse in the implementation of the family therapy method is that one-to-one discussions should not take place between the nurse and members of the family; the nurse should serve mainly as the facilitator and instigate

---

[42] Nathan W. Ackerman, Frances L. Beatman, and Sanford N. Sherman, *Expanding Theory and Practice in Family Therapy,* Family Service Association of America, New York, 1967, pp. 4–5.

[43] Penny Kossoris, "Family Therapy," *American Journal of Nursing,* 70(8):1730–1733, August 1970.

[44] Virginia Satir, *Conjoint Family Therapy,* 2nd ed., Science and Behavior Books, Inc., Palo Alto, Calif. 1967, pp. 182–183.

interaction of family members with each other. If family members will direct open, honest statements to each other, communication patterns are more congruent and the nurse can interpret the intent behind the statements in such a way that they are nonthreatening and understandable to the other family members. Also, in this climate the presence of a third party, the nurse, often helps some family members to say things that they are unable to utter usually.

Whether or not the nurse actively participates in the family therapy method or acts as a coworker with a qualified family therapist, dysfunctional family interaction patterns as described by Satir should be identified. These families should be directed or guided toward treatment with family therapists or family counseling facilities. Much of the work of community health nurses is of a preparatory nature and consists of helping dysfunctional families to become aware of ineffective or destructive interactional patterns and motivating them to seek expert help, since they are often unhappy families and have multiple health problems.

For nurses who have not practiced any form of family therapy or counseling, it feels risky to gather family members together to talk about their interactions. Oftentimes, it seems less threatening to call the meeting a family conference and to have the reason for the conference clearly labeled as helping the family member who seems to be the "obvious" one in trouble. Once the family is together in a comfortable setting with the nurse who is acting as the therapist, the procedure of managing the counseling session is outlined as follows:

1 The nurse should introduce herself or himself to each member of the family first, shake hands, or exchange a pleasantry in recognition of each individual family member in the group.

2 Efforts should be made to assist all members of the family to feel comfortable and relaxed.

3 The nurse should state the purpose of the family conference clearly and ask family members to correct or add to the information according to their individual perceptions.

4 In getting the family to "work," the nurse should talk directly to and individualize each member of the family in a way that communicates that each one is valued.

5 Clear questions must be asked and family members expected to give clear answers. When answers are fuzzy or "gray," the nurse should seek clarification until the answer is made clear.

6 The nurse must always be in charge of the meeting and should be a "model of confidence" whether feeling so or not. By maintaining control, the nurse may have to interrupt, firmly silence a family member, rearrange the seating of the family, request family members to do a task such as drawing pictures, or provide a distraction of some sort.

7 When concluding the conference, it is facilitative to give the family an assignment or homework tasks which they are willing to do. It must be of such a nature that it makes sense to each family member, is fun, and gets them started in the direction of the goal toward which they are striving. The assignment can be quite simple, such as eating *one* family meal without arguments. If a family can function without arguing one time, it reveals to them the possibility that with one step at a time, future desired goals may be attainable.

Questions that are helpful and sometimes illuminating for the nurse to ask the family during the conference are as follows: "What would you like different in this family?" "What would you like for yourself in this family?" "In what way do you let other people know how you feel?" "How do you let another family member know that you are pleased with them?"

Satir described the use of "family-system games" based on her classification of interaction patterns as either open systems or closed systems. *Closed systems* are those in which every participating member must be very cautious about what he or she says. The principal rule seems to be that everyone is supposed to have the same opinions, feelings, and desires, whether or not this is true. In closed systems, honest self-expression is impossible and if it does occur, the expression is viewed as deviant or "sick" by other members of the group or family. The *open system* permits honest self-expression for the participating members. In such a group or family, differences are viewed as natural and open negotiation occurs to resolve such differences by "compromise," "agreement to disagree," or "taking turns." In open systems, the individual can freely express feelings and thoughts and can negotiate for reality and personal growth without destroying the self or the others in the system.[45] By the use of simulated games, Satir helps families to see and understand the nature of their own family system and experience the movement from a pathologic system of interaction to a growth-producing one. She elicits the family's feelings, responses, and body reactions to the games, each other, and the interactions. She urges family therapists to be open, flexible, enthusiastic, and innovative.[46] By being knowledgeable about Satir's approach to families and willing to try some of the suggested exercises, the community health nurse can adapt and improve the style of interacting successfully with families. When the nurse initiates role-playing games in the family setting, unexpected insights are gained by all participating members. Often the games are fun and stimulating and create a lighthearted atmosphere, which is therapeutic in itself. New approaches and ideas are often received with enthusiasm by families, particularly if they are implemented skillfully and appropriately and if the results bring forth new insights.

The Transactional Analysis Approach Transactional analysis offers a systematic, consistent theory of personality and social dynamics and an actionistic, rational form of therapy which is suitable for, easily understood by, and naturally adapted to the great majority of clients.[47] Its goal is to help people to be their true selves. Transactional analysis identifies three ego states inherent in each person. The ego states are systems of feelings which motivate a related set of behavior patterns.[48] They are called the parent, adult, and child ego states within each individual. The child ego state is represented by spontaneous, rational, and irrational feelings. The child expresses genuine feelings of joy or anger and speaks in words and thoughts saying "*I am.*" The child can be a good or bad child. The parent ego state is represented by fixed feelings

---

[45] Ibid., p. 185.
[46] Ibid., pp. 188–189.
[47] Eric Berne, *Transactional Analysis in Psychotherapy,* Grove Press, Inc., New York. 1961, p. 21.
[48] Ibid, p. 17

of right or wrong behavior, acceptance of traditional values. The parent moralizes and judges others and speaks in words and thoughts, saying "*you* are." The parent can be a good or bad parent. The adult ego state is represented by responsible, rational, and predictable feelings. The adult is nonjudgmental and always in the process of learning. The composition of each person's ego states varies according to past and early child-hood experiences, but perceptible predominant characteristics can be identified by other persons when they take note of verbal transactions and nonverbal behavior. When people do not interact openly and make use of "games," these cues suggest that they are masking their true selves and are possibly unaware that they have a distinctive identity. For the person who consistently and spontaneously acts according to feelings, the child ego state is dominant. When the person tends to be inflexible and judgmental, the parent ego state is dominant.

Transactional analysis classifies four possible life positions that can be held with respect to oneself and others. They are interpreted in detail by Harris in a book which is easy reading for nurses and consumers.[49] The life positions are:

1 I'm OK–You're OK.
2 I'm not OK–You're OK.
3 I'm not OK–You're not OK.
4 I'm OK–You're not OK.

The life position "I'm OK–You're OK" is the healthy situation and is the goal toward which all persons in transactional analysis therapy strive. However, the predominant majority of people hold the life position "I'm not OK–You're OK." As explained by Harris, this is the universal position of early childhood, being the infant's logical conclusion from the situation of birth and infancy. Since all infants are naturally dependent and *must be* cared for by adults, the not-OK-ness is a natural conclusion about themselves. In this position the person feels at the mercy of others and seeks recognition and approval from others.[50] It is the people who hold the life position "I'm not OK–You're OK" of whom the community health nurse must be cognizant. By explaining the simple interpretation of the three ego states and the life positions that the majority of people hold, new insights often are gained which help people to understand a great deal more about themselves. They are naturally drawn to remember their early childhood, the role of parents in their lives, and the conclusions they reached about certain emphasized beliefs which had been accepted at face value once upon a time, yet later were questioned after weighing the facts rationally and thought-fully. For example, a child may have been told by a parent that handling frogs would cause warts to appear on the hands. However, upon observing other children handling frogs and eventually venturing to pick one up, it was discovered that warts did not appear. Consequently, the child no longer believed a statement which had been ac-cepted at face value formerly.

The belief is held by transactional analysts that each individual is responsible for

[49] Thomas A. Harris, *I'm OK–You're OK*, Harper and Row, Publishers, Incorporated, New York, 1969.
[50] Ibid., pp. 43–45.

her or his own feelings. Feelings are internal and cannot be manipulated by external forces unless the person allows and responds to the outside forces. The individual *chooses* feelings. When the going gets rough, each person runs back to familiar territory or familiar feelings which were used in early childhood. A necessity for all persons is "stroking," recognition, or attention. As infants and children, any stroking, positive or negative, was sought as long as attention of some kind was gained. Most persons are well aware of negative strokes, since the present society tends to be negatively oriented and criticisms are much more easily given by others than praise or recognition. As adults, symbolic positive strokes are solicited and acquired by receiving compliments, recognition of achievements. Positive strokes are better than negative ones or conditional ones. Conditional strokes are those that imply, "I'll approve of you *if*." When interacting with individuals and families, positive strokes, not conditional ones, designed to strengthen the recipients should be used at every appropriate opportunity by the nurse.

Transactional analysts make use of another idea which is practical and catches the interest of the consumer. The idea is that of trading stamps, which are collected daily in order to obtain an object or reward that one desires. The trading stamps in transactional analysis represent feelings; good feelings are identified as gold stamps, and bad, hurt, or resentful feelings are brown stamps. Gold stamps are collected by giving and receiving tangible positive recognition and earning desirable achievements. Brown stamps are collected by giving and receiving insults, feeling injured or put upon. Brown stamps can be collected dishonestly and are often accompanied by a feeling of triumph. When a book of brown stamps or an accumulation of angry feelings is collected, a person is entitled to have a temper outburst free of guilt, or with several books of brown stamps, a divorce or extramarital affair can be claimed free of guilt. For those persons familiar with the trading stamp idea in transactional analysis, the labeling of a behavior as gold or brown stamping has lasting meaning and can often be conveyed in a nonthreatening manner. For the community health nurse who chooses to use a modification of the transactional analysis method with families, the interpretation of the basic beliefs and language are easily conveyed and understood and provide a nonthreatening climate for growth-promoting interaction. The goal toward which the nurse would work in using this method is assisting the client or family to become their true, genuine selves and rely less on behaviors which mask their identity.

The Parent Effectiveness Training Approach In developing parent effectiveness training, Gordon wanted to provide a preventive program helping parents to communicate facilitatively with children. He was convinced that adolescents do not rebel against parents, but against certain destructive methods of discipline almost universally employed by parents.[51]

All parents have feelings about the behavior of their children which can be defined into an area of acceptance and nonacceptance. The acceptability of behavior as defined by the parent may change from day to day, may vary in terms of the individual child

[51] Thomas Gordon, *Parent Effectiveness Training,* Peter H. Wyden, Inc., Publisher, New York, 1970, p. 3.

performing the behavior, or may show inconsistency dependent upon the parent's mood or the situation in the home. Parents cannot be wholly consistent regardless of their determination to be so because parents are people who, if they are real, have a variable area of acceptance. When parents "seem" to accept a behavior but are not genuine about it, the child invariably knows the true feelings of the parent. For parents who want to facilitate the growth and actualization of their children to the fullest potential, they must communicate their acceptance in such a way that the children *feel* the acceptance. They must learn the language of acceptance which is communicated verbally and nonverbally and incorporates the skill of *active listening*. Active listening requires the listener to suspend personal thoughts and feelings in order to attend exclusively to the message of the speaker. It forces accurate receiving. To listen actively the listener must (1) *want* to hear what the speaker has to say, (2) genuinely *want* to be helpful to the speaker, (3) genuinely be able to accept the speaker's feelings, (4) trust the speaker's capacity to handle personal feelings and find solutions for problems, (5) appreciate that feelings are transitory, not permanent, and (6) see the speaker as separate from the listener. The skills of active listening may seem almost impossible for parents to practice with their children, but it can be learned and effectively utilized if earnestly practiced.

Another aspect of parent effectiveness training is problem ownership. When an individual has a need that is not being satisfied, that individual owns a problem. For children, the problem can be feeling rejected by a friend, getting angry when losing a game with a friend, feeling inadequate because of acne. When the child owns the problem, the parent can assist by "active listening." For parents, the problem is owned when children's behavior potentially threatens a need of theirs. For example, when the child is tugging and interrupting while the parent is on the telephone, the child's toys are scattered all over the kitchen floor, or the child does not care properly for equipment belonging to the parent. When the parent owns the problem, the parent can try to modify the child directly, modify the environment, or modify himself or herself. However, inevitably parent-child conflicts occur, and the "no-lose" method of resolution must be employed. This is essentially a problem-solving method in which both parents and children participate. The goal is to solve their unique conflicts by finding their own unique solutions acceptable to both. This method tends to be effective because the child is a participant in arriving at a unique solution, has been required to think about possible solutions, and feels less resistant to carrying out the agreed-upon solution. Relationships between parents and children tend to be more satisfying with the use of the "no-lose" method.[52]

Community health nurses can explain the concept of parent effectiveness training to parents and children and serve as educators, consultants, and arbiters in the implementation of the method. Since nursing students are so well versed in the problem-solving method, the role of "expert" is easily assumed.

The Epidemiologic Approach   Epidemiology has often been considered the study of factors determining the occurrence of communicable diseases in populations. How-

[52] Ibid., pp. 15–264.

ever, the study has broadened to include *all* diseases, whether communicable or not, and health behavior of groups of people. Epidemiology consists of a methodological investigation of disease or health behavior occurring in human groups for the purpose of discovering factors essential to or contributing to disease occurrence or unhealthy behavior and developing methods for prevention of disease or unhealthy behavior. The epidemiologic method is closely related to the problem-solving method, which is generally used with individuals rather than with groups. Epidemiology is more a method than a body of knowledge and in essence is similar to the detective approach of gathering clues or data, making hypotheses or deductions, and finding solutions. The epidemiologist mainly uses two methods for study of data, observational and experimental. By observation the investigator simply makes note of circumstances and events in the normal pattern of life. By analysis the investigator searches for association between disease occurrence or unhealthy behavior and the possible causative influences.[53]

Customarily, the community health nurse serves as an associate with epidemiologists in the study of diseases and investigation of all related data. However, by using the epidemiologic approach on a small scale with families or groups, it is proposed that the community health nurse play the role of principal investigator in seeking out solutions for diseases or health behaviors occurring in a given family or group and stimulate family or group members to serve as associates in bringing out related data. For example, a small but effective epidemiologic study could be done of a family or group who are faced with the problem of obesity or a high incidence of home accidents. In dealing with the obesity problem, a detailed history of amounts and types of food ingested by the family or group members for a period of 3 days to 1 week would provide data that could be analyzed thoroughly in terms of nutrients and calories. In addition, characteristic habit patterns associated with mealtimes and snacktimes could be studied, and antecedent events which seem to cause undesirable consequent behaviors could be observed. If the group or family members are participating as associates in the epidemiologic study, they may be encouraged to bring out facts related to eating, such as the ingestion of more food following hostile interactions with others or early childhood training which taught them to clean up their plates rather than waste food. When all participants are alert for possible causative factors of eating, a great amount of significant data can be secured, which will lead to ideas of possible hypotheses to be tested. The nurse serves as the detective or agent in search of significant clues from all possible perspectives, including physical, emotional, and social. By playing the role of detective, the nurse must have a comprehensive knowledge about the variety of factors which may lead to obesity. When a definition of the nature and significance of the problem is obtained about all the participants and all important data are collected, classified, and appraised, a hypothesis can be tentatively formulated for testing. Future practical activities based on the hypothesis can be planned and implemented for a determined time period and ultimately, an evaluation of the results of the study can be decided. For the group studying the causation of obesity, the testing of a hypothesis focusing on mealtime practices and habits may lead to more

[53]John P. Fox, Carrie E. Hall, and Lila R. Elveback, *Epidemiology, Man and Disease,* The Macmillan Company, New York, 1970, pp. 7–16.

successful results than one related to ingestion of superfluous calories. By involving all family or group members in the detective game, curiosity is stimulated and motivation to change behavior is often self-induced.

In the case of a family or group having a high incidence of accidents, the nurse can introduce the idea that accidents don't happen, they are caused by what people do or by what they fail to do.[54] This idea alone may arouse the group to do some reflective thinking and serve as a stimulus for further study. If the family or group responds with the desire to lessen the occurrence of accidents, each person can be asked to determine the frequency of individual accidents and describe completely the events occurring before and during the last accident in which she or he was involved. Environmental, psychological, and stress factors representing hazards in each described situation can be elicited and studied by the group in search of commonalities. They may formulate a hypothesis based on the relationship of stress to personal psychological characteristics which culminate in accident proneness in individuals. By becoming more knowledgeable by means of references about the characteristics of persons who seem to be accident-prone, by attempting to reduce the number of stress- or risk-producing life events, and attempting to control unsafe reactions, acts, and behavior, the group may test their hypothesis by tabulating the frequency of accidents occurring to them after four weeks of discussion and study compared to their first frequency estimates. By accepting the fact that accidents occur when alertness, efficiency, skill, or judgment of persons is temporarily impaired, subsequent behavior can be made more conscious and perhaps "safe." The epidemiologic method provides a more interesting approach to accident prevention than lectures about safety. The nurse when acting as a stimulator of ideas and promulgator of learning has more satisfactions and is more apt to see learning internalized by the family or group.

The Paradoxical Communication Approach The community health nurse may make use of paradoxical communication as a last resort when all other approaches have failed or as a mode of communication to which a specific type of client will respond best. A *paradox* is a term describing a directive which qualifies another directive in a conflicting way, either simultaneously or at a different moment in time.[55] For example, in order to persuade a client to change undesirable symptomatic behavior, she or he must be told to do something and that activity should be related to the problem in some way. For a person complaining of persistent insomnia, a directive can be given to spend each night reading books that the client has put off reading and, to ensure against falling asleep, to stand up at the mantle and read all night. After several nights of reading standing up, the insomnia problem may be cured, and this was accomplished by the client. The emphasis of treatment was placed on the client's activity rather than on the symptomatic behavior.[56] By directing the client's attention to activities which must be accomplished and avoiding the suggestion of ceasing the

---

[54] Albert Chapman, "The Anatomy of an Accident," *Public Health Reports,* 75:630–632, July 1960.
[55] By permission of Jay Haley, *Strategies of Psychotherapy,* Grune & Stratton, Inc., New York, 1963, p. 17.
[56] Ibid., p. 49.

symptomatic behavior, the therapist poses a paradox in the client's mind of retaining the symptomatic behavior or following directives that are not always attractive to the client. This method of giving action-type directives related to symptomatic behavior commits the client to either giving up the symptom or following the directives as given by the therapist. The paradoxical communication method has interesting implications, particularly for childlike persons who want to change symptomatic behavior but cannot resist the desire to rebel when told or ordered to do something. If the nurse utilizes the paradoxical communication approach, the client must be known well enough for the nurse to predict the client's response to a direct suggestion. If the nurse is almost certain that the client cannot resist rejecting an order, a directive can be given which is the reverse of the goal wished for the client. This method often works with small children.

A student nurse accidentally stumbled upon this method of communication with the mother of a child who was diagnosed as needing a tonsillectomy to alleviate a hearing loss. The nurse had made repeated weekly visits to persuade the mother to make an appointment for the surgical procedure. Upon each home visit the mother had some legitimate excuse which had caused a postponement in scheduling the surgery. At last the frustrated nurse gave up and told the mother to forget the whole thing. In all probability the child would manage all right without the tonsillectomy. The following week the nurse visited the home and learned that the child had had the surgery and was recuperating nicely.

The Force Field Analysis Approach When planning any kind of change with a client or family, a multitude of factors characteristic of the nature and dynamics of the family system must be considered. Every client and family operates in a state of quasiequilibrium. Careful assessment of the factors contributing to the existing equilibrium must be noted before major changes are proposed. Lewin developed a model called force field analysis which can be used as the basis for proposing change, analyzing the dynamics of a difficult situation, or solving recognized problems. As explained by Lewin, quasiequilibria can be changed in either of two ways: by adding forces in a desired direction (driving forces) or by diminishing opposing forces (restraining forces).[57] In other words, when a client is faced with an unresolved problem, there are two equal and opposing sets of forces that counterbalance each other. For example, a 45-year-old woman recently has noticed a lump on her breast and asks the community health nurse to check it. The nurse feels a small, hard nodule which is not freely movable. The client admits she just noticed the lump while showering and has no idea how long it has been there or if it seems to be growing in size. When the nurse suggests that an immediate visit to the physician is highly advisable, the woman responds in horror and says, "What if the doctor says it's cancer? I don't want to see the doctor." The following figure depicts some of the factors contributing to the dilemma of the client and nurse. A graphic picture of the force field analysis approach illustrates how the forces affect the quasi-equilibrium line of the client (see Fig. 6-2).

[57]Kurt Lewin, "Group Decision and Social Change," in Theodore M. Newcomb and Eugene L. Hartley, (eds.), *Readings in Social Psychology,* Holt, Rinehart and Winston, Inc., 1947, pp. 340-344.

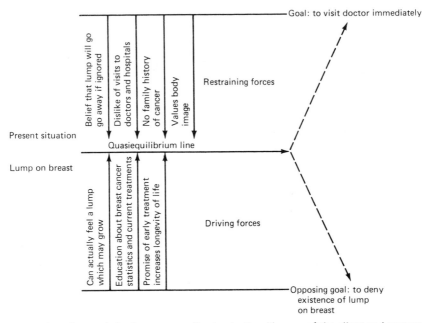

Figure 6-2 Some of the factors contributing to the dilemma of the client and nurse when the client is faced with being examined for breast cancer.

As the variety of factors contributing to the behavior of the client are assessed, the nurse can decide to add or strengthen a force which is designed to modify the client's equilibrium in the direction of the goal—to visit the physician. Convincing evidence regarding the success of early treatment of cancer of the breast may be the driving force that changes the direction of the client's equilibrium toward the desired goal. Or, the nurse may decide to eliminate or weaken a force as the best strategy for removing resistance to the desired goal. In an exploration of the client's experiences with doctors and hospitals, distortions of client perceptions can be discussed and clarified. Offers to assist the client in finding an expert physician who will be considerate of her needs will give needed support to the client and possibly weaken a restraining force.

In using the force field analysis approach it's important to:

1   Analyze the problem situation accurately and well.
2   Determine which forces can be altered with the most likelihood of reaching the desired goal. Driving forces are those forces or factors which are "pushing" a situation in a particular direction; they tend to initiate a change and keep it going. Driving forces have the possibility of increasing resistance toward a goal. Restraining forces can be characterized as walls or barriers. They prevent or retard movement toward them or toward a goal. Having a client identify restraining forces which prevent a change of behavior has been found to be more effective in facilitating change than reinforcing driving forces.
3   Make changes indicated only after a thorough analysis of the situation. Changes will occur as the most appropriate forces for the client are modified, thereby changing the direction of the equilibrium line.

4 Stabilize the new situation so that it will be maintained at a level comfortable for the client.[58]

The support of the nurse in reinforcing all positive behaviors on a continuing basis until the client is completely stabilized and at peace with self is essential.

Planning Care and Coordination with Others

As a member of the health team serving the client and family, the community health nurse must be constantly alert to the necessity for conferring with the other interested members of the team. These members include the physician, social workers, nurses in other settings, teachers, and any number of allied community workers and health aides. By initiating communication by means of the telephone, prearranged personal discussions, or scheduling a multidisciplinary conference, all team members can be made cognizant of agreed-upon, common objectives by which all will abide in their work with the client and family. Planning a successful intervention with and for the client and family involves teamwork, maintenance of an open exchange of information, sharing of resources among team members and ultimate goals toward which all are working. Planning with other professional and nonprofessional workers is essential and requires time and effort expended to maintain open channels of communication. By following a carefully designed plan of action which has been individualized for the client and family, successful interventions and satisfying relationships are more likely to be attained by all persons involved.

THE NURSING PROCESS: IMPLEMENTING

Implementing a nursing care plan implies that a careful assessment and planning process has been accomplished and activities for or in behalf of the client and family are now available which will contribute to their comfort and well-being or facilitate their coping behaviors as related to their specific health problems. Implementation is an ongoing activity or series of activities which necessitates evaluation in order to determine the effectiveness of nursing care. Action is taken with the expectation that if the planned action is followed, an expected result will occur. The evaluation process may indicate a need for reassessment and replanning or a modification of the plan of care. Implementation of nursing care includes all the activities of the nurse in carrying out the nursing care plan designed to enhance the well-being of the client and family.[59] It is essential that the nurse continue to involve the client in decisions regarding changes in the plan of care so that both parties comprehend the focus of each nursing visit.

While carrying out a plan of action, the nurse must be constantly aware of (1) a therapeutic use of self with the client and family; (2) the nurse's affect on the client

[58] David H. Jenkins, "Social Engineering in Educational Change: An Outline of Method," *Progressive Education,* 26:193–197, May 1949.

[59] Mildred Wesolowski, "Implementation of the Nursing Care Plan," in Yura and Walsh, op, cit., pp. 78–79. Helen Yura and Mary B. Walsh (eds.), *The Nursing Process: Assessing, Planning, Implementing, and Evaluating,* The Catholic University of America Press, Washington, D.C. 1967, pp. 78–79.

and family (and the client and family's affect on the nurse); (3) knowledge of physical, psychological, and social manifestations of pathology, deviance, or wellness; (4) opportunities for teaching, supervising, or guiding persons toward better coping patterns of health; and (5) evaluation of the total effect of the implementation activity.

The Process of Effecting Change

A persistent goal to which all nurses are committed is to influence change in clients or families in the direction of improved health or wellness. However, what motivates people to change? Will they change when they see no reason to do so? Will they change when others want them to do so? Will they change when they believe they want to do so but cannot resist the pull of forces compelling them to pursue old habit patterns? Effecting change is much more easily talked about than accomplished. According to Wheelis, *we are what we do*. The actions that we *do* describe our character to others. The fact that the action is repeated over and over reinforces the description that others have ascribed to us. When we *say* that we are one thing but *behave* or *act* in opposition to what we say, others take note of the behavior and believe the behavior rather than the words. Because we tend to maintain behavior or actions that are familiar and customary, we resist change.

All persons have potential for change and can change when they *choose* to do so. Therefore a person who is suffering or uncomfortable with a health problem, must recognize that it is a problem that is causing her or him to suffer or be uncomfortable, and must be ready and willing to do something about the problem before a change can be effected. Since we are what we do, if we want to change what we are, we must begin by changing what we do. A new mode of action is often difficult, unnatural, unpleasant, or anxiety-provoking, and in order to sustain the change, a considerable effort of will is required. Change will occur only if such action is maintained over a long period of time.[60] Consequently, the role of community health nurses in assisting clients or families to effect change can be enumerated as follows: (1) reach an agreement with the client or family about the health problems that are causing difficulties and that they desire to change; (2) assist the client or family in determining the new behavior or action which will help them to attain their goal; (3) provide constant reinforcement for the client's or family's behavior or actions which have been adjusted in the direction of meeting their goal; and (4) maintain contact with the client or family for an extended period of time and continue to encourage and strengthen them in their new behavior until their goal has been attained and maintained to the satisfaction of all concerned. At the same time as working with the client or family to effect change, the nurse must also be utilizing relationship skills, cognitive knowledge about the particular health problems which are the focus of attention, interactional skills, and predictive skills in anticipating the probability of success in the venture undertaken by the client, family, and nurse.

Barriers to Change

Some barriers which may be encountered by the nurse attempting to effect change with clients or families may be: (1) faulty perception regarding the clients' or families'

---

[60] Allen Wheelis, *The Desert,* Basic Books, Inc., Publishers, New York, 1970.

readiness to change. The nurse may believe that the client desires to change when in reality the client is only being momentarily compliant to the nurse's persuasiveness or wishes to appear worthy of the nurse's attention. (2) The language used by the nurse may be unfamiliar to the client or family and rather than ask for an explicit interpretation, the consumer may elect to pretend an understanding of the issues involved. (3) The emotional content of the messages between the client or family and the nurse may be missed, avoided, or inaccurately interpreted as being irrelevant to the issue under discussion. When detecting an emotion in the consumer that is not completely understandable in terms of the words being spoken, the nurse must verbalize uncertainty about what she or he is sensing or perceiving. For example, the nurse may say to a client who is using bullet-like speech and staring pointedly out the window, "You seem disturbed about something and I am not sure if I understand the message you are giving me. Are you angry with me?" By so doing the client is given the opportunity to express or interpret her or his emotion, whether it is directed at the nurse or another target. (4) Too many suggestions for change may be offered by the nurse, resulting in an overload of information for the consumer to manage. (5) The timing may be poor, inconvenient, or incomprehensible to the consumer. (6) The client or family may misinterpret the messages of the nurse, or vice versa. To avoid misinterpretations of messages it is good practice to request the consumer to give feedback on what she or he has heard from the nurse. This is called perception checking. When a verification of the message received is indeed the message intended by the sender, then the communication is clear to both parties. (7) The client or family may arbitrarily desire the right to refuse, regardless of the idea, because of the element of power. If able to accept this type of consumer and assess her or his behavior characteristics, the nurse can engage in an encounter in such a way that the consumer retains control but is provoked to *think*. Nothing is gained if the nurse enters the game of superiority with the consumer.

Stress and Crisis

An emotionally healthy person is one who has dealt and is dealing in a satisfactory manner with the conflicts inherent in each stage of human development. Inherent in this description is the implication that all persons have conflicts, problems, or stresses. In other words, life is not a bowl of cherries but a roller coaster with highs and lows. By acknowledging that all persons experience stress and crisis, the complicated task of the community health nurse is to determine when to intervene with individuals and families in need of assistance.

Stress is commonly associated with the rate of wear and tear on the body or the burden under which the individual is struggling. Rapoport referred to stress as the relation of the stressful stimulus, the individual's reaction to it, and the events to which it leads.[61] The state of crisis occurs when an imbalance between an important problem and the resources immediately available to deal with it are unsuccessful. In other words, the person in a state of crisis is unable to cope adequately with the im-

---

[61] Lydia Rapoport, "The State of Crisis: Some Theoretical Considerations," in Howard J. Parad (ed.), *Crisis Intervention: Selected Readings,* Family Service Association of America, New York, 1965, p. 23.

mediate problem. The essence of crisis is struggle—a struggle to master an upsetting situation and to regain a state of balance.[62] For health professionals who utilize crisis theory, a crisis is an opportunity for respondents to try new actions or new coping mechanisms which will strengthen adaptive capacities and raise levels of emotional health.

In community health nursing, the systems approach helps the nurse to view the family as an integral unit and as made up of individuals who are influenced by all occurrences within the family. The family is seen as a source of strength or a source of stress, dependent upon the constructive or destructive influences in operation within it. When a family is in crisis, they are at a turning point. They are faced with problems for which their coping mechanisms seem inadequate, they feel helpless and frustrated and are uncertain of how to act effectively to solve the problems.[63] It is at this point that the intervention of the community health nurse can be most effective. If interaction occurs during the period of crisis, the nurse has an optimum opportunity to guide the family toward improved coping mechanisms, which will successfully restore a state of balance within the family system and promote them toward a higher level of emotional health.

There are two types of crisis which families undergo, developmental and situational. As described by Robischon, *developmental* or *maturational crises* are those which human beings experience in the process of their psychosocial growth. They are considered stages of the normal life cycle. For families, some examples of these crises occur when a new baby is born, when the children reach adolescence, or when retirement occurs. *Situational* or *accidental crises* are external events or stresses. They are often more sudden, unexpected, and unfortunate.[64] For example, these crises occur when a member of the family dies, a handicapped child is born, a debilitating disease is diagnosed and seen as inevitable, or a serious accident maims a family member.

As stated by Leighton, there are three universal kinds of behavior with which individuals react to authority when subject to forces of stress that are disturbing to the emotions and thoughts of the individual. They are cooperation, withdrawal, and aggressiveness. The nurse who is watchful for these behaviors is better able to assess the dynamics involved in each family situation. Relief from excessive stress is assisted by the utilization of a sense of humor, observable facts, reasoned thinking, and new opportunities to achieve security and satisfactions.[65]

Some of the activities which the community health nurse can use in crisis intervention with an individual or family are:

1 Help the troubled person to confront the crisis by helping to verbalize and to comprehend the reality of the situation.

[62] Donald G. Langsley and David M. Kaplan, *The Treatment of Families in Crisis,* Grune & Stratton, Inc., New York, 1968, p. 3.
[63] Donna C. Aguilera, Janice M. Messick, and Marlene S. Farrell, *Crisis Intervention, Theory and Methodology,* The C. V. Mosby Company, St. Louis, 1970, p. 1.
[64] Paulette Robischon, "The Challenge of Crisis Theory for Nursing," *Nursing Outlook,* 15(7):28–32, July 1967.
[65] Alexander H. Leighton, *The Governing of Men,* Princeton University Press, Princeton, N.J. 1945, pp. 252–286.

2 Help the person to confront the crisis in manageable doses. By observing the individual's nonverbal cues, the nurse may facilitate verbalization of feelings which the client had considered to be taboo but were contributing to the state of tension.

3 Help the client to find the facts of the situation and explore all possible ways of coping. Proceed at the client's pace. When exploration is done mutually, the client is helped to think and may devise solutions which are highly original and made possible because of the stimulus of another person helping with the problem-solving process.

4 Help the client by recognizing strengths and encouraging the use of capabilities.

5 Help the client accept assistance from others as needed and as she or he is ready, until the client's personal resources have been mobilized.[66]

By being available, patient, willing to listen, and supportive of strengths, the nurse can enable individuals or families in a state of crisis to move toward resolution of difficulties in an acceptable manner and promote their sense of responsibility and well-being at the same time.

The Social Readjustment Rating Scale

Stress affects all ages and can be measured in terms of the magnitude of life changes. A rating scale developed by Holmes and Rahe measures the intensity and length of time necessary to accommodate to a life event, regardless of the desirability of the event. The scoring technique which has been tested for reliability indicates the level of stress or life changes experienced by individuals. When the number of life changes clusters, the score is high. This means that an individual with a high score has had to cope with many changes within a specified time period and is therefore likely to become sick. It does not seem to matter whether the change has desirable or undesirable aspects. By reviewing forty-three items on the rating scale reflecting life-changing events and scoring as instructed, an individual can determine the amount of recent stress experienced, and the likelihood of becoming ill or having an accident within the next year. The tool is best used by community health nurses not for prediction purposes but to give some clues to families about what activities to avoid or modify if one wants to reduce a high score with subsequent chances of illness. If presented as an interesting tool with which to measure stress, family members can be encouraged to think of preventive measures and manipulate their plans so as to lessen their total life-event scores.[67] The scale and method of scoring is shown in Table 6-3.

Homework

When working with individuals in the implementation phase of the nursing process, a simple activity or assignment is frequently accepted with keenness and ambivalence— eagerness to be doing something that may help themselves and uncertainty about their ability to carry out the assignment. These tasks or activities are called "homework," a term used by David Kupfer, a transactional analyst who stated that people like to be given homework. The assignment given must be reasonable, fairly easily accomplished,

---

[66] Robischon, op. cit., pp. 28-32.

[67] Thomas H. Holmes and R. H. Rahe, "The Social Readjustment Rating Scale," *Journal of Psychosomatic Research,* **11**:213-218, 1967.

Table 6-3 Social Readjustment Rating Scale*

Rank	Life event	Life crisis units
1	Death of spouse	100
2	Divorce	73
3	Marital separation	65
4	Jail term	63
5	Death of close family member	63
6	Personal injury or illness	53
7	Marriage	50
8	Fired at work	47
9	Marital reconciliation	45
10	Retirement	45
11	Change in health of family member	44
12	Pregnancy	40
13	Sex difficulties	39
14	Gain of new family member	39
15	Business readjustment	39
16	Change in financial state	38
17	Death of close friend	37
18	Change to different line of work	36
19	Change in number of arguments with spouse	35
20	Mortgage over $10,000	31
21	Foreclosure of mortgage or loan	30
22	Change in responsibilities at work	29
23	Son or daughter leaving home	29
24	Trouble with in-laws	29
25	Outstanding personal achievement	28
26	Wife begins or stops work	26
27	Begin or end school	26
28	Change in living conditions	25
29	Revision of personal habits	24
30	Trouble with boss	23
31	Change in work hours or conditions	20
32	Change in residence	20
33	Change in school	20
34	Change in recreation	19
35	Change in church activities	19
36	Change in social activities	18
37	Mortgage or loan less than $10,000	17
38	Change in sleeping habits	16
39	Change in number of family get-togethers	15
40	Change in eating habits	15
41	Vacation	13
42	Christmas	12
43	Minor violations of the law	11

*Social Readjustment Rating Scale Instructions:
Add up value of life crisis units for life events experienced in a 2-year period.
Score of 0 to 150—No significant problems.
Score of 150 to 199—Mild life crisis and a 33 percent chance of illness.
Score of 200 to 299—Moderate life crisis and a 50 percent chance of illness.
Score of 300 or over—Major life crisis and an 80 percent chance of illness.

Source: Adapted with permission from T. H. Holmes and R. H. Rahe, "Social Readjustment Rating Scale," Journal of Psychosomatic Research, 11:213–218, 1967.

and within the context of the goal toward which the client is working. For example, for the person who has low self-esteem, an assignment can be given for that person to write down 100 personal strengths and to show the list to the nurse on the next visit. Or the client may be assigned a pamphlet to read and jot down questions for discussion on the nurse's return visit. The client may be requested also to tally on a chart the number of times a prescribed set of exercises was performed, and the nurse will anticipate examining the chart on the next visit. The performance of an assignment sometimes relieves tension, gives a sense of movement toward a desired goal, and a feeling of accomplishment that is satisfying. The achievement of the assignment, whether partial or complete, must always be recognized and reinforced positively by the nurse.

In a study reported by Geismar and Krisberg, it was found that families respond most favorably to communication which is focused on problem solving. The approach very frequently sought by families was the quick solution. However, when family members were encouraged to think through the problem-solving process and their strengths were reinforced, movement toward their goals was more apt to be realized.[68] The assignment of homework which is individualized to fit the situation and gives the family something to do can be one of the methods used to reinforce family members about their existing strengths and latent capacity for problem solving.

The Nursing Bag

For the nurse who gives bedside care in the home, the nursing bag has always been a necessary accessory. Historically, its contents have included equipment needed to perform the nursing functions. The equipment has varied dependent upon the period of history that nursing care was given. In the early 1800s, the nurse carried a satchel which contained black currant jelly for the parched throat and racking cough, Irish moss to be made into a soothing drink, chicken jelly for a nourishing broth, and perhaps an orange or a lemon.[69] In the 1900s, the nurses in New York City carried heavy "telescope" bags containing more than a dozen bottles and porcelain jars.[70] From 1900 to the present era, the bags that have been used are familiar to most nurses because of their shape and black color. The contents include equipment for handwashing, taking temperatures, giving injections, doing occasional dressings, and performing other nursing skills necessary to carry out a physician's orders. Frequently the equipment is disposable and entails a careful daily scrutiny of the bag to ensure that all needed articles for the services to be performed on that day are included, are sterile or clean, and are intact.

The manner with which the supplies in the nursing bag are used communicates

---

[68] Ludwig Geismar and Jane Krisberg, "The Family Life Improvement Project: An Experiment in Preventive Intervention," Parts I and II, *Social Casework,* 27:9, November 1966 and 28:10, December 1966.

[69] Alfred Worcester, *Nurses and Nursing,* Harvard University Press, Cambridge, Mass., 1927, p. 40.

[70] Mary M. Roberts, *American Nursing, History and Interpretation,* The Macmillan Company, New York, 1954, pp. 3-4.

to families much nonverbal data about the nurse's behavior, attitude, and skill. If the family members like what they see, their respect, confidence, and acceptance of the nurse as a skilled practitioner are increased. They may adopt unconsciously some of the practices of asepsis and cleanliness. By routinely using nursing skills which include vital signs, the nurse conveys professionalism and a genuine concern for the client's welfare. Many opportunities for teaching clients can be realized through the use of the nursing bag—and the teaching is often not on a verbal or a demonstration basis. The most effective teaching may be accomplished purely on the nonverbal basis, during which the nurse is performing unconsciously as a role model.

A nursing student who did a ministudy on nurses' attitudes about the bag asked the question, "Is the nursing bag a symbol of the community health nurse?" From a very small sample of practicing community health nurses, four out of five answered, "no." The fifth nurse said that the bag was "whatever the nurse makes of it." Two nursing students out of a sample of three stated that the bag was a symbol of the community health nurse.

In view of the ongoing technological advancements in medical and nursing care, it is difficult to predict if nursing bags will continue to retain the shape, color, and size that they currently have. However, a means for carrying necessary equipment which aids in the administration of nursing care in the home will always be required.

Casefinding

Inherent in every community health nursing visit are the possibilities for casefinding and referral. These are important functions of each member of the community health team and are carried out in the home, the school, the clinic, and in places of employment. While providing nursing care and health counseling during the home visit, the nurse has unusual opportunities for casefinding. In discussions with the family, the nurse must be alert to and observant of early symptoms of such conditions as cancer, diabetes, communicable diseases, birth injuries, and mental and emotional disturbances. The nurse must be perceptive and alert to what the client and other family members are saying or doing and to objective and subjective symptoms that may be revealed.

A nurse calling on a migratory farm worker's family noted that Judy, a 3-year-old, had a definite limp as she walked across the bare floor. The nurse questioned the mother about it, and possible symptoms, suggestive of bone tuberculosis, came to light. A referral to a children's orthopedic clinic brought a diagnosis of bone tuberculosis. Further study of the family revealed that the father had active tuberculosis.

An ostensible purpose of community health nursing service is the early finding of pregnancy and the referral of prospective mothers for medical care. At this time, i.e., early in pregnancy, the nurse can place the mothers under nursing supervision also and teach them care of themselves and their babies. This teaching can often be related to the health needs, e.g., nutritional needs, of other members of the family.

Referral

Closely allied to casefinding during the home visit is referral, i.e., the referral of the client or family to the community agency best suited or equipped to help meet the particular problems recognized by the nurse. These might be of a health, welfare, social, or recreational nature.

Often, the major task of the nurse is not referring a family to an appropriate community agency, but getting the family *ready* to accept the services of the community resource as needed and desired. The process involved in preparing a family includes the initiation of an effective relationship with the family, the recognition that problems are existing and must be resolved, and a time period during which an exploration of problems and possible solutions can be discussed with the family. The time during which the family is searching for appropriate solutions may be extended into weeks or months, dependent upon their readiness to act. In the meantime, the nurse can be utilizing methods or ideas which will reveal the discomfort the problems are causing for the family, will communicate indirectly the family's inability to resolve the problems without competent assistance, will give promise that ultimate solutions are possible and available, and that a referral to an appropriate community resource is indeed necessary to attain a desired goal. An interpretation of the services of a designated community resource and the manner in which the personnel will work with the family must be made. Also, when the family is ready to visit a selected community resource, they should be taught how best to present their desires and goals to the agency from whom they are requesting help. Sometimes the process of preparing a family for a referral to a community resource is a lengthy one and requires a patient and persistent nurse.

In making a referral, the nurse must be well aware of the services and contributions of the community's health and social agencies. Usually lists are available of recognized agencies and their services. Some agencies have developed interagency referral forms. The simplest is a card that includes the name of the agency, its address, telephone number, and the hours that the agency is open. This is signed with the name of the nurse's agency and given to the family. Other types of referral forms may include more details. The nurse as a professional practitioner has an obligation to the client to follow up on referrals made to other agencies. Nurses must be aware of services currently offered by community agencies. If not aware, the nurse should contact the agency by phone or letter to assure that services available are appropriate for the type of referral. There is no quicker way to have clients distrust health professionals than to be shuffled from one agency to another, only to find that they have been abandoned with no one available to coordinate their care. Nurses can make a follow-up telephone call or visit after a referral is made to assure that the family received the necessary assistance. In certain instances, the nurse may send the agency a notice with some pertinent information that the client or family have been referred. Some agencies arrange to return these forms to the nurse with the findings and recommendations that were made to the family. The nurse can utilize this information on future visits. A workable referral system is basic to any communitywide program of continuity of care of the client.

Closing the Visit

The community health nurse terminates the visit with a brief review of the important points covered during the visit. Stressing the positive aspects and emphasizing family strengths, the nurse reiterates the plans the client and family will carry out in the nurse's absence. Together the nurse and the family plan for the next visit, establishing a date and approximate time convenient for family and nurse. Summarizing the visit can be a learning experience for the client and family and will give the nurse an opportunity to organize her thoughts in preparation for recording the visit.

Recording the Visit: Problem-Oriented Recording

Community health agencies are continuously seeking ways to improve their family records by eliminating the writing of unnecessary detail or duplication and focusing on a succinct accounting of important information. Because the search for a satisfactory record form is elusive, community health nurses must be flexible and adapt to whatever record form is in use in the particular agency for whom they are working. By concentrating on writing only essential information, nurses can limit their recording of family situations to a few well-stated sentences, phrases, or brief paragraphs which convey the current situation and plans for future visits. This ability takes continuous effort and self-discipline.

Adaptations of problem-oriented recording as originally introduced by Weed have appeared in many agencies as the recording of choice. The features making this form of recording useful and desirable are its systematic approach to the recording of pertinent facts, the easy accessibility of information in an orderly and logical arrangement, and the capability of evaluating the effectiveness of services given.

The components of a problem-oriented record consist of a database, a problem list, problem assessment and plan formulation, and progress notes and flow sheets. The contention of the problem-oriented recording system is that with the delineation of a client's or family's multiple problems at a level which is understood and can be managed, a structural framework is provided for the planning and delivery of health care. When each problem is identified and recorded and has an explicitly formulated plan for investigation and management of the problem, the result is a logically organized documentation of the course of each problem. Such a record provides easy access for a methodical analysis of a family's total health needs and services provided.[71]

Database In giving comprehensive care to a family, all health-related problems must be ascertained, including potentially threatening problems, resolved or controlled problems, socioeconomic problems and emotional problems. To elicit a complete database, the assessment and screening process of each family and its members should be as systematic and thorough as conceivable. A list of the problems that are assessed by the nurse should be jotted down. The data that describe the family's perceptions of problems, their strengths, and their limitations should be included. In securing a history regarding each family member, the nurse should be cognizant of and inquire about risk factors for certain age levels, such as frequency of upper respiratory infections in infants, accessibility of household poisons for preschool youngsters, susceptibility of school-age children to peer pressures related to drug abuse, diet patterns of middle-

[71] Lawrence L. Weed (major contributor), Jay S. Wakefield and Stephen R. Yarnall (eds.), *Implementing the Problem-Oriented Medical Record,* Medical Computer Services Association, Seattle, Wash., 1973 pp. 1–15.

aged persons, and medication usage of elderly citizens. As much as possible, the database should be explicit, more so than wordy.

The problem of eliciting a useful database and not acquiring volumes of interesting but irrelevant data is a difficult one for many community health agencies. Some have written guidelines for data considered to be essential; some have devised database sheets for specific health situations which suggest data considered pertinent for various assessments—family, individual, social, and environmental, mental health, antepartum, postpartum, and newborn. Other agencies have allowed the nurse to be the judge of what information is essential to the database regarding the assessed family.

In many instances, the nature of the visit and contract with the family spells out the extent of information recommended for the preliminary database. When episodic care is given, the nurse starts with the problem list which specifies the presenting complaint of the family. To aid in determining how to manage the problem, a minidatabase is secured. In other words, information which is relevant for the specific complaint is collected and carefully analyzed before treatment measures are instituted.

Problem List A problem is some aspect of the client that disturbs or endangers health (mental or physical). It is something that requires further attention for diagnosis, treatment, or just observation. A problem list should contain legitimate problems to the client, for which the nurse has a legitimate plan, for which a legitimate goal has been set, and for which legitimate progress notes can be written. The problem list can contain currently active problems, those which have been resolved, potential problems, chronic problems, psychological problems, socioeconomic problems, and others.

One difficulty that some nurses have in determining a problem list for families is the family's denial that they have problems. Many families reject the word "problem" when it is used to judge their methods for managing activities of daily living. They can accept words like concern, difficulty, or worry, but the word problem conveys the meaning that they are not coping satisfactorily. For many individuals, even though problems are present, it is generally conceded that each person can manage her or his own problems. When the use of the word "problem" is a deterrent to eliciting the concerns of families, use different words which connote less judgmental inferences regarding their current mode of living.

Another difficulty that nurses face in making a problem list is assigning priority to problems according to the way the nurse or family sees them. For many multiproblem families, the nurse is able to make a lengthy and legitimate problem list but the family will not accept a contract with the nurse dealing with the obvious problems, such as lack of immunization for children, unsanitary living conditions, and abusive disciplinary measures used with children. Instead, the family will accept a contract which is more satisfactory to their desires such as eliminating the enuresis of a preschool child, getting the children into a headstart or preschool program, and/or securing dental care for the children. Each nurse or agency must determine how problems should be itemized. However, if problems that the family recognizes and accepts are dealt with first, the more obvious ones that are disturbing to the nurse can be managed later as the relationship between family members and nurse develops into one of trust.

Problem Assessment and Plan Formulation Within the body of the record, the problem is referred to by number or title. Some agencies incorporate the problem assessment and plans within their progress notes. When this is done, each note is dated and signed. Recording is structured to include information classified under the categories of subjective, objective, assessment, and plan (SOAP) with each progress entry.

S Subjective data consists of statements or concerns as elicited from the family's point of view. A direct quote conveying the family member's perception of the problem may be helpful.

O Objective data includes direct physical findings, vital signs, blood pressure readings, behavioral descriptions and observations, and test or screening results if available.

A Assessment is the nursing diagnosis, a summary statement or conclusions regarding the subjective and objective findings, any changes in the client's status and prognosis in terms of the identified problem. If the nurse initially is unable to write an assessment in all honesty, then write "Don't know."

P Plan includes the plan and goal for each problem and can be written in behavioral terminology if this seems helpful for the nurse. The plan can be written in several different contexts, depending upon the status and nature of the problem. It can be immediate plans related to the problem, a plan for collecting further information and data, a plan for outlining a specific methodology or initiated procedure, a plan for educating the family as to the nature and management of the problem, a plan for measuring the progress of the family in terms of follow-up of an implementation, or a plan for stating an intent to refer to an appropriate resource. Short-range plans can be variable and recorded from visit to visit.

Progress Notes and Flow Sheets Depending upon the requirements of the agency, progress notes are incorporated with the problem assessment and plans, or they are written separately. Each progress note must be dated and signed. Each problem does not have to be written about unless important changes have taken place. For rapidly developing problems, a flow sheet is used to display data of a progressive nature, such as a graphic display of temperature, pulse and respiration, blood pressure, fluid intake and output, or a tabular display of medication self-administration, listing of nutritional intake, or fulfillment of task assignments.

Summary reports should be written in the progress notes in SOAP fashion at periodic intervals. These reports should summarize all pertinent factors related to a problem, the actions taken, interpretation of flow sheet information, the outcome, and the plans for the future.

The problem-oriented record system is a tool which facilitates evaluation of services given. Problems, plans, implementation of nursing services, flow sheet data, evidence of progress or lack of it, consistency of services, resolution or nonresolution of problems—all contribute information evaluating the efficacy of nursing intervention with a family.

Other Factors to Remember when Recording When a correction is necessary, the nurse lines out the erroneous statement, writing the correct statement below it and initialing it. The confidentiality of client and family records must be maintained at all times. As in the hospital, the community health record is considered a legal document and, as such, is subject to court order. Elements of good record keeping include accuracy, conciseness, legibility, promptness, and the use of standard abbreviations only.

The appropriate use of the client and family record enables the nursing staff to provide continuity of nursing care. Because of vacation relief, emergencies, and staff absences, it is not always possible for the same nurse to visit the client each time. However, a clear, concise, and accurate record, always complete to date, makes it possible for a different nurse to make an effective home call without disturbing the sense of security the client had in the former nurse or interfering with the general relationship between the agency and family.

The community health nursing record is used frequently as a supervisory tool. It is helpful to both supervisor and staff nurse to review it from time to time in order to trace the nurse's growth and development and to determine where additional help may be needed in the nurse's work with families. The agency also reviews the records as a basis for program planning and in consideration of budgetary needs.

When visual aids have been used during the visit, the name of the pamphlet or guide should be given, either underlined or in quotes. This will help in the planning for future visits by the nurse or another staff member who assumes the responsibility for the case load. It is frustrating to a nurse who has selected a pamphlet for use in teaching to be told during the visit, "The other nurse brought me that last time."

In recording plans for the next visit, the nurse notes what she or he believes the family will be ready to accept and carry out. The plan should include a memorandum to see how much and how well the client and family learned from the teaching done at the previous visit and how they have been able to use what they learned. The plan may include calling the physician for additional orders and listing teaching aids that might be helpful.

There is a difference of opinion among agencies as to the most appropriate time for staff nurses to write their records. Some agencies wish the nurse to complete the records before leaving the home; others prefer to have this done immediately following the visit but not in the home; still others wish the recording to be done either at the end of the day or on the following morning before the nurse returns to the community. Some agencies, particularly in rural areas, provide tape recorders or dictaphones to be used by the nurse following the home visit.

In summary, skillful written records to ensure continuity of agency contact and nursing service must be accurate, complete, concise, and promptly done as is shown in Table 6-4. They should include a database, an up-to-date problem list, progress notes written according to the SOAP categories, the plan for the next visit, the signature of the nurse, and the current date. The same principles apply in writing referrals, memorandums, and letters to professional workers in other agencies.

THE NURSING PROCESS: EVALUATING

Evaluating the intervention of a community health nurse with an individual or family requires careful appraisal of the nurse's performance and behavior and the individual's

Table 6-4 Sample Recording of Ms. B., Age 25

	Database

Subjective	"I want to lose weight. I'm trying not to eat candy and potato chips. I have been drinking diet pop but I'm not losing any weight. I snack a lot, particularly at night."

Objective	Height:	5 ft 2 in	Eats three meals a day.
	Weight:	189 lb	An alert and active young woman who does no
	Temperature:	Not taken	prescribed exercises. Has not had a PE
	Pulse:	72 regular	for a year.
	Respiration:	20	
	Blood Pressure:	130/82	

Assessment	Overweight woman who seems committed to losing weight. Financial resources limited.

Plan	Client to visit local clinic for PE. Client will keep food diary for 1 week. Request consultation from dietitian and ask about low cost foods. Return in 1 week. (initialed) T. K., PHN

	Problem list		
	Number	**Problem**	**Date resolved**
7/7/76	1	Ms. B. wants to lose weight	

	Progress notes

7/15/76 No. 1	**S** "I was shocked when I saw how many slices of bread I eat. Keeping a food diary was not easy!"

	O Diet high in carbohydrates.
Weight: 189½ lb	Supplements with a candy bar almost every day.
Bust: 38 in	Takes second helpings.
Waist: 30 in	Eats 6 to 8 slices of bread a day.
Hips: 40 in	T.C. to clinic re. PE—Normal findings.
	OK for client to lose weight.

	A Recording of food diary complete for 1 week. Client good candidate for weight reduction.

	P Client willing to eliminate candy bars and second helpings for 1 week. Will snack on carrot sticks. Client will exercise daily for 10 minutes: was given some simple exercises to do. Will weigh and measure client every week. Goal: lose 8 lb in a month. (initialed) T. K., PHN

7/22/76 No. 1	**S** "I didn't eat any candy, but I don't think I lost any weight. I simply cannot eat another carrot stick!"

	O Kept food diary voluntarily for a second week.
Weight: 188 lb	No candy.
Bust: 37½ in	Exercised every day.
Waist: 30 in	Pleased with loss of 1½ lb.
Hips: 40 in	Recipes given for low cost, low calorie meals.

Table 6-4   Sample Recording of Ms. B., Age 25 (*Continued*)

Progress notes
A Client follows through well with suggestions. Has a good chance for reaching her goal.
P Client to continue same regimen. Will snack on celery sticks and eat less bread. Client willing to replace diet pop with water. Show food diary to dietitian and request suggestions. Weigh and measure in 1 week.
(initialed) T. K., PHN

and family's responses in terms of a temporarily or permanently changed mode of behavior. The nurse constantly must be watchful for evidences of change in individual or family behavior as an index that the plan of nursing care is indeed of value and beneficial to the client and family. If the nurse decides that the implementation approach is not showing any desired effects based on her or his appraisal of the client's response, the plan of care can be changed in hopes that a new approach will produce clues indicating a desired change of response or behavior on the part of the client or family. Changes in the nursing care plan should be in the record to assure evaluation of goals and currency of approach to the problem. By accepting the fact that evaluation is an ongoing activity that is constantly present in every phase of the nursing process, the nurse indicates a realization of how crucial evaluative skills must be in order to intervene effectively with a client or family.

Evaluation involves measuring behavior and interpreting the results in terms of the desired behavior change—which is complicated by the fact that all such measurement contains error.[72] Since the purpose of evaluation is to predict how the individual or family will behave in the immediate future, it is advantageous to write behavioral objectives (see Chap. 3) preceding any nurse or client action and *with* the client's agreement. When behavioral objectives have been written outlining desired behaviors to be attained within a specified time frame, these behaviors serve as criteria for determining the extent of the achievement of desired outcomes. Evaluation and discussion of outcomes is facilitated when objectives serve as the basis for examination.

Current evaluative methods utilized by nurses in community health nursing are suggested as shown. Nurses are strongly encouraged, however, to have specified behavioral objectives individualized for each client before utilizing an evaluative method. Evaluation presumes a legitimate purpose for asking for feedback or examining behavioral changes, and clients must be cognizant of nurses' intentions. Evaluative methods include direct observation of client behavior by means of tangible results or attainment of desired goals, questionnaires or rating scales designed to elicit opinions or attitudes of consumers regarding effectiveness of health services, anecdotal notes jotted down on a sequential basis by the nurse, process recording or tape recording of interactions on an intermittent basis, or written family analyses. By making use of combinations of

[72] Barbara Klug Redman, *The Process of Patient Teaching in Nursing,* The C. V. Mosby Company, St. Louis, 1968, p. 106.

several measuring tools, an evaluation of the results of the nursing intervention tends to be more reliable. As yet, there are too few measurement tools for determining the effectiveness of nursing intervention with clients and families. Many complex factors contribute to behavior change and the endeavor to evaluate the effect of nursing intervention alone is elusive.

Observation of Behavior

Direct observation of the client's change of behavior or attainment of desired goals is easy in some instances but not always possible for all situations. For example, when a client loses 20 lb and maintains the weight loss according to the plan of care, this result represents successful accomplishment of a desired goal and tangible evidence of a change. When a mother of a family accepts a suggestion by the nurse to perform a prescribed task consistently and several weeks later exhibits the change of behavior on a routine, casual basis, this observation may be taken as evidence of successful learning by the mother. Sometimes a sensitive observation of the client's behavior, attitude, or action will reveal clues that alert the nurse to think about the effectiveness of the approach. An example is cited as written by a nursing student:

> At first I thought it very easy to see what were the needs of this family. As a community health nurse, I saw my roles to be very obvious. I saw myself helping the mother to get appointments for herself and the children for their medical care. I also saw my role to be one of a health teacher, especially to the mother concerning her condition. I began to do these things. My first two or three visits were dedicated to carrying out these objectives. Mrs. S. would listen very patiently to everything I said. She would promise to make appointments for herself and the children. However, after three visits, I evaluated my progress and found that I was really getting nowhere. I would encourage her to make appointments, which she would do, but I found that most of them she was unable to keep for a variety of reasons. Actually, other than a medical checkup for Sammy, I had accomplished nothing.
>
> It was at this point that I realized that my diagnosis and plan were all wrong. I was looking at the family from my point of view, which was that of an inexperienced community health nurse. I also realized that I had placed my values on what should be done and what was not necessary. I saw that although we had developed somewhat of a good relationship, I was not meeting Mrs. S.'s needs as she saw them. So in my future visits, I decided to sit and listen to her and find out what her needs were. I knew it was vital that she realize my interest and concern not only in her health problems but also in the family and its relationships. Mrs. S. saw her family's two main problems to be marital and financial. Health problems were secondary. She felt the need to talk with someone about these problems because she knew so few people in whom she could confide.

When the nurse feels that observation of behavior change in the individual or family is insufficient or intangible, other measurement tools can be used.

Questionnaires or Rating Scales

Brief questionnaires or rating scales can be used occasionally or on an intermittent basis to elicit the opinions or attitudes of consumers about the health services they are

Table 6-5   Some Information to Obtain from the Consumer

1   I always learn something new about health when the nurse visits me.   ☐ Yes   ☐ No

2   It helps me to be able to talk to the nurse about things that concern me.
    ☐ Strongly disagree
    ☐ Disagree
    ☐ Uncertain
    ☐ Agree
    ☐ Strongly agree

3   I would like to talk about the latest ideas in:
    ☐ Low-cost buying
    ☐ Birth control
    ☐ Nutrition
    ☐ Developmental problems of preschool children
    Other _____

receiving or would like to receive. The use of a questionnaire or rating scale differs from a face-to-face oral evaluation by allowing the consumer to respond to questions or statements when the nurse is not present and providing time to think about the questions before expressing an honest opinion. The consumer can be requested to mail the completed questionnaire or rating scale to the nurse or the nurse's supervisor or teacher, whichever course of action is desired. Examples of information that the nurse may wish to obtain from the consumer may consist of statements such as those in Table 6-5.

By carefully constructing the statements or questions, the nurse can elicit and receive information and ideas from the consumer regarding attitudes about the health services already experienced or receptivity to more comprehensive health services. When requesting completion of questionnaires it is important for the consumer to understand the purpose of such a request. Occasionally, families feel the need to be very positive on evaluations so as not to "lose" services and may indicate responses they feel are expected rather than their true feelings.

Anecdotal Notes

By jotting down casual notes in a notebook from time to time about observations of the client or family, specific levels of client or family activity; attitudes of the client, family, or nurse; or goals of the client, family, or nurse; an examination of the notes at prescribed time intervals will frequently reveal minute changes that have occurred over the course of time. After becoming absorbed with interest in the client or family, the nurse all too often forgets the initial assessment of the situation. Consequently, the nurse is unable to determine the changes that have taken place until reminded to compare the status of the client and family with the anecdotal notes written on the first visit. It is strengthening for the nurse to be able to evaluate changes that have occurred during a specific time period and to realize the role he or she has played in effecting a change. If the changes are discussed with the family as evidence of progress (as revealed in the anecdotal notes), the client and family members are also strengthened and motivated positively to continue to work toward desired goals. Anecdotal notes can also be shown to instructors or supervisors as evidence of a client's or family's progress.

Process Recording: Tape Recording

By doing a process recording or tape recording of an interaction during a visit, the nurse is enabled to evaluate her or his interpersonal relationship with clients and families by gaining sensitivity to interviewing skills, follow-up of cues, phrasing of questions and statements, and the family's responses. If electing to do a tape recording of an interaction, the nurse must obtain permission from the client or family to do so. Frequently, a signed permission form which indicates the client's or family's willingness for the use of the tape recorder and the purpose for which the interview will be reviewed simplifies the procedure. Many families respond affirmatively to the request to do a tape recording of a visit.

When choosing to do a process recording of a visit, the nurse must be cognizant of the desirability of writing the content of the interaction as soon as possible. Its value lies in its prompt recording, and therefore it should be written immediately after the visit, as recall of the verbal and nonverbal behavior lessens as the time interval lengthens.

Process recording has been described as a verbatim recording of all recallable verbal and nonverbal communication between the nurse and the client or family member. The record includes introductory statements describing the family constellation and the purpose of the visit; the verbatim recording of the verbal and nonverbal communication between the nurse and the client or family member; comments and analysis of feelings the nurse experienced and those the nurse may have noticed on the part of the client or family member; evaluation and analysis of the interaction that took place during the visit; a summary statement evaluating the visit and making plans and objectives for ensuing visits.

Table 6-6 An Example of a Process Recording Form

Family
Address
Date of visit
Purpose of visit
Introduction

Client-nurse verbal and nonverbal exchange and interaction	Nurse's comments and analysis

Summary

Process recording requires considerable time to write, analyze, and review. To become skillful in the method requires a great deal of effort, practice, and experience on the part of the nurse. Table 6-6 is a form employed by one agency in the use of this method; other agencies use variations of this form.

Family Analysis

The best description of a family analysis was written by a nursing student as follows:

> During a home visit the community health nurse is involved with the nurse-client interaction to the extent that it is impossible to separate out the different components of the interaction. Often recording of the home visit back at the office does not provide the nurse with insight of the changes that are going on in the family. Webster's definition of *analysis* is an examination of a complex, its elements, and their relations. Thus, a *family analysis* could be defined as an examination of the complex which is a family, the different elements (persons) that compose it, and the relations between the elements.
>
> The value of a family analysis lies in its potential to improve client care. Through doing a family analysis, the nurse is able to get a grasp on what changes are going on within the family and to see her or his role in relation to the initiation of support of these changes. It is exciting for the nurse to get this overview of the family to see in what areas she or he has been effective, how, and what further needs should be concentrated on.

An analysis gives a comprehensive view of the family under study and can be done whenever such a study seems expedient. It requires a thoughtful review of all components of the nursing process, a knowledge in depth of the family, and deliberate study of the effect and direction of the nursing intervention. A guide for writing a family analysis is suggested as follows:

I Assessment
  A Identify health factors.
    1 Physical factors.
      a Chronological age and physical level of growth and development.
      b Past and present physical problems.
      c Special physical abilities.
      d Utilization of medical resources.
      e Nutritional status.
    2 Mental factors.
      a Achievement in school.
      b Ability to solve problems.
      c Presence of sense of humor.
      d Special mental abilities.
      e Sense of self-esteem.

         3 Social-cultural factors.
           a Nationality and cultural influences.
           b Religious beliefs.
           c Interaction with family members.
           d Dominant attitudes toward health, education, and life.
           e Child-rearing skills.
         4 Environmental factors.
           a Characteristics and atmosphere of home, car, and neighborhood.
           b Safety hazards.
           c Attitude of community toward family.
           d Beauty in environment.
         5 Socioeconomic factors.
           a Annual income of breadwinner.
           b Occupation and employment of family members.
           c Management of money.
     B What are the interfamily relationships?
         1 What are the dynamics?
           a Interactional style of communication of family.
           b Decision-making skills.
           c Relationship of family members in seriousness and in fun.
         2 What are the strengths?
  II Nursing diagnosis
     A Identify the needs of the client or family which were focused upon. List them in order of priority. Were the family members in agreement with these needs?
     B Were behavioral objectives written with outcomes agreed upon by the family?
     C State the contract that the family and nurse made mutually.
III Nursing plan and implementation
     A Describe your plan of action to fulfill the contract.
     B What was your rationale for the plan? State nursing principles or theories used as a basis for your actions.
IV Evaluation
     A Were written behavioral objectives utilized as the basis for discussion about outcomes with the family? Did the achievement of objectives concur with fulfillment of the contract? How has the family indicated that they have achieved a higher level of health?

TERMINATING WITH FAMILIES

Many nursing students recognize that separating or terminating with families is difficult and sometimes traumatic for the family and for the nurse. When a caring, therapeutic relationship has evolved in which family and nurse trust each other, have seen and taken joy in distinct progress, and feel a genuine impending distress when the time for terminating arrives, an open talk about the feelings of both parties must take place. For many families, separation by the nurse means rejection—regardless of how well it is explained. For many nurses, it is hard to "give up" a family with whom one has worked effectively and seen excellent results. A mutually agreed upon contract allows both nurse and family to monitor progress and facilitates the termination process through the recognition of goal achievement. By sharing feelings openly, the nurse encourages family members to speak openly and creates the opportunity for explanations of the termination process. Nurses can maintain a friendly relationship with families if they so desire by sending birthday cards, accepting special invitations, and/or occasionally engaging in friendly pursuits. However, the professional relationship in which the nurse was assisting the family toward accomplishment of desired goals must be terminated and released for the next nurse to carry on. Explanation of the difference between friendly and professional relationships must be explained understandably and acceptably to the family.

In the final analysis, all relationships with significant persons have a beginning, a maintenance period, and an ending. Families and nurses must learn to give and to "release" when growth has reached a maturity that helping is no longer indicated. For nursing students, the termination frequently occurs *before* the family's growth has stabilized. In this instance the nursing student must trust that the next nurse will carry on the program with the family. In order to ensure the probability, the student must discuss her or his contract with the family, the implementation of plans, and evaluation of results with the family and with the succeeding nurse. If the family and the succeeding nurse are prepared properly, continuity can be carried on and adjustments made, even though the next nurse is a different person from the first one. It is helpful for the succeeding nurse, who has already been informed and is prepared to deal with the family, to request and listen to the family's explanation of their situation, their interpretation of the helpfulness of the services of the previous nurse, and their sense of accomplishment regarding their growth. In so doing, acceptance is communicated and the new relationship is facilitated.

SUMMARY

Working with families is most easily done by a visit, either in the home or in another convenient setting. The components that must be considered in all visits include activities such as preparation for the visit, meeting the family, setting up an agreeable contract with the family, assessing, planning, implementing, evaluating, and recording. The objective of the nurse is consistently directed toward assisting the family to advance toward wellness.

Assessing the needs of the client or family is a continuous process, during which flexibility and willingness to redirect goals in keeping with the family's desires are essential. Use of assessment tools is important to confirm the accuracy of nurses' perceptions. Planning the nursing intervention includes the determination of methodology and techniques required to meet the assessed and distinctive needs of the client and family. A variety of methods can be used with families, dependent upon their needs. Implementing the plan of care consists of taking action to meet the assessed need. By taking action, the nurse must be aware of the elements influencing behavior during the change process and stress and crisis periods. The nurse must be cognizant of factors affecting the referral process. Evaluating the implementation of a plan consists of determining outcomes in terms of success and family and nurse satisfaction. Evaluation is an ongoing activity, which can be measured and judged more easily with the use of behavioral objectives. Some suggested evaluative techniques include direct observation of client and family behavior, utilization of questionnaires or rating scales, writing anecdotal notes, doing process recordings or tape recordings, and writing family analyses. Recording the nursing activities of the visit succinctly on the appropriate record form completes and summarizes the nursing process.

SUGGESTED READING

Aradine, Carolyn R., and Margaret Guthneck: "The Problem-Oriented Record in a Family Health Service," *American Journal of Nursing,* 74(6):1108–1112, June 1974.

Atwood, Judith, and Stephen R. Yarnall: "The Problem-Oriented Record," *The Nursing Clinics of North America,* 9(2):215–302, June 1974.

Auerbach, Aline B.: *Parents Learn through Discussion,* John Wiley & Sons, Inc., New York, 1968.

Austin, Barbara Leslie: *Sad Nun at Synanon,* Holt, Rinehart and Winston, Inc., New York, 1970.

Axline, Virginia M.: *Dibs, In Search of Self,* Houghton Mifflin Company, Boston, 1964.

Bach, George R., and Peter Wyden: *The Intimate Enemy,* William Morrow & Company, Inc., New York, 1968.

Barnard, Kathryn: "Teaching the Retarded Child Is a Family Affair," *American Journal of Nursing,* 68(2):305–311, February 1968.

Bates, Barbara, and Robert A. Hoekelman: *A Guide to Physical Examination,* J. B. Lippincott Company, Philadelphia, 1974.

Becker, Wesley: *Parents are Teachers,* Research Press Company, Champaign, Ill., 1971.

Bennis, Warren G., Kenneth D. Benne, and Robert Chin: *The Planning of Change,* Holt, Rinehart and Winston, Inc., New York, 1961.

Berne, Eric: *Games People Play,* Grove Press, Inc., New York, 1964.

Berne, Eric: *What Do You Say after You Say Hello?* Grove Press, Inc., New York, 1972.

Bloch, Doris: "Criteria, Standards, Norms: Crucial Terms in Quality Assurance," *Journal of Nursing Administration,* September 1977, 7(7):20–30.

Burr, Wesley R. et al.: *Contemporary Theories about the Family,* The Free Press, New York, 1979.

Chinn, Peggy L., and Cynthia J. Leitch: *Child Health Maintenance,* The C. V. Mosby Company, St. Louis, 1974.

Coletta, Suzanne Smith: "Values Clarification in Nursing: Why?" *American Journal of Nursing,* 78(12)2057–2063, December 1978.

Committee on Ways and Means, *National Health Insurance Research Book,* Government Printing Office, Washington D.C., 1974.

Gebbie, Kristine, and Mary Ann Lavin: "Classifying Nursing Diagnoses," *American Journal of Nursing,* 74:250–253, February 1974.

Gersh, Marvin J.: *How to Raise Children at Home in Your Spare Time,* Fawcett Publications, Inc., Greenwich, Conn. 1966.

Ginott, Haim G.: *Between Parent and Child,* The Macmillan Company, New York, 1965.

Glasser, William: *Reality Therapy,* Harper & Row, Publishers, Inc., New York, 1965.

Gordon, Marjory: "The Concept of Nursing Diagnosis," *The Nursing Clinics of North America,* 14(3):487–495, September 1979.

Gordon, Thomas: *Present Effectiveness Training*, Peter H. Wyden, Inc., Publisher, New York, 1970.

Haley, Jay: *Uncommon Therapy*, W. W. Norton & Company, Inc., New York, 1973.

Harris, Thomas A.: *I'm OK—You're OK*, Harper & Row, Publishers, Inc., New York, 1969.

Hart, Nancy A., and Gladys C. Keidel: "The Suicidal Adolescent," *American Journal of Nursing*, **79**(1)80–84, January 1979.

Holmes, Thomas H. and R. H. Rahe: "The Social Readjustment Rating Scale," *Journal of Psychosomatic Research*, **11**:213–218, 1967.

James, Muriel, and Dorothy Jongeward: *Born to Win*, Addison-Wesley Publishing Company, Inc., Reading, Mass., 1971.

Johnson, Orval G. and James W. Bommarito: *Tests and Measurements in Child Development: A Handbook*, Jossey-Bass, Inc., Publishers, San Francisco, 1971.

Johnson, Vernon E.: *I'll Quit Tomorrow*, Harper & Row, Publishers, Inc., San Francisco, 1980.

Lair, Jess: *"I Ain't Much, Baby—But I'm All I've Got,"* Doubleday & Company, Inc., Garden City, N.Y., 1972.

Langsley, Donald G. and David M. Kaplan: *The Treatment of Families in Crisis*, Grune & Stratton, Inc., New York, 1968.

Levine, Myra E.: "The Pursuit of Wholeness," *American Journal of Nursing*, **69**(1): 93–98, January 1969.

Lippitt, Gordon: *Visualizing Change*, University Associates, Inc., La Jolla, Calif., 1973.

Lippitt, Ronald, Jeanne Watson, and Bruce Westley: *The Dynamics of Planned Change*, Harcourt Brave Jovanovich, Inc., New York, 1958.

Loustau, Anne: "Using the Health Belief Model to Predict Patient Compliance," *Health Values: Achieving High Level Wellness*, **3**(5)241–245, September–October 1979.

Mager, Robert F., and Peter Pipe: *Analyzing Performance Problems*, Fearon Publishers, Belmont, Calif., 1970.

Malasanos, Lois et al.: *Health Assessment*, The C. V. Mosby Company, St. Louis, 1977.

Marram, Gwen D.: "Patients' Evaluation of Their Care—Importance to the Nurse," *Nursing Outlook*, **21**(5):322–324, May 1973.

Marriner, Ann: "Planned Change as a Leadership Strategy," *Nursing Leadership*, **2**(2): 11–14, June 1979.

Meister, Susan: "Charting a Family's Developmental Status—For Intervention and for the Record," *Maternal Child Nursing*, **2**(1):43–48, January–February 1977.

Menninger, Karl: *The Vital Balance*, The Viking Press, Inc., New York, 1963.

Munichin, Salvador: *Families and Family Therapy*, Harvard University Press, Cambridge, Mass., 1974.

Montagu, Ashley: *Touching*, Columbia University Press, New York, 1971.

Murray, Ruth, and Judith Zentner: *Nursing Assessment and Health Promotion through the Life Span*, Prentice-Hall, Inc., Englewood Cliffs, N.J., 1975.

Nierenberg, Gerald I., and Henry H. Calero: *How to Read a Person Like a Book*, Pocket Books, New York, 1971.

Oelbaum, Cynthia Hastings: "Hallmarks of Adult Wellness," *American Journal of Nursing*, **74**(9):1623–1625, September 1974.

Otto, Herbert A.: "A Framework for Assessing Family Strengths," in Adina Reinhardt and Mildred Quinn (eds.), *Family-Centered Community Nursing: A Sociocultural Framework*, The C. V. Mosby Company, St. Louis, 1973.

Parad, Howard J. (ed.): *Crisis Intervention: Selected Readings,* Family Service Association of America, New York, 1965.

Patterson, Gerald R.: *Families: Applications of Social Learning to Family Life,* Research Press, Champaign, Ill., 1971.

Phaneuf, Maria C.: *The Nursing Audit: Profile for Excellence,* Appleton-Century-Crofts, Inc., New York, 1972.

Price, Mary Radatovich: "Nursing Diagnosis: Making a Concept Come Alive," *American Journal of Nursing,* **80**(4):668–671, April 1980.

Rezler, Agnes G., and Barbara J. Stevens: *The Nurse Evaluator in Education and Service,* McGraw-Hill Book Company, New York, 1978.

Roy, Sister Callista: "A Diagnostic Classification System for Nursing," *Nursing Outlook,* **23**:90–94, February 1975.

Samuels, Mike, and Hal Bennett: *The Well Body Book,* Random House, Inc., New York, 1973.

Satir, Virginia: *Conjoint Family Therapy,* Science and Behavior Books, Inc., Palo Alto, Calif., 1967.

Schutz, William C.: *Here Comes Everybody,* Harper & Row, Publishers, Inc., New York, 1971.

Sommer, Robert: *Personal Space,* Prentice-Hall, Inc., Englewood Cliffs, N.J., 1969.

Wright, Beatrice A.: *Physical Disability—A Psychological Approach,* Harper & Row, Publishers, Inc., New York, 1960.

Wu, Ruth: *Behavior and Illness,* Prentice-Hall, Inc., Englewood Cliffs, N.J., 1973.

Yura, Helen, and Mary B. Walsh: *Human Needs and the Nursing Process,* Appleton-Century-Crofts, New York, 1978.

Chapter 7

Working with Groups

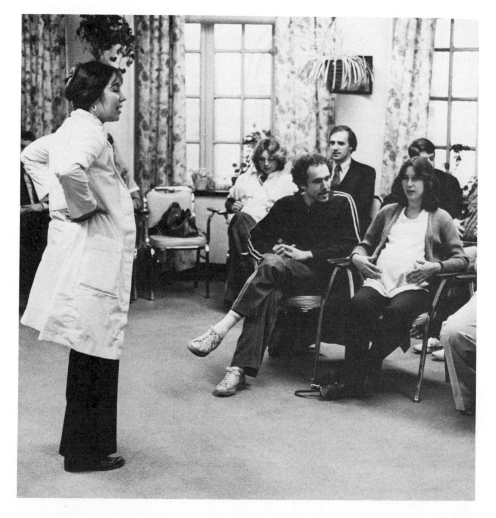

With reduction of home visits which have been primarily directed toward health education and preventive health practices, community health nurses have started utilizing group approaches to reach consumers who want to learn more about content of a specific nature. In a study of McNeil and Holland, it was found that the cost of nurses serving as leaders of groups of postpartum mothers was one-third less per contact than each nurse making home visits to a comparable number of mothers.[1] The cost economy of working with groups is recognized. The added advantages of group work include the support that members give one another, the sharing of ideas and experiences, increased problem-solving capabilities and stimulation of ideas, improved reality testing, greater awareness of the universality of common problems, increased understanding and sensitivity toward others, and opportunity to test new behavior with limited consequences coming from other members of the group.

Community health nurses are learning that group work is an efficient means for facilitating growth of all consumers with whom they come in contact, for giving health education, for teaching about prevention, treatment, and rehabilitation, and for meeting other consumer needs and problems. As nurses become increasingly comfortable and confident in leading or facilitating groups, they can reach out and encourage many more people with common problems to come together to grow, learn, combine forces, give support, and resolve problems. "Nurses must know what benefits can be expected from group experiences and how to intervene in a meaningful therapeutic manner to ensure that these benefits are operant for the individuals in groups."[2] Consequently, nurses must actively seek experiences in group work, and take advantage of the vast opportunities in the community for groups of many kinds, such as prenatal, weight-watching, relaxation, mental health, child discipline, special disease conditions, geriatric, discussion, and many other groups. The opportunity for the nurse to be truly creative is potentially inherent in community group work.

The community health nurse generally has a range of membership in different professional groups such as staff, team, or in-service education meetings in agencies and multidisciplinary meetings with persons from other professions. However, the nurse should become much more involved in community health meetings in which many of the participating members are lay people or nonprofessional representatives. By attending these meetings, the nurse will be exposed to a variety of people with a variety of expectations. The nurse must know *why* she or he is a member of the group and what is to be her or his role and purpose. Specifically, a group may be defined as a plurality of individuals who are in contact with one another, who take one another into account, and who are aware of some significant commonality. It is essential that members have something in common and that they believe that what they have in common makes a difference.[3] Olmsted stated that there are two groups, primary and secondary. Primary groups are composed of members who are warm, intimate, and have personal ties with each other. They are usually of a small face-to-face sort, spon-

---

[1] Helen Jo McNeil and Susan Spangler Holland, "A Comparative Study of Public Health Nurse Teaching in Groups and in Home Visits," *American Journal of Public Health,* 62(12): 1629–1637, December 1972.

[2] From Gwen D. Marram, *The Group Approach in Nursing Practice,* The C. V. Mosby Company, Saint Louis, 1973, p. 5.

[3] Michael S. Olmsted, *The Small Group,* Random House, Inc., New York, 1959, pp. 21–22.

taneous in their interpersonal behavior, and often have common goals. The family, gang, or friendship groups are examples. Generally a primary group is "fun," brings enjoyment of some kind, and functions in a training or supportive capacity. Secondary groups are made up of persons who are apt to be impersonal, rational, contractual, and formal. Members of these groups participate in special capacities and not necessarily as whole personalities. The groups are gathered together as a means to some end and have intermittent contacts. Examples include a range of associations which include professional, office, community, or bureaucratic interests.[4] It is membership and functioning in secondary or community groups for which the nurse needs to become knowledgeable.

PROBLEMS IN ENTERING A NEW GROUP[5]

When entering a new group, whether it is a professional or a community group, the nurse is faced with four issues which must be resolved before she or he can be comfortable. The first is that of *identity*. The nurse must decide on a comfortable role which is acceptable with the group. "What role should I play that is acceptable to me and to the group?" The choices include that of an aggressive talker who wants to gain attention, a quiet listener who avoids all risks, a logical thinker who asks pertinent questions, the obstructionist who finds fault with all suggestions, the humorous person who gives a "light touch" to the conversation at appropriate times, and any number of other possible roles. The second issue involves *control, power,* and *influence.* Who are the persons in the group with the most power and control? Which individuals will influence me or vice versa? Therefore, initial group dialogue may be characterized by individuals' testing and experimenting with different forms of influence until they feel acquainted and have come to terms with the basic structure of the group. *Individual needs* and *group goals* are the third issue with which the group member is concerned. "Will the group goals be such that my own personal goals are met? Can I be committed to work toward a group goal if my own need is not attended to?" In many groups where group goals are decided but little action evolves, the explanation often lies in the fact that the group's needs as a whole were not requested or discussed; therefore, little member commitment was obtained. Early in a meeting group members often take a "wait and see" attitude until the direction of group activity develops, which reveals that personal interests will be met in some way. Then the new members get on the bandwagon. The fourth issue that concerns the new member is *acceptance* and *intimacy.* "Will I be liked and accepted by others in the group? Can I be comfortable and respectful of the others? Is the environment conducive to formal or informal behavior?"

With respect to the four issues involved in entering a new group, there are generally three basic kinds of coping patterns which the membership of the group demonstrate. They are (1) the basically tough, aggressive coping, which is characterized by arguing, cutting down another's points, deliberate ignoring of others, or barbed humor. These behaviors may be manifested in an open, assertive manner or in a subtle, polite

---

[4] Ibid., pp. 17–19.
[5] Adapted from Edgar H. Schein, *Process Consultation: Its Role in Organization Development,* Addison-Wesley Publishing Company, Inc., Reading, Mass., 1969, pp. 32–37.

manner. Members who are resisting the authority or chair of the group can demonstrate aggressive coping by setting up the situation with, "Let's find out what the chair wants and then *not* do it." (2) The basically tender, support-seeking coping is demonstrated by those members who try to form an alliance with another group member or who avoid conflict by being supportive of each other. Their support may be based on genuine understanding or a blindly dependent response to the person in authority, to whom they look for guidance or solution of their problems. (3) The withdrawal behavior based on denial of any feelings is characterized by the passive, indifferent kind of response. The attitude of these group members is that feelings are inappropriate in a group discussion, and they withdraw when feelings become apparent. They let others fight an issue while they sit blandly on the sidelines. However, feelings *are* a reality, and until they are brought out into the open, group tasks representative of the entire group cannot be accomplished.

When groups have worked through the four issues described and reached the point where all members realize that they are a contributing part of the group, they begin to relax and are willing to pay closer attention to each other. Their cooperation as a group becomes apparent and they are ready to attend to group tasks.

Content of Group Meetings

When an individual focuses on what the group is talking about, that is *content*. Members of the group may be working toward accomplishing some task or goal which they have established and will demonstrate specific behaviors that facilitate this end. The behaviors which aid in the group's fulfillment of its *task* include the following:

1 *Initiating* A member proposes a task or goal, succeeds in defining a group problem, suggests an idea for solving the problem, or sets target dates for fulfillment of a task.

2 *Seeking information or opinions* Someone requests facts, asks for an expression of feelings, or seeks suggestions or ideas.

3 *Giving information or opinion* An individual offers facts, provides information which is relevant to the discussion, or gives suggestions and ideas.

4 *Clarifying and elaborating* A member attempts to interpret ideas and suggestions in order to clear up confusions, defines terminology, or indicates alternatives open to the group.

5 *Summarizing* Someone pulls together related ideas, restates suggestions more succinctly, reviews points that have already been considered, or offers a conclusion for the group to accept or reject.

6 *Consensus testing* An individual may ask, "Are we ready to decide?" to test if the group is ready to make a decision.[6]

Behaviors which enable the group to service, maintain good working relationships, and also permit maximum use of the resources of the members are called *maintenance functions*. These include the following:

[6] Ibid., pp. 38–40.

1 *Harmonizing* A member attempts to reconcile disagreements, reduces tension, or attempts to help people to explore their differences.

2 *Gatekeeping* Someone tries to keep communication channels open or suggests procedures that will permit sharing remarks.

3 *Encouraging* An individual will maintain friendly, warm responses to others or will indicate acceptance of others' contributions by nonverbal means (nodding, facial expression).

4 *Compromising* A member whose original idea was not totally acceptable will offer a compromise, will admit an error, or will modify an idea in the interest of group cohesion.

5 *Standard setting and testing* Someone will test whether the group is satisfied with its procedures or will suggest procedures that are available for testing.[7]

In all groups both kinds of behaviors are observed to some degree and are needed in order to get the job done and to keep the group in good working order. Through increasing familiarity with group work, the nurse will be able to identify each behavior as it occurs.

Group Process

When an individual focuses on how the group is handling its communication, i.e., who talks how much or who talks to whom, that is *group process*. It refers to the "here and now" of what is happening within the group. Many groups do not wish to look at group process because they are reluctant to analyze their own and others' behavior. If individuals do not wish the group process to be studied, it should not be urged. However, if a group is willing to take 5 or 10 minutes at the conclusion of their meeting to discuss *only* the group process as it occurred, it facilitates understanding and openness and promotes cohesion of the group. If group process is to be studied, an observer should be selected whose function is to remain objective and carefully observe the group interaction. When the group is ready to examine and reflect on their process, the observer reports personal observations to the group and discussion ensues. The observer does not provide a summary of the discussion, is free to participate in the discussion, and only reports on *process* that facilitated or inhibited the group.

Leading or Facilitating a Group

All nurses have had exposure to several group theories, such as the interpersonal framework of Sullivan; the communication framework of Watzalawick, Jackson, and Satir; the group dynamics and group process framework of Cartwright and Zander, Knowles and Knowles; and the existential and gestalt frameworks of Perls, Maslow, and Rogers. As a result, most nurse leaders possibly have an eclectic theoretical orientation which, if so, is advantageous in providing flexibility and freedom for interventions with groups. The nurse leader who works with a variety of groups in a variety of settings has the opportunity to adapt and apply the most suitable theory with the group and intervene at the level of skill and understanding which she or he has mas-

[7]Ibid., pp. 40–41.

tered.[8] After continuously studying and practicing group work, an understanding of the concepts, principles, and assumptions of each theory becomes internalized, and the nurse's effectiveness as a leader increases. In many groups the entire responsibility for leadership is expected to be taken by the chairperson. However, if the chairperson wishes to involve all members in any group, she or he can do so. By virtue of their presence in the group, all members can be seen as possessing some degree of responsibility or resourcefulness which must be ferreted out and revealed by the leader. All members ideally need and want to have a commitment toward fulfillment of the task for which the group was organized. Therefore, it is up to the leader to set the stage. Rather than acting as an authoritarian leader, the leader can consciously act as a *facilitator,* a person who makes sure that the task and process function of the group are carried out effectively. By doing so, the group process moves smoothly and members are reminded to continue moving toward clearly defined and mutually set goals. The leader does not dominate but encourages or facilitates all members of the group to assume responsibility for accomplishing the group goals.[9]

The task of facilitating a group takes preparation and forethought. Some of the factors and questions that must be considered by the leader are preparation, getting the group started, defining the group's purpose and objectives, and concluding the group meeting.

Preparation "Why is this group being formed? Will the members become interested and motivated to work toward purposeful goals? What can I say or do that will catch their attention?" When the leader prepares for the meeting by thoroughly studying appropriate readings, reference materials, and audiovisual aids, ideas for presenting the material in an interesting and provocative way to group members can be the focus. Sometimes a short, appropriate film or tape recording will be effective or, depending on the group, a game or exercise may be the initial way of "warming up" a group and gaining their attention.[10] The ability of the leader to be resourceful, original, or creative in the beginning enhances the possibility for gaining the group's attention and ultimate commitment.

Getting Started What physical set-up will be most conducive to establishing a comfortable environment? Sometimes the chairs are best arranged around a table or in an intimate circle. The environment should be such that the temperature, light, and ventilation are adequate. If a blackboard, charts, or audiovisual apparatus are needed, they should be set up before the meeting begins. The leader should arrange the room so that it communicates the climate intended.

When the group members enter the meeting room, the leader should greet each individual with friendliness and make each feel welcome. When all members are gathered together, the leader should start the meeting by introducing herself or himself and the overall purpose for being together. Time should be taken for all to become acquainted and feel a pleasant friendly atmosphere. An effective method for enabling

[8]Marram, op. cit., pp. 123-124.
[9]Elwin C. Nielsen, "Process Groups for Self-Learning and Problem Solving," (unpublished) paper presented at "Accent on Creative Nursing" workshop, Park City, Utah, 1969.
[10]William C. Shutz, *Joy,* Grove Press, Inc., New York, 1967, pp. 117-186.

others to relax and feel free to express their ideas is to state that a way for getting better acquainted is for all members in the group to introduce themselves and tell something about themselves. The leader should always start the introductions with a personal description and whatever information she or he wishes the group to know. Dependent upon the length and extent of the leader's self-introduction will be the contribution of each succeeding member's description of self. Groups tend to conform to the norm established by the leader. If the leader divulges quite a bit of appropriate information, group members will feel more at ease in following the lead and revealing pertinent information about themselves, and general group comfort will be facilitated. Sometimes, it is a good idea to have name cards until the members are well acquainted.

Purpose and Objectives   The general purpose for which the group was formed should then be expressed or reiterated by the leader, and the plan to involve the members should be executed, whether it is a game, a film, or something deliberately provocative. When the time arrives for the group members to discuss, react, or present their thoughts, the leader should ask for an expression of ideas and *facilitate* discussion from that time on. The facilitator's task involves (1) getting an expression of ideas from all members, (2) keeping the conversation centered on the issues of the meeting, (3) promoting the establishing of objectives or goals that are agreeable to all members, (4) encouraging the divulgence of each member's resources or skills, and (5) promoting a commitment to the group's goals by all the members. When words or terminology are not clear, the facilitator can ask group members for clarification. If the members of the group expect the facilitator to solve an issue, she or he can return it to the group by rephrasing or reinterpreting the issue at stake. At periodic intervals summarizing statements of the discussion or important points can be phrased for the purpose of clarifying the progress of the discussion. Tolerance, patience, open-mindedness, and flexibility are important for successful meetings. As all persons in the group are encouraged to speak their ideas, thoughts are formulated and crystallized, are spread to others contagiously, and the group inevitably progresses toward new, sometimes exciting conclusions. By being willing to hear different viewpoints expressed, a flexibility and open-mindedness is facilitated and each member learns.

Concluding the Meeting   The facilitator must be aware of the passage of time and stay within the scheduled limits. It may be advisable to warn the group that only 5 or 10 minutes are remaining. Or the facilitator may summarize the progress of the discussion and ask "What have we decided to do?"; "Have we included everything?"; "What assignments or tasks do we need to do before the next meeting?" or "When shall we meet again?" If all members have participated verbally in the issues of the meeting or have demonstrated nonverbal interest, there will be a general aura of purposeful activity and involvement that denotes a successful meeting.

Criteria for Group Growth

To determine if the group is developing into an effective, workable unit which functions smoothly, the following questions can be asked.

1   Does the group have the capacity to deal realistically with its tasks?
2   Is there basic agreement within the group about ultimate goals and values?
3   Does the group have a capacity for self-knowledge?
4   Is there an optimum use of the resources available within the group?
5   Does the group learn from its experience? Can it assimilate new information
and respond flexibly to it?[11]

A successful and satisfying group is one in which all members participate and
assume responsibility for functioning in an integrated fashion. Facilitation of such a
group is a stimulating learning experience for the leader. The composition of the group
does not affect the process of leading or facilitating a group. Professional groups or
community groups can be facilitated by a skillful leader who consciously draws out
the resourcefulness of the members, whether they have lay, nonprofessional, or professional identities. Much of what happens in groups can be attributed to the leadership, particularly if it is creative and flexible.

COMMUNITY GROUPS

Multiple groups exist in communities and can be studied from a variety of perspectives,
depending on the nature of the group. Marram has identified and described the characteristics of several community groups; the ones of special interest to community health
nurses include the therapeutic groups, self-help groups, growth groups, and reference
groups. Other community groups with whom community health nurses are acquainted
are community action groups, in-service training groups, and others.

Therapeutic Groups

Therapeutic groups are concerned with promoting emotional health and educating
individuals to adjust as normally as possible to situational and developmental crises.
These groups are made up of essentially "normal" people who are in need of primary
prevention measures and education. They are faced with a particular crisis and can
profit from learning about more satisfactory methods of coping. Community therapeutic groups are made up of individuals with special interests, common problems,
or developmental similarities, such as juvenile delinquents, elderly persons, mothers
and children, school-age children, individuals with concern for mental health, family
services, chronic diseases or diagnoses, rehabilitation, cultural deprivation, and similar
groups.[12]

Self-help Groups

Self-help groups are "organized and operated by group members themselves without
the supervision, guidance, or leadership of professionally trained group leaders." They
"solve problems of members as defined by members." They are "groups of, for, and
by the client."[13] Benefits in belonging to a self-help group include support and em-

[11] Schein, op. cit., pp. 61–63.
[12] Marram, op. cit., pp. 24–36.
[13] Ibid., p. 39.

pathic understanding from others, an impetus to change which is promoted through the use of role models who have successfully changed their lifestyle, and a knowledge of how to "work the system" from role models who have incorporated the essentialities required of the new lifestyle or environment. Examples of self-help groups are numerous and reveal the effectiveness of peer or consumer supportive systems which is not gained through other means. Successful self-help groups include Alcoholics Anonymous, Alanon groups, Parents Anonymous, Synanon, Weight Watchers, TOPS (Take Off Pounds Sensibly), Ostomy groups (colostomy, laryngectomy, etc.), Recovery, Inc., and many others.[14]

Growth Groups

Growth groups were designed originally "to help learners incorporate the values of (participatory) democracy into their own processes of personal and collective decision making and problem solving."[15] Emphasis on experimentation, feedback, and collective deliberation continues to be promoted in an environment which is purposely democratically free and permissive. Goals of growth groups are of an educative or therapeutic nature relating to self-awareness, self-discovery, self-enhancement, and self-actualization. Many groups directly or indirectly aim toward increasing members' ability to achieve greater skill and insights so that "take-home" knowledge will be synthesized into greater effectiveness on the job. In growth groups, the opportunity and freedom to express oneself in new ways is frequently experienced with immediate feedback from the group participants. Members often become aware of inhibitions and innate hidden capacities and gain greater sensitivity regarding their ability to relate with others. The benefits of growth groups for all participants are not easily identifiable or documented. Individual reports can be found reflecting both pro and con attitudes regarding the practices of such groups. Examples of growth groups are rampant. They include T groups, sensitivity training, group dynamics, encounter, marathon, human potentiality, self- and body awareness, assertiveness training, and many, many others.[16]

Reference Groups

Reference groups designate groups which are real or imaginary and serve to influence the individual regarding perception and judgment of others, objectives, and principles which occur within her or his life sphere. As a member of a reference group, the individual behaves according to a perception of the real or anticipated beliefs and values of that group. Reference groups include religious, racial, ethnic, familial, and occupational groups. The individual can be responsive to several reference groups, but often will utilize one group in particular for evaluating behavior. Reference groups can change as the individual grows and develops through the total life process. " 'Membership' in a reference group involves a vague, yet all-encompassing identification with others in the group."[17] The individual uses reference groups as a pervasive influence

[14] Ibid., pp. 39–53.
[15] Ibid., p. 55.
[16] Ibid., pp. 55–72.
[17] Ibid., p. 75.

throughout life and allows them to play an important role in a concept of self. It is through the eyes of referent others that a person determines who she or he is and what she or he should do.

People can be active participants of a group, but it will not be a reference group for them until they allow the group to decide for them about goals worth seeking, the manner in which to proceed, and the values and standards worth attaining. Reference groups provide individuals with positive sources of identification and security and play a role in formulating distinct identities. They give individuals a sense of belonging, a continuity and sameness with the outside world which is like others in the group but, at the same time, provide a sense of autonomy and separateness as a distinct member. Reference groups can be classified in two ways in terms of their effect on members. They can be constructive or destructive for individuals in influencing identity formation, role adjustment, and self-concept.

Destructive reference group affiliations divide the self, instill a low self-esteem, or cause an imbalance in the satisfaction of needs for homonymy and autonomy. "Certain ethnic, racial, occupational, and religious groups have acquired a negative image in our society. Being a member of these groups elicits certain prejudices from others."[18] In Chap. 5, an explanation of identity conflicts for some ethnic minorities is explored. Constructive reference group members assist individuals in integrating self-perceptions, affording a balance of autonomy and homonymy, and increasing self-esteem. Members of constructive group affiliations experience feelings of knowing who they are, where they are going, and suffering few self-doubts. They are goal directed, self-assured, and self-directive. They are frequently leaders in the community.[19]

ROLE OF THE NURSE LEADER

A frequent goal of nurses who are leaders of groups "is to foster the development of the group as a whole and to enhance the growth of individuals in the group."[20] This is true particularly of therapeutic and growth groups. For self-help groups, nurses should know about them and be supportive of them. They should not expect to be members of such groups unless they are experiencing the problems common to the specified group. If called in as a consultant, they should elicit the desires of the group asking for assistance and provide information or resources as requested. Knowledge about the influence and identification of reference groups in the lives of individuals serves to broaden the assessment perspective of nurses and aids in understanding the basis for some observed behaviors.

In facilitating a climate that is nonthreatening and growth-producing for members of a group, the nurse must be knowledgeable about group dynamics, sensitive to the meaning of body language, perceptive of the behavior of each member of the group, confident in directing the activities of the group, capable in moving the group toward its stated objectives, neutral in the event an argument occurs, supportive of positive contributions or changes of behavior that occur with individual group members who

[18] Ibid., p. 80.
[19] Ibid., pp. 75–84.
[20] Ibid., p. 193.

are visibly anxious, knowledgeable about specific content if acting as a resource person, reinforcing of the group's successful activities, and aware of timing for summarizing and concluding meetings. For nurses who wish to become effective group leaders, frequent practice with groups must be sought, even though inner self-confidence and assurance is hesitant. The composition of all groups is different, regardless of the type of group, and learnings gained in acting as a group leader are invaluable and contribute toward development of seasoned leadership characteristics.

CO-LEADING GROUPS

For nurses who feel unprepared to assume complete responsibility for leading a group, the option of being a co-leader is often available. A co-leader can be in the position of a subordinate to a professional leader who is recognized as having theoretical knowledge and expertise, or the co-leader can have an equal participatory role with a primary leader and share knowledge and insights from a perspective different than that of the primary leader. Co-leading combinations are numerous, such as physician, psychologist, or social worker with nurse, female with male, superior with subordinate.

Advantages in co-leading with a professional leader are dependent upon the nurse's needs and capabilities. Learning takes place when the expertise, technical abilities, and theoretical knowledge of the professional leader are observed and critically analyzed. Group participants are enabled to observe interactions between the master teacher and learner and translate the meaning of the behavior in terms applicable to their own situations. Opportunity for role-playing or simulating a dyad can be used for learning purposes. When ready, the learner co-leader can assume primary responsibility for leading the group under the supervision of the professional leader. Analyses of group process, interactions, behaviors, and decisions can be studied and discussed evaluatively following group sessions.

For the nurse who elects to co-lead on a participatory equal basis with the designated leader, experience is gained in learning to work together cooperatively. Goals, procedures, process for intervening, interrupting, and making decisions must be mutually understood between the two leaders before convening the group. With the two leaders, each has an individual perspective in observing group members, encouraging interactions, and providing direction toward the stated purpose of the session. When one leader is interacting with the group, the second leader has the opportunity to observe, actively listen, seize cues as they become apparent, intervene, and give the first leader time to reflect while temporarily relieved of the intense "heat" of responsibility for the direction of the interaction. The manner in which the co-leaders interact with each other whether in agreement or disagreement can be an excellent demonstration for group members to observe and imitate. Open, honest, spontaneous communication can be releasing and therapeutic when demonstrated well. For co-leaders who are a female and male combination, the opportunity for group members to observe instrumental and expressive roles, and modeling of interaction dynamics between a female and male, is beneficial. Also, viewpoints, insights, and supportive statements based on a sexual perspective can be freely expressed by the participatory leader of the same or opposite sex as appropriate within the context of the group discussion. Following group sessions, the two leaders can analyze their theoretical framework and share their thoughts from two perspectives regarding the dynamics that occurred, can give feedback to each other regarding their leadership characteristics and behavior, and can mutually evaluate and contribute ideas for future meetings of the group.

Frequently female nurses who co-lead with a male whether from the same or another discipline, tend to be quiet and wait for the male to extend the opportunity to participate before they intervene. As co-leaders, female nurses must practice the experience of taking the initiative and interrupting when they believe the interaction can benefit from such an intervention. Nurses must gain increasing self-assurance as leaders of groups and must practice behaviors that seem initially uncomfortable (e.g., aggressiveness) if they truly desire to become effective group leaders and co-leaders.

GETTING THROUGH TO GROUPS

People behave differently when they are members of a group than when they are alone. Individuals join groups for a variety of reasons and are generally members of several different groups. The motivation to belong to a particular group is apparently related to an individual's sense of isolation. Individuals want to gain the security, economic and socialization advantages, sense of belonging, or sense of strength (since the group is bigger and more powerful and less vulnerable than the individual is) that a group may give. Members are exposed to the group's beliefs, values, jargon, way of dress, and other identifiable characteristics and adopt the group norm on a continuum of complete acceptance to little acceptance according to individual needs.[21] If the acceptance of a particular group is complete, the members sacrifice their own individuality and identity, and frequently are unaware that they have made such a choice. Many individuals have a more moderate commitment to groups, behaving in a given group in relationship to the benefits they derive personally. Some persons reflect the group norm only while in the presence of the group.

With the composition of groups made up of individuals who are either wholly or partially committed, or have hidden motives or personal reasons for belonging, the nurse cannot realistically expect to get through to *all* members of a group. All that can be done is to make the best effort possible. When presenting an idea or activity to a group for the purpose of getting them involved, the nurse must accept and/or welcome resistance or opposition. Opposition is a sign of involvement! In order to persuade individuals to accept a new idea or activity, they must pass through a stage of resistance first—that of readjusting or giving up some of their own ideas associated with their current thinking about that subject. When people feel pressured to change their current thinking, some resistance will always be aroused.

There are three levels of listening when someone else is speaking. There is (1) the nonhearing level, where receivers are not listening at all. They may have eye contact with the speaker and give appropriate responses at right intervals such as "I see," "Mm," but their thoughts are elsewhere. (2) There is the level of hearing where

[21] Earnst G. Beier, *The Silent Language of Psychotherapy*, Aldine Publishing Company, Chicago, 1966, pp. 152-154.

individuals remember and are able to repeat the sentences the speaker said; however, there is no real absorption of ideas. (3) There is the level of hearing where listeners *think* about what the speaker is saying. Thinking means doing mental work—evaluating, comparing the thought with something else, analyzing, predicting likely outcomes, making decisions.[22]

For third-level listeners who are thinking and feeling an inner pressure in response to the speaker's ideas, resistance is inevitable. Something within them is responding to the speaker's ideas—saying that the speaker is making sense, yet they do not want to let go of their own ideas without fighting. Their resistance and struggle to convince the speaker of their own point of view means they are fully involved in considering the speaker's position. They are open to persuasion. If or when the opposition becomes intense, it is best for the speaker to become neutral, objective, and no longer press the new point of view. By so doing, these listeners are given time to think about and reflect on their own and the speaker's positions, and will come to terms later with their final decision regarding the issue.[23]

In talking with groups, the nurse must be cognizant of several obstacles that impede assimilation of ideas. Members of groups have varying interests, and all are not listening equally attentively. As a group member, it is easy to release responsibility for listening and responding to the speaker when other group members are known to be consistently responsive and articulate. As a consequence, there is unequal participation and feedback from members in a group. Some individuals may take the opportunity to make an irrelevant statement or ask an irrelevant question. When doing this, they are meeting personal needs, and other members of the group lose interest if the interruption becomes prolonged. Individual group members frequently have to suppress or control emotions which are innately aroused dependent upon the issues under discussion. When this happens, attention is temporarily distracted from active listening. Invariably within every group, there are members who respond in their unique styles and capitalize on the opportunity to perform before an "audience." There always seems to be an inhibited shy person who is afraid of saying the "wrong thing," so says nothing. For the extrovert, the temptation to talk and impress is irresistable, and the purpose of the group session is subordinated to that individual's personal needs. Or there may be group members who desire to attack the speaker as an authority figure and can generally depend on getting support from the group, either actively or passively.[24]

Awareness of the possible obstacles that can occur in groups and having a clear idea of the intended goals for group meetings helps the nurse to manage group sessions. It is frequently facilitating to orient the group's thinking at the beginning of each session. Group members should know the purpose of the meeting and what the leader intends to do. Examples should be given at every opportunity so that multiple interpretations are reduced, and feedback from group members should be encouraged. To be sure that the participants are listening and understanding, the speaker must request

[22] Jesse S. Nirenberg, *Getting through to People,* Prentice-Hall, Inc., Englewood Cliffs, N.J., 1963, p. 109.
[23] Ibid., pp. 124–144.
[24] Ibid., pp. 179–181.

their ideas at intervals. This is best done with questions from the speaker designed to stimulate thought or with the encouragement of questions coming from the group. Instead of answering a group member's question immediately, it is often strategic to ask that person to elaborate further regarding personal thoughts on the subject, or wait for another group member to respond to the original question. In this way, group participation is encouraged and an environment of "freely expressed" ideas is fostered.

A certain amount of irrelevancy should be allowed during each group session since the various group members are mentally traveling along their individual routes of associated ideas at different paces. The leader can always terminate digressions whenever necessary. It is advisable to reiterate ideas by means of new applications or new examples at periodic intervals and to summarize at the conclusion of the meeting. In this way, the leader assists group members to assimilate the expressed ideas and allows time for the reinforcement of ideas to take root.[25]

SPECIAL TECHNIQUES FOR USE WITH GROUPS

Introducing new ways of dealing with the content of each meeting attracts the attention of group members, maintains interest and/or control, and "gets through" to most individuals much better than the sole use of words. Introductory statements or overviews of the subject material can be presented with the use of special films, slides, graphs, statistics, or fact sheets. Short plays, skits, or short stories can be used to dramatize a problem. Poems, songs, role-playing, and psychodrama can also be utilized, or a variety of exercises or techniques can be initiated which involve the participation of group members and accelerates the process of gaining their attention.

Strengthening Exercise

An exercise that nursing students seem to need or that awakens their consciousness about personal self is Otto's personal inventory of strengths. This exercise requires each group member to write all the personal strengths which can be thought of. Usually a brief time limit for writing is given. In every group, there are always one or two participants who can think of only a minimal number of strengths. Follow this exercise with a similar one in which group members are asked to pair; the directions require each partner to write all the strengths about each other that come to mind, then share verbally with each other what was written. When the partners share, the environment becomes relaxed and much pleasure, laughter, and camaraderie is expressed. This exercise seems to have an impact of positive force with particular individuals (those who probably need it the most), and builds self-confidence and belief in one's capabilities.

Active Listening Exercise

An exercise which offers group members the opportunity to experience what "active listening" is consists of pairing, e.g., having one person talk about herself exclusively

[25] Ibid., pp. 179–188.

for 3 minutes and requesting the second person to listen attentively but nonverbally throughout the entire 3 minutes. In this exercise the listening person becomes aware of the difficulty of actively listening—particularly when unable to respond verbally in any way. The talking person learns how easy or how difficult it is to talk about self and may learn some new insights about self.

Many exercises or experiments described for families are contained in the book, *Peoplemaking*, by Virginia Satir. Trying these experiments in a learning situation for nursing students or for families who are willing to receive new ideas causes individuals to reflect and become consciously aware of family dynamics. Learning to cope in a structured situation differently and positively takes time, a conscious behavior change, a determination to change, and repetitive practice.

With all exercises, the leader must elicit the thoughts of the group regarding their reactions and observations while the exercises were being enacted. Experiential insights of group or family members, whether positive or negative, are valuable for the entire group to hear, consider, and discuss. When exercises and/or techniques are used, the length of time, purpose, and appropriateness must always be carefully planned by the leader. Group or family discussions can be directed sensitively toward learnings intended to be attained by the use of the exercise. Often a group or family will bring out the points desired without specific intervention of the leader. Insights gained by individual members through experiential exercises are not perceptible or known to exist unless the member shares his or her thoughts with the group. The leader must accept that insights occur differently with individuals—some are spontaneous and some germinate, waiting for the right time to sprout.

ASSERTIVENESS TRAINING

Enrolling for assertiveness training in a class or group has been an activity which many individuals have considered essential in recent years. The incorporation of the principles of assertiveness training in the content of classroom lectures for nursing students has been received enthusiastically by many of the students. The quiet and passive students have responded, knowing that they need the training, but are frequently frightened to try it.

As stated by Bakker, all people need a territory, a place to live, a field of action, a stage on which to act out the story of their life. In the daily practice of everyone's life from birth until death, all persons' borders are disputed in one way or another. To maintain territory which they regard as their own, individuals have to exert steady outward pressure. In daily human affairs the territorial boundaries of individuals are continually under stress; borders can move outward or inward, and the pressure on each side can be increased or decreased. Persons attempting to expand their territory and consequently move in on another person's territory are labeled as exhibiting aggressive behavior. In the context of territoriality, *aggression* means any act which results in the extension of the territory that a person holds.[26] *Assertiveness* is an act of

---

[26]Cornelis B. Bakker and Marianne K. Bakker-Rabdau, *No Trespassing: Explorations in Human Territoriality*, Chandler & Sharp Publishers, Inc., San Francisco, 1973, pp. 49–52.

independence whereby people maintain control over all parts of their territory. In other words, the defense of one's territory is assertive when it is direct and specific to the area under attack. Assertive persons rely on feelings of adequacy and strength. Defensive persons give the appearance of weakness because they are unsure of their borders or their ability to defend them. Consequently, they do not convey self-assurance to others.[27]

In learning how an individual defends or acquires territory, the word "weapon" is used to signify the means that is used for aggressive or assertive purposes. Every person uses weapons, uses the ones best known and which have been effective on previous occasions. For example, to resolve an interpersonal conflict, there must be a clear understanding of the issue involved. Whose territory has been invaded? What weapons were used by the aggressor? There are a great variety of weapons used to take over another's territory, and frequently, they are not obvious ones, are not recognized as weapons, and are successful in distracting the defender from the primary issue.

Assertiveness training classes deal with the concepts of human territoriality, assertive behavior, and ways to handle selected situations assertively. Recognition of subtle fighting techniques or weapons and learning to defend one's territory consciously, honestly, and successfully has value in achieving the objectives that one desires. Also, a keen insight into techniques used in interpersonal conflicts leads one to evaluate the consequences of any selected behavior. On occasion, an individual may choose to consciously acquiesce to an aggressive behavior because of the secondary undesirable consequences of assertiveness. Consciousness of one's own behavior and weapons, and another's behavior and weapons when an issue is at stake—whether assertive or aggressive, overt or very subtle—is the desired goal.[28]

When nurses have studied, practiced, and feel well acquainted with the concepts of human territoriality, assertive behavior, and weaponry, they can teach assertiveness training to groups of citizens desiring to learn. Lists of weapons and how they are used and successfully counteracted can be role-played and practiced in a variety of practical situational contexts.

COMMUNITY ACTION GROUPS

There are times when nursing students come into contact with citizens who are dissatisfied with their immediate conditions and want to do something about them. It is helpful to assess where the citizens are, listen to the issues that bother them, elicit all the facts of the situation, inquire regarding obstacles that may interfere, and investigate if participation from "outsiders" will be accepted. If the citizen group is willing to incorporate the various skills of nursing students, a number of valuable activities can be implemented. Students can act as informal leaders, consultants, data-gatherers, active participants, facilitators, advocates, investigators, instructors, or in capacities where action and/or knowledge are required. Many of the activities are opportunities for experiential learning and prepare students for future citizen and/or professional leadership activities.

[27]Ibid., pp. 59–62.
[28]Ibid., pp. 169–172.

Self-Perpetuation of the Community Action Group

The principles of community organization practices must be remembered and reviewed with the citizen group if necessary and appropriate. After the issue for which action is deemed essential is decided and objectives determined, other factors bearing consideration by community action groups include recruiting additional interested citizens, gaining support from recognized power structures, fund raising, informing through publicity, and campaigning through legislative or political channels.

Recruiting To recruit additional interested citizens, it is necessary to talk to various individuals in the community informally. The ideas and opinions of those who may be interested in the issue should be elicited in one-to-one informal conversations. Whenever a citizen seems to have a conviction about an issue, an invitation should be extended to attend a planned meeting which will convene at a well-known and easily accessible location in the local community. The suggestions of various citizens should be integrated and implemented as feasible. Personal invitations to attend meetings which fit the schedules of citizens get best results. If transportation or baby-sitting facilities are needed in order to persuade citizens to attend, arrangements should be made for these resources. Citizens should be reminded before scheduled meetings by telephoning, sending postcards, or canvassing door-to-door. When the meeting is held, the chairperson should be a recognized and well-liked leader of the local community. After the purpose for the meeting has been explained, all persons attending the meeting should have the opportunity to speak and participate in formulating plans. Assignments or short-term action projects can be designated and divided among group members so that each is involved and feels a part of the group. A meeting that is well-placed and purposeful is the responsibility of the leader. If all participants feel they have contributed in some way, the meeting is generally considered successful, and additional citizens are recruited.

Support from Power Structures Support of an identified issue from certain key leaders or recognized establishments in the community is always helpful. To determine which leaders are sympathetic to an identified issue requires initiative and risk-taking behavior of citizen participants. Visiting recognized influential citizens or talking to representatives of the news media, government, schools, professional organizations, labor unions, and other recognized establishments takes preparation. The organizational structure of each establishment should be requested in advance so that preparation for entering the bureaucratic system with a formal hierarchy of authority can be made. Desired results are best attained when correct procedures for entering a system are followed and the appropriate persons representing the chain of command of the bureaucratic institution are approached. Facts, logic, and straight-forward arguments about the identified issue should be well-formulated in the mind and easily articulated. It is good strategy to listen to the position of the community leader first, agree on points when there is agreement, and be ready to question or answer points with which there is disagreement. It is always wise to be objective, friendly, and respectful in manner. When support from a community leader is obviously unavailable, the visit should be terminated and other leaders consulted from whom to request support.

When a community leader is sympathetic to an identified issue, the form of support which she or he is able to give should be requested directly. This may be a signature, request for money, use of a building, equipment, an advertisement, or active membership in the citizen group.

Fund Raising Solicitation for funds can be done through mailings, advertisements, pledge groups, parties, garage sales, bake sales, dinners, dances, special events, fairs, canvassing, or by writing a grant proposal. For the citizen participants who are involved with planning for and raising money, the method decided upon for soliciting funds requires knowledge about details ensuring successful implementation. Small fund raising can be fun, such as organizing a raffle, garage sale, dinner-dance, and similar functions. If the citizen group decides that a grant proposal has distinct possibilities for procuring the needed funds, a committee can be assigned the task of writing and submitting a proposal. Organizations from whom funds can be solicited should be identified and the required explanatory documents obtained regarding correct procedures to follow. Usually guidelines are available for writing a formal application for funds. The guidelines must be read carefully and followed exactly. The written proposal must make use of clear, succinct language, contain documentation of facts, objectives, evaluative methods, a bibliography, and a reasonable budget. Writing a grant proposal is an excellent learning experience for citizen participants since the process consolidates the purpose, objectives, planning, implementation, and evaluation of a project into a complete whole. The act of writing a proposal tends to increase the commitment and conviction of participants.

Informing through Publicity Communicating about an identified issue to the general public can be achieved by various means. Whatever method is selected, it is necessary initially to catch the public's attention, be explicit about the content of a message, and have all necessary details included in a message. If the message addresses itself to immediate concrete problems that citizens are experiencing, attention will be easily secured. Pictures, cartoons, phrases, and colors are noticed if they show humor, emotion of some type, or timeliness. It is advisable to know the selected target population—what they are thinking and feeling—and address the content of the message within a context that has meaning for the target population.

The means for informing the public include leaflets, newsletters, newspapers, posters, television media, slide shows, films, exhibits, and letters to the editor. Organizing a speaker's bureau is another way of informing community groups. The choice of the publicity method must be carefully planned. Learning to prepare an attractive poster, leaflet, or newsletter may require consultation from local community artists and publicity experts. Knowing the strategy for approaching a local newspaper or writing an acceptable article has advantages toward getting desired results. Slide shows can be created by citizens committees and be "right on target." If films are used, they must be previewed and carefully selected in terms of the intended message. Canvassing on a door-to-door basis is a grass roots method which can be done for some projects. It tends to broaden one's perspective of human behavior and is best done in selected neighborhoods. (See Chap. 4.)

Organization is Key to Political Influence

Becoming thoroughly knowledgeable about the political process is advantageous for all nurses in behalf of themselves and their clientele. Health care and politics go hand in hand. Government funds support the vast majority of health care programs. To become familiar with the legislative process at the local, state, and national level and play a participative role in influencing changes favorable for selected health care issues, it is wise to know how a bill becomes a law, how to lobby most effectively for the passage of a bill, and how to communicate with legislators. When an organized group (e.g., nurses, health professionals, community action groups) supports a health issue and actively lobbies for its adoption, the chances for influencing its passage are greatly enhanced if they understand the process a bill goes through before becoming a law. The example in Fig. 7-1 is written at the state level. Note how many committees study each bill, the number of readings before the legislature, and the number of opportunities for amending the bill or rewriting it. Also, note that the bill as amended or rewritten must be accepted by *both* legislative houses before it is passed. In addition, after a bill has been processed through both houses, it still can be vetoed by the governor. Bills that are passed and signed by the governor into law have one more obstacle before they can be implemented. Funds must be appropriated by the legislature. This involves study by the appropriations committee and a similar procedure taken within the legislature before funds are finally approved and money allocated.

To have the greatest impact on a health care bill, education of the legislators regarding the merits or inadequacies of the bill is essential. For the most part, legislators are not totally familiar with the intricacies of the health care field. They welcome letters with well-presented facts regarding the pros and cons of each bill under study. They want to know how their constituencies are viewing bills being processed. Getting to know the names of the legislators of your state and communicating regularly regarding specific health care issues has influence on how the legislators vote.

Lobbying is the direct personal presentation of citizen views to government representatives. Interests of nurses and health care issues of particular interest to nurses are represented on the local, state, and federal levels by lobbyists employed by the American Nurses' Association. Additional tactics employed by small groups of nurses organized to support or defeat a particular bill, however, also have influence and must not be disregarded. It is important to know the local state legislators' records regarding positions on various issues. The legislators should be supplied with facts about identified health issues for which support is desired. All studies, articles, statistics, data, and research with which to persuade legislators should be made available to them. The best arguments are individualized personalized ones whether delivered in person or in a brief yet convincing letter.[29] When hearings are held by legislators on identified health issues important to a group of nurses or citizens, as many supporters as possible should be gathered to attend the hearings and speak in support of the bill. Evidence of enthusiasm, conviction, and commitment from an organized group has an influential impact on legislators.

[29] The O. M. Collective, *The Organizer's Manual,* Bantam Books, Inc., New York, 1971, pp. 170–172.

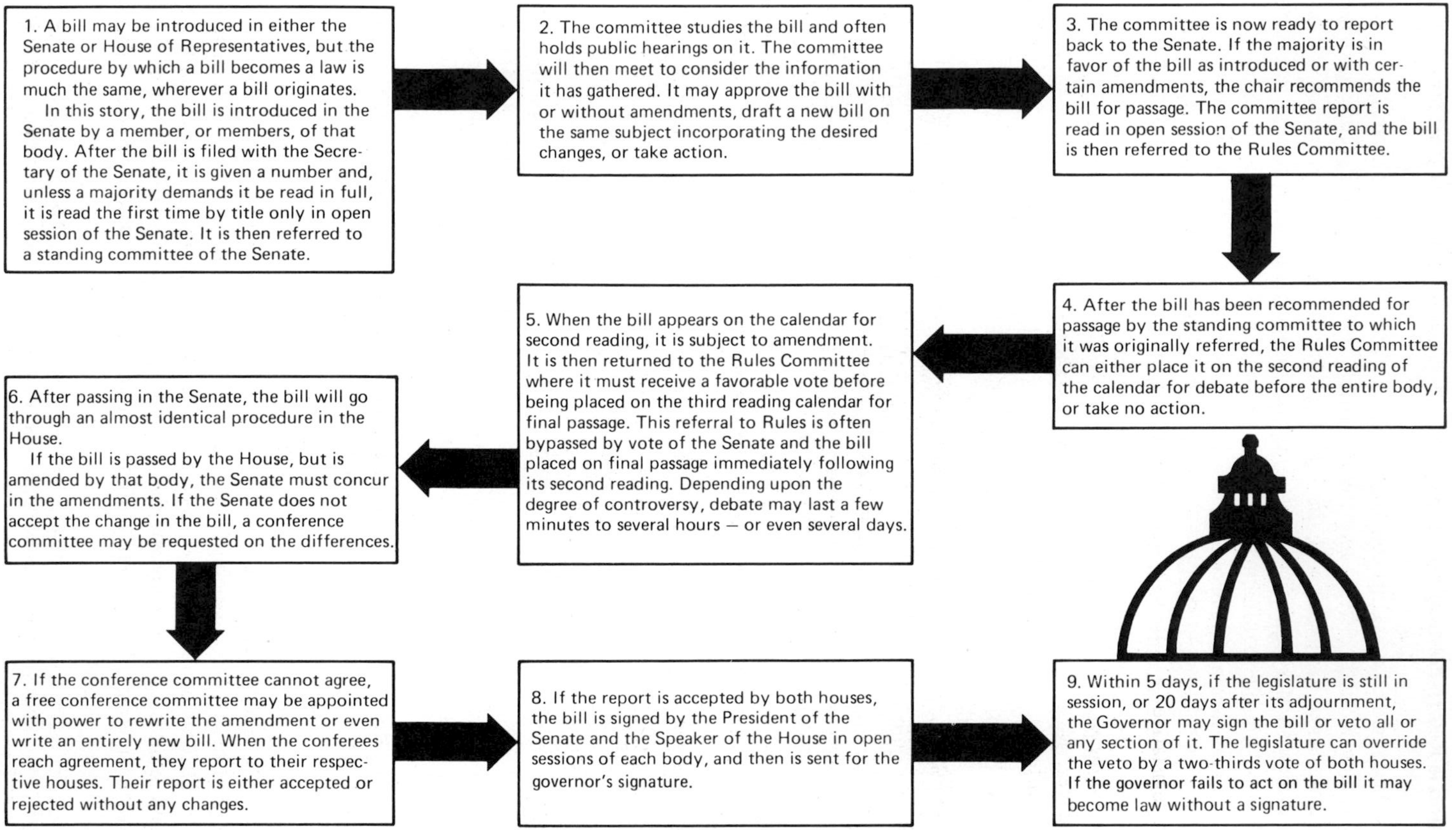

1. A bill may be introduced in either the Senate or House of Representatives, but the procedure by which a bill becomes a law is much the same, wherever a bill originates.
   In this story, the bill is introduced in the Senate by a member, or members, of that body. After the bill is filed with the Secretary of the Senate, it is given a number and, unless a majority demands it be read in full, it is read the first time by title only in open session of the Senate. It is then referred to a standing committee of the Senate.

2. The committee studies the bill and often holds public hearings on it. The committee will then meet to consider the information it has gathered. It may approve the bill with or without amendments, draft a new bill with the same subject incorporating the desired changes, or take action.

3. The committee is now ready to report back to the Senate. If the majority is in favor of the bill as introduced or with certain amendments, the chair recommends the bill for passage. The committee report is read in open session of the Senate, and the bill is then referred to the Rules Committee.

4. After the bill has been recommended for passage by the standing committee to which it was originally referred, the Rules Committee can either place it on the second reading of the calendar for debate before the entire body, or take no action.

5. When the bill appears on the calendar for second reading, it is subject to amendment. It is then returned to the Rules Committee where it must receive a favorable vote before being placed on the third reading calendar for final passage. This referral to Rules is often bypassed by vote of the Senate and the bill placed on final passage immediately following its second reading. Depending upon the degree of controversy, debate may last a few minutes to several hours — or even several days.

6. After passing in the Senate, the bill will go through an almost identical procedure in the House.
   If the bill is passed by that body, but is amended by that body, the Senate must concur in the amendments. If the Senate does not accept the change in the bill, a conference committee may be requested on the differences.

7. If the conference committee cannot agree, a free conference committee may be appointed with power to rewrite the amendment or even write an entirely new bill. When the conferees reach agreement, they report to their respective houses. Their report is either accepted or rejected without any changes.

8. If the report is accepted by both houses, the bill is signed by the President of the Senate and the Speaker of the House in open sessions of each body, and then is sent for the governor's signature.

9. Within 5 days, if the legislature is still in session, or 20 days after its adjournment, the Governor may sign the bill or veto all or any section of it. The legislature can override the veto by a two-thirds vote of both houses. If the governor fails to act on the bill it may become law without a signature.

Figure 7-1 How a bill becomes a law. *Note:* The title of this chart could also be *How to Prevent a Bill from Becoming Law.* Every step is a potential chance for the bill to be defeated as well as passed. Generally it's easier to defeat a bill than it is to pass one. (*From* How a Bill Becomes Law, *The Senate and House of Representatives, State of Washington, Olympia, Wash., 1980*)

Target Lobbying Impact on the political decision-making process occurs when:

1 It comes from organized activity.
2 It is done by a specific group.
3 It is for a specific purpose.
4 It is aimed at a specific target.
5 It is done at the appropriate time.[30]

Additional information congruent with these five critical factors interprets how best to achieve legislative outcomes desired by an organized group.

1 *It comes from organized activity.* Few individuals can lobby effectively acting by themselves. Most political change occurs through organized groups who have a *continuing* interest in a problem area. A major tactic of an organized group is not only to organize itself into a political interest group, but to form coalitions with other interest groups having mutual legislative goals.

2 *It is done by a specific group.* A legislative network is the organizational vehicle for achieving desired goals. If members are broadly representative of the community located in two-thirds of the state's legislative districts, it is possible to achieve contact with most of the state's legislative leaders.

3 *It is for a specific purpose.* The legislative goals of an organized group can be established each year by the Board of Directors and reflect the highest priority goals to be achieved by legislative action. The number of issues being actively lobbied should remain at one or two so as to concentrate existing resources. Legislators are faced with understanding thousands of bills each session.

4 *It is aimed at a specific target.* The key to target lobbying is to focus the lobbying activity of the organized group only on those individuals or committees who are able, at a given point in time, to move (or kill) the bill of interest. Much energy and effectiveness can be dissipated if this simple precept is not followed.

5 *It is done at the appropriate time.* There are four times when lobbying is effective. In order of priority those time periods are: (a) Before the primary election; (b) Between the primary and the general election; (c) Between the general election and the legislative session; (d) During the legislative session. Political effectiveness is enhanced when lobbying is done *before* the legislative session begins.

Communicating with legislators in state capitols can be done by letters and postcards, a telephone hot line, telegrams, mailgrams, night letters, and straight wires. When a letter or postcard is written, mail it directly to a legislator in the state capitol. Address the legislator by title and name (Senator John Doe or Representative Jane Doe), State Legislature, name of capitol city, name of state, and zip code number. During legislative sessions, a toll-free public opinion hot line will be in operation in most states. Dial the number, when the operator comes on the line, give your name and address and a brief message intended for a specific legislator. There is no charge and the messages are promptly delivered to the intended legislator. *If the line is busy,*

---

[30] *Legislative Advocates Guide of the Puget Sound Health Systems Agency,* National Health Planning and Resources Development Grant No. 10P 55000204, U.S. Department of Health, Education, and Welfare, 1980.

call back. The Public Opinion Message (POM) provides the fastest and least expensive form of telegraphing a legislator. Mailgrams are also sent over a network that is received directly in the legislative building. Mailgrams will accommodate longer messages. Night letters or straight wires can be sent but are more expensive forms of communication.

Tips on Communicating with Your Legislators

1 Sit down and do it! A message to a legislator can make the difference. Your legislators are *elected by you.*
2 Address members of the legislature with due respect. Make sure that full name, initial, and title are correct.
3 Be vocal. Tell how the matter under consideration affects you, your organization, or your community. Your message is your lobby.
4 Be brief.
5 Be specific. Let them know what you want. Identify the bill or specific issue. To you there is the one interest. Legislators must deal with hundreds of bills and maybe even several on the general topic you are contacting them about.
6 Be as factual as possible.
7 Ask for an answer. You have made your views known. It is now the legislator's turn to say where she or he stands.
8 Be sure to leave your name and address.
9 Be polite. A nasty message or threat can easily work to your disadvantage.
10 Remember to say thanks. After your legislator has pushed for your bill, a note of thanks will go a long way toward building goodwill the next time you want something—and there is always a next time.

Seven Pressures to Which Legislators Are Regularly Subjected[31]   When it comes to the manner in which legislators make decisions on bills and related matters, there are seven different pressures to which legislators are regularly subjected. These are

1 *Personal convictions*   These are self-imposed through personal experience. This in turn is largely the result of personal contacts, personal education, personal background and close family, personal friends, and campaign helpers.
2 *Constituency pressures*   These result from the legislators' perceptions of what their constituency believes, wants, or needs.
3 *Interest groups' lobbyists*   These are the persons, employed or not, whom special interest groups send to the state capitol to represent their legislative views.
4 *Legislative peer group pressures*   These are the pressures to which legislators are subjected (or which they seek) from fellow elected members of their caucuses, legislative committees, or the general legislative body.
5 *The executive branch of government*   These are pressures which the governor or executive department heads and staffs exercise on the legislative branch.
6 *Political party pressure*   This pressure occurs in strong-party states or where the political party has taken an instrumental role in the legislators' elections.
7 *Legislative staff pressures*   Increasingly, staff members of the legislators

---

[31]C. Montgomery Johnson and Associates, 501 Securities Building, Olympia, Wash. 98501, 1980.

themselves or of legislative committees or caucuses influence the shape of legislative proposals originating with special interest groups or individual legislators.

Normally, the most effective pressures on members of the legislature are personal convictions and constituency pressures, followed closely by legislative staff members in whom legislators place great trust.

For groups wanting to play a participative role in influencing health care legislation, knowledge about the legislative process, when, where, and how to lobby and/or communicate with legislators is essential. Organized activity can make a difference in legislative outcomes, and the experience for members of the group is invaluable.

EVALUATING GROUP MEETINGS

In a study done by Chopra which evaluated the ingredients contributing to successful groups, the primary characteristic was found to be their high degree of motivation. Concurrent with the motivation are the attributes of enthusiasm, a high level of interest, and commitment. He found that the nature of the group task is not as significant in motivating as the fact that members of such groups are *motivated to work with each other.* He concluded that the factor which is critical to the success of a group is the way members interact with each other and treat each other's ideas. In successfully motivated groups, when an idea is disclosed by one member, other group members will spend a lot of time and energy trying to fully understand the idea, exploring its implications, and suggesting ways to overcome its limitations. In other words, members of a motivated group work *with* the person who offered the idea and try to help strengthen it. All too often, this kind of strengthening behavior is not common in community groups. The reversal is more apt to be practiced—that of immediately raising objections and reasons for why an idea will not work. As a consequence, the person who suggested the idea, regardless of her or his overt reaction and behavior, feels "put down," and the meeting goes on and on.[32]

When evaluating group meetings, factors to consider for analysis include the following:

1 *Goals* Were the goals explicit? Were the group members interested and involved in attaining the group goals? Was the interaction goal-directed?

2 *Leadership* What were the interpersonal influences of the leader? Was leadership distributed and participatory in nature or was it obviously controlled by one or two individuals? Was there evidence of a coalition of power?

3 *Psychosocial environment* Was the psychosocial climate warm, friendly, spontaneous, informal, cold, threatening, etc? Were group members generally responsive and considerate of each other?

4 *Physical environment* Were the arrangements (seating, chairs, table, blackboard, equipment) suitable? Were the temperature of the room, lighting, acoustics satisfactory?

[32] Amarjit Chopra, "Motivation in Task-Orientation Groups," *Journal of Nursing Administration,* 3(1):55–60, January–February 1973.

5 *Mechanics of meeting* Was the meeting well-paced? Was the agenda followed? Were all reports included? If a group decision was made, was this managed satisfactorily?

6 *Skills of group members* Which members attended to the task functions of initiating, seeking information or opinions, giving information or opinions, clarifying and elaborating, summarizing, and checking for consensus? Which members performed the maintenance functions of harmonizing, gatekeeping, encouraging, compromising, and setting standards? Did all group members interact and/or participate? Were communication skills used such as paraphrasing, perception checking, giving "I" messages? Was there evidence that nonverbal behavior was noted?

7 *Problem-solving skills* Were all group members cognizant of the issues? Was the group productive? Did they listen to each one's ideas in a constructive fashion?

8 *Other factors* Were there other factors that were generally helpful or upsetting in terms of the group's behavior and productivity?[33]

Evaluation is a necessary ongoing process and, when done conscientiously, assists in improving future meetings. In every community, group meetings are convened with little thought directed toward evaluation. One such community council meeting which met regularly was observed by a nursing student and described as follows:

> Group dynamics showed a loosely knit group purposelessly meandering toward a vague goal. There were poor habits of communication, little verbal expression of feelings, and an underlying atmosphere of tension. There was little cooperative effort, give and take, and limited efficiency.

The above group description occurs all too frequently in community meetings. Group participants do little to change or improve meetings, and general deterioration and dissatisfaction occurs. For groups convened by nurses, evaluation must always be considered essential if success and goal attainment is the desired end product.

COORDINATION OF INTERDISCIPLINARY PERSONNEL

Nursing is a highly diversified occupation and there are some tasks which nurses undertake that are noted to be their function exclusively. One such task for community health nurses is that of *coordination* of client care. When working intensively with families, community health nurses learn of a variety of agencies or personnel who are communicating with one or more members of the family constellation and often arrange for a conference of all interested personnel or call the representative of each discipline individually in an effort to coordinate the services given to the family. This particular task is essential and must be *stressed* as an important, vital attribute of community health nurses.

When people are drawn together to combine their efforts for a given purpose, this is coordination. *Coordination* is the orderly arrangement of group effort to

---

[33] Jack R. Gibb, Grace N. Platts, and Lorraine F. Miller, *Dynamics of Participative Groups*, National Training Laboratories, Washington, D.C., 1951.

provide unity of action in the pursuit of a common purpose.[34] In community health nursing, the common purpose that is focused upon by the various health representatives is the integration of community health services to the client or family. Communication among personnel of all community health facilities is essential to share information and discuss what is involved in sustaining or improving the health status of the given client and family. All too often coordination of health personnel is not initiated spontaneously and duplication or overlapping of services to a family occurs. By assuming the task of coordination with responsibility, the community health nurse contributes to the assurance that continuity of client care will be achieved.

Health Teams

In community health nursing the composition of health teams varies according to the purpose for gathering the group and the nature of the personnel attending. Community health teams can consist of professional persons or a combination of lay and professional persons. Some examples of health teams include: (1) a group of community health nurses working in an agency; (2) a group of community health nurses, licensed practical nurses, home health aides, and community aides working in an agency; (3) a community health nurse representing a health department, a social worker representing the department of public assistance, a physician, a school principal, a school nurse, an individual representing the housing authority, etc.; (4) a community health nurse and paraprofessional personnel representing a clinic service such as family planning; (5) a community health nurse, a medical nurse representing the hospital, a family member, a family counselor, a school teacher, and other involved personnel; (6) a community health nurse and a group of lay volunteers getting ready to execute a screening test for vision, hearing, or a related health measure.

As a member of any health team, the nurse must know her or his purpose for being included as a participant and must be willing to assume responsibility for leadership when it is needed or implicit. The preceding discussion about working with groups is applicable to developing effective health teams, particularly if the team meets on a regular basis. The emphasis of health teams should always be focused on their mutual purpose: action directed toward agreed-upon goals, and effort expended toward maintaining working relationships which facilitate satisfactory progress. Sharing of information in a noncompetitive fashion enables all team members to function in a responsible, satisfying manner and expedites the purpose for which the group was brought together.

Multidisciplinary Conferences

When the community health nurse initiates a plan for a conference of professional persons representing several community agencies to discuss a care plan for a specified family, she must call all the professionals serving the family and invite them to a stated place at a specific time for the purpose of pooling their information about the family. All too often representatives of the various community agencies working with

[34] James Mooney, "The Coordinative Principle," in Joseph A. Litterer (ed.), *Organizations: Structures and Behavior,* John Wiley & Sons, Inc., New York, 1963, p. 39.

a given family are not called together to unify their purposes and goals in giving assistance. If the conference is to be one in which confidential information is disclosed, the nurse should clear the exchange of such information with the client by asking him to sign a release-of-information form. In so doing, the client is made aware that such a conference is in the planning stages and realizes the purpose is to facilitate the integration of health services in her or his behalf. When talking to the professionals who are being invited to the conference, the nurse should state that the client has signed a release slip, indicating that it is permissible to bring confidential records and reports. The nurse should also state expectations of the contribution the professional person will make to the conference. If the professional wishes to bring printed materials that will aid in the group's understanding, this would be desirable. If it seems expedient to invite the professional worker's supervisor to the conference, the correct procedure for doing so should be requested. By being knowledgeable about the organizational structure of allied community agencies and complying to their modus operandi, coordination is facilitated.

A review of the four points in the discussion of leading or facilitating a group will give the nurse ideas regarding the plan of procedure for the conference. It is important to remember that all group members should be introduced. Too often in professional groups, the assumption is made that everyone knows each other, and this is not necessarily so. Another essential point to realize is that the initiator of the conference must act as the leader or facilitator. When the group is composed of community professional leaders, it is often tempting for the nurse to transfer the leadership of the conference to another person who holds a more imposing position. However, when the nurse is the initiator, she or he *must* perform responsibly as the leader or facilitator. If refreshments will serve the function of relaxing the group members, the leader should plan for and offer coffee and cookies early in the conference. If a blackboard is available and the listing of issues coming out in the discussion seems indicated, the leader should feel comfortable about writing the ideas on the blackboard or asking someone else to do so. Regardless of the composition of the group, whether it is made up of more important persons professionally than the leader, the nurse leader should perform the tasks of facilitation with confidence and responsibility.

Coordination with Other Community Professionals

It is essential that the community health nurse keep open lines of communication with the family physician at all times. This may require several telephone calls or a visit to the physician's office. When the nurse's function with the family is interpreted to the physician, the nature of the nurse's role as a coordinator can be emphasized. The nurse can explain how she or he was referred to the family, and the contract agreed upon with the family for continued service. The nurse can describe her or his assessment of the family situation and identify the need for validation of specific information given or activities prescribed by the physician. By bringing out omissions, misperceptions, or incompletions of the family's health knowledge or practices in the home, the nurse can demonstrate the efficacy of her or his role as a coordinator. By working *with* the physician, making the physician knowledgeable about the obstacles hindering the family's implementation of stated recommendations, and stating the nursing goals, the essentiality of the nursing function with the family is communicated.

It is equally important for the nurse to keep open lines of communication with all allied professionals representing different community facilities who are serving commonly known families. For example, if the family receiving public assistance is on the active roster of the housing authority's and family counseling service, those workers representing allied disciplines should be made aware that the nurse is also serving the family. The main objective for keeping open lines of communication is to work toward common, unified goals in serving a family. Otherwise, families are given the opportunity to exploit the services of several community facilities in a number of ways or become confused about the multiplicity of professionals who are communicating varying suggestions. When starting work with a family, the nurse should inquire about the possibility of other community facilities to whom the family is known. A point should be made of requesting the names of other workers who are serving the family currently and explain that she or he wishes to talk to them. If it is necessary for the family member to sign a release-of-information slip, the form should be made available and signed at the time of the visit. The nurse can then arrange for a multidisciplinary conference or talk to each professional individually. It is vital that all community workers, professional and nonprofessional, discuss their contact with the family so that common goals are determined and methods of working toward goals are synchronized. Attitudes toward a given family are concomitantly revealed, discussed, and adjusted toward the purpose of accomplishing the mutually accepted goals. To reiterate, the community health nurse is in the best position to initiate and implement coordination of community health services to the client and family whenever several professionals are involved.

Coordination with Other Community Nonprofessionals

The utilization of nonprofessionals or paraprofessionals in the medical and nursing ranks is increasing rapidly in our society. With the advent of a wide selection of trained and untrained community workers, it is essential that all community professionals relate in a manner that enhances and enriches the capabilities of these people. The term *nonprofessional* refers to those persons whose tasks are mainly of a technical nature, i.e., licensed practical nurses, nurse's aides. Paraprofessionals refer to those persons within the community who are unskilled, have little formal education but are being trained successfully as assistants in some capacity to professionals, i.e., home health aides, community aides, nutritional aides. Studies have shown that locally selected trainees or paraprofessionals living in impoverished neighborhoods have a strong desire to work and earn a decent living. When they have received on-the-job training, they contribute effectively to a given program because they know a great deal about the persons living in the "hard to reach" neighborhoods who have need for health services. The paraprofessionals can be genuinely open, empathic, supportive, and persuasive of people they serve because they have lived through very similar circumstances. They can overcome barriers of cultural differences, communication difficulties, and lack of motivation and understanding which have often interfered when professionals have dealt with the disadvantaged groups.[35]

[35] Wilbur Hoff, "Older Poor Adults Trained as Home Health Aides," *Public Health Reports,* 83(3):184–185, March 1968.

Because nonprofessionals and paraprofessionals are demonstrating their effectiveness in the health field, it is essential that professionals recognize and utilize their services to a maximum degree, promote the idea of teamwork, and take advantage of the extra time to perform professional functions which they alone can best fulfill, i.e., managerial tasks or research studies. Relating effectively to nonprofessionals is no different from relating to any other group of people. Nonprofessionals want to be seen and heard, deemed worthy, and considered a part of the team. They generally know their assets and limitations, appreciate recognition of their strengths, and are honest about their limits. They appreciate and want supervision when their competencies are uncertain. Even though they are not so well educated academically as professionals, they have knowledge and attitudes about the local community which are valuable for the professional to know. Often they have an intuition and compelling warmth for the consumer which the professional may not possess. In team meetings, the skilled, effective nurse is one who provides a comfortable environment and encourages all members to contribute their ideas whether they have a professional, nonprofessional, or paraprofessional status. It behooves the nurse leader to recognize all the team members, regardless of their professional standing, as worthy of her or his respect and interest. By working *with* the nonprofessionals and paraprofessionals and not *over* them, the performance of the team as a whole is enhanced and satisfying.

It is not unusual for professionals to demonstrate lack of enthusiasm toward the skills of nonprofessionals. When a negative reaction of professionals is perceived, it often results from a lack of understanding and acceptance of paraprofessionals in any field of nursing. One way to counteract negative attitudes is to provide the opportunity for professionals to talk openly about their feelings and attitudes in a series of closed sessions. When it is appropriate and timely, their special strengths and capabilities as professionals should be pointed out in conjunction with the paraprofessional's requirement for competent supervision, and a new relationship which is reality-based and very much needed may be started. Emphasis on the responsibility for directing or supervising other personnel to give skilled health services to consumers is highly important and demanding. When done well, the professionals can take pride in the fact that they played an essential role in facilitating expert care to the client, which restored the client's dignity, worth, and health.

Interdisciplinary Teams

Interdisciplinary coordination implies team-centered leadership which is based on the nature of tasks to be completed and usually connotes an extended period of time. An interdisciplinary team is made up of several persons, each representing a specific discipline, who agree to work as a group toward a common purpose with mutually acceptable goals. The interdisciplinary team differs from the multidisciplinary team in its commitment, mode of operation, and shared responsibilities.

Working as a member of an interdisciplinary team requires an understanding of the goals, roles, tasks, and communication processes of the group. Each member must have respect for and accept all other members of the group. A team composed of several persons representing different disciplines and professions does not always exemplify what is commonly considered "team spirit." For the group who has consented to be a team, effort, commitment toward common goals, understanding of the role boundaries of each discipline, willingness to learn each other's language and viewpoints in problem-solving and decision-making sessions, patience, and persistence must be realized.

Initially when an interdisciplinary team comes together, they have limited knowledge about each other. They must assess the level of education each member possesses in terms of each one's discipline; interpret and clarify the capacities, territories, and roles of each discipline, including functions which seem to overlap or duplicate; and feel comfortable about communicating openly so that viewpoints and assumptions can be questioned and criticized. In getting acquainted, sometimes members show deference to particular individuals—a reaction representative of the caste system in each profession. Or relationships with persons of the opposite sex are such that a characteristic superior-subordinate manner is apparent. If this happens, the behavior must be consciously changed before a true team-centered leadership can evolve. It takes time and patience to understand about the territories, limitations, and extensions of roles of other disciplines. When there is role ambiguity or role conflict, negotiations must be made eventually about who will do what. It helps to develop ground rules for governing the communication process and operation of the team. As necessary, the rules can be cited when contradictions or stalemates take place. The process of solving problems and making decisions as a team is a shared responsibility which, practically speaking, differs considerably from practicing independently, an activity which each individual is accustomed to doing. Learning to share, coordinate, and integrate with others takes time, patience, and persistence but can be rewarding, eventually, when the many inevitable obstacles have been ardously overcome and the goals of the endeavor have been attained. Experimentation with interdisciplinary teamwork is on the increase and when the demonstration of collaborative relationships has shown that the provision of health care is superior in terms of efficiency, efficacy, quality, and satisfaction to all concerned, these new interdisciplinary models may well be accepted and emulated.[36]

USE OF CONSULTATION

There are many times when a community health nurse needs consultation. Because the nurse is a generalist, consultation in specialized fields of nursing and closely allied disciplines such as nutrition, social work, psychology, community development, and others is essential and edifying in improving the quality of services given to the consumer. Consultation can be gained from many sources, such as nursing supervisors, clinical specialists, physicians, social workers, nutritionists, specialists for specific disease categories or social conditions, and others.

The consultation process involves the following three features: (1) the consultee, an individual who has defined a need—something she or he wishes to know; (2) the consultant, the person with the expertise to fulfill the need; and (3) the problem area with which the consultee wants help. The problem can be a health need of a client or a community activity in which the consultee is involved. The assumption is made by the

[36] Robert A. Hoekelman, "Nurse-Physician Relationships," *American Journal of Nursing,* 75(7):1150–1152, July 1975.

consultee that the consultant can fulfill the need, and the consultant assumes that the consultee will be prepared with all the data relevant to the problem.

When the consultee desires help in regard to a problem, she requests an appointment with the appropriate consultant and gathers all data she believes will be pertinent to the consultation. This may involve making a summary of all essential information from the family record and forwarding a copy of the summary to the consultant prior to the appointed time. Or, it may involve reading more-inclusive references pertinent to the problem to enable the consultation to be on a sharing, knowledgeable basis between two professionals.

The success of the consultation is dependent on several factors listed as follows: whether the consultee (1) has correctly diagnosed the needs, (2) is adequately prepared with all essential data, (3) has adequately communicated the needs to the consultant, (4) has selected the appropriate consultant, and (5) has thought through the consequences of implementing ideas or changes that may be recommended by the consultant.[37] The conversation between consultant and consultee should be two-way, not in one direction only. Ideas suggested by the consultant should be thoroughly explored by both parties as to their feasibility in relation to the specific problem area being studied. Since the consultee is personally acquainted with the problem area, its idiosyncracies and complications, she or he alone can suspect if an idea will work. When the consultee is helped to see a problem area more comprehensively and is actively involved in reaching realistic conclusions regarding the next steps, there is a greater likelihood for satisfaction with the consultation process and subsequent demonstration of successful learning. Rather than expecting the consultant to provide answers, the consultee should anticipate the problem-solving approach to be used, during which the consultant aids in sharpening the diagnosis of the problem area and suggests ideas or alternatives that have not already occurred to the consultee. It is up to the consultee to make the ultimate decision as to what action to take, since she or he is fully acquainted with the uniqueness of the problem. Inherent in the consultation process is the requirement for openness in discussion, a comfortable, sharing environment, and a bond of mutual respect which facilitates a helping relationship between the two participants.

While learning to make use of a wide selection of available consultants within the community, the community health nurse develops an expertise in becoming an exceptional generalist who is recognized by all community specialists. The nurse gains recognition as the individual who has a grasp of the wholeness of health practices occurring within her or his particular community.

SUMMARY

Community health nurses have started utilizing group work as an efficient means for reaching out and facilitating growth of consumers with whom they come in contact. In conducting group work they must know the problems of entering a new group— how to focus on the content of meetings, how to utilize the communication process, how to lead or facilitate, and how to evaluate group growth.

[37]Schein, op. cit., p. 5.

Some community groups with whom community health nurses should be knowledgeable were identified as therapeutic groups, self-help groups, growth groups, reference groups, assertiveness training groups, and community action groups. Nurses must seek out opportunities to act as leaders, co-leaders, consultants, data-gatherers, facilitators, advocates, instructors, or in any capacity where action and/or knowledge is required. Group work provides excellent experiential learning for professional leadership roles and activities.

The coordination role of the community health nurse is vital to ensure that health services to a family are integrated and purposeful. Someone must bring into a common focus all of the elements of the health care system which are directly or indirectly involved in giving services to individuals, families, or groups. This means teamwork with professionals, nonprofessionals, and paraprofessionals who are working in the various health facilities in a community. Being a generalist, the community health nurse must be prepared to use consultation, which will result in increased expertise for self and beneficial activities for consumers.

SUGGESTED READINGS

Bakker, Cornelis B., and Marianne K. Bakker-Rabdau: *No Trespassing: Explorations in Human Territoriality,* Chandler & Sharp Publishers, Inc., San Francisco, 1973.

Beckhard, Richard: *Organization Development: Strategies and Models,* Addison-Wesley Publishing Company, Inc., Reading, Mass., 1969.

Beier, Ernst G.: *The Silent Language of Psychotherapy,* Aldine Publishing Company, Chicago, 1966.

Berne, Eric: *Principles of Group Treatment,* Grove Press, Inc., New York, 1966.

Bradford, Leland P., Jack R. Gibb, and Kenneth D. Benne: *T-Group Theory and Laboratory Method,* John Wiley & Sons, Inc., New York, 1974.

Bradford, Leland, Dorothy Stock, and Murray Horowitz: "How to Diagnose Group Problems," in Sandra Stone et al., (eds.), *Management for Nurses,* The C. V. Mosby Company, St. Louis, 1976.

Bumbalo, Judith A., and Delores E. Young: "The Self-Help Phenomenon," *American Journal of Nursing,* **73**(9):1588–1591, September 1973.

Brown, Barbara (ed.): "Politics and Power," *Nursing Administration Quarterly,* 2(3):1–96, Spring 1978.

Cartwright, D., and A. Zander: *Group Dynamics,* 3rd ed., Row, Peterson & Company, Evanston, Ill., 1968.

Clark, Carolyn Chambers: *The Nurse as Group Leader,* vol. 3, Springer Publishing Company, New York, 1977.

Jacobson, Sylvia R.: "A Study of Interprofessional Collaboration," *Nursing Outlook,* **22**(12):751–755, December 1974.

Janis, Irving L.: "Groupthink," *Psychology Today,* **5**(6):43–46, November 1971.

Johnson, David W.: *Reaching Out,* Prentice-Hall, Inc., Englewood Cliffs, N.J., 1972.

Johnson, David W., Frank P. Johnson: *Joining Together: Group Theory and Group Skills,* Prentice-Hall, Inc., Englewood Cliffs, N.J., 1972.

Knowles, M., and H. Knowles: *Introduction to Group Dynamics,* Association Press, New York, 1969.

Lewis, Howard R., and Harold S. Streitfeld: *Growth Games,* Harcourt Brace Jovanovich, Inc., New York, 1970.

Lippitt, Ronald, Jeanne Watson, and Bruce Westley: *The Dynamics of Planned Change,* Harcourt Brace Jovanovich, Inc., New York, 1958.

Marram, Gwen D.: *The Group Approach in Nursing Practice,* The C.V. Mosby Company, Saint Louis, 1973.

Maslow, Abraham: *Toward a Psychology of Being,* D. Van Nostrand Company, Inc., Princeton, N.J., 1972.

Nirenberg, Jesse G.: *Getting Through To People,* Prentice-Hall, Inc., Englewood Cliffs, N.J., 1963.

The O. M. Collective: *The Organizer's Manual,* Bantam Books, Inc., New York, 1971.

Redman, Eric: *The Dance of Legislation,* Simon and Schuster, New York, 1973.

Rogers, Carl: *On Becoming a Person,* Houghton Mifflin Company, Boston, 1961.

Satir, Virginia: *Peoplemaking,* Science and Behavior Books, Inc., Palo Alto, Calif., 1972.

Schein, Edgar H.: *Process Consultation: Its Role in Organization Development,* Addison-Wesley Publishing Company, Inc., Reading, Mass., 1969.

Schmidt, Cheryl Klouzal: "Five Become a Team in Appalachia," *American Journal of Nursing,* **75**(8):1314–1315, August 1975.

Sedgwick, Rae: "The Role of the Process Consultant," *Nursing Outlook,* **21**(12):773–775, December 1973.

Sullivan, Harry Stack: *The Psychiatric Interview,* W. W. Norton & Company, Inc., New York, 1954.

Thomstad, Beatrice, Nicholas Cunningham, and Barbara H. Kaplan: "Changing the Rules of the Doctor-Nurse Game," *Nursing Outlook,* **23**(7):422–427, July 1975.

Veninga, Robert, and Delphie J. Fredlund: "Teaching the Group Approach," *Nursing Outlook,* **22**(6):373–376, June 1974.

Watzlawick, P., J. Beavin, and D. Jackson: *Pragmatics of Human Communication,* W. W. Norton & Company, Inc., New York, 1967.

Chapter 8

Promoting Health and Self-Care Practices

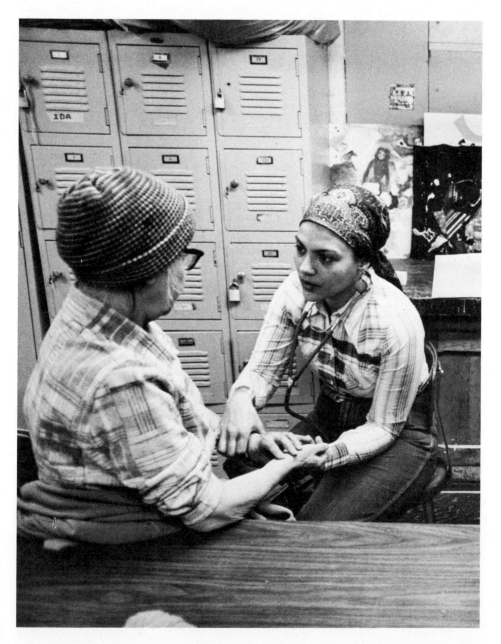

Wellness as defined by Dunn is an integrated method of functioning that is oriented toward maximizing the potential of which the individual and family are capable, within the environment where they are functioning.[1] All individuals have the capacity to become more well because all individuals participate in their own health at all times. This is done through their beliefs, their feelings, and their attitudes toward life as well as in more direct ways, such as exercise, relaxation, diet.[2] As proposed by the Simontons, "the mind and body are to be viewed as an integrated system"[3] and must be dealt with as such. No longer can the body be seen separately as a physical entity only. The whole person consists of a body, mind, and emotions and all are unified into an end product which becomes the nurse's challenge of assessment. In what way can this client (whole person) be stimulated to desire more wellness?

Wellness is a concept upon which community health nurses can capitalize! Moving toward positive states of health may require complete reeducation of some clients, encouragement, and/or reinforcement of wellness behaviors of others. Since community health nurses are interested in improving the health of population groups as well as individuals, commitment to health promotion practices is essential. To promote ideas of wellness, methods utilizing group work and formal and informal health education classes reach the most people. Many classes or beginning groups may have to be instigated by the nurse until individuals recognize and accept that tactics promoting positive states of health are within the repertoire of health professionals' expertise. More and more nurses and physicians are integrating holistic health care measures into treatment regimens.

RATIONALE FOR PROMOTING HEALTH

What are the risks of doing nothing about your health? Risks exist in every facet of our lives. When individuals are unaware of or ignore risk factors, illnesses can occur without warning or can become manifest insidiously after exposure for prolonged periods of time. It is important for clients to be aware of risk factors. They need to know that they are at risk biologically when stress levels are high and health practices are inadequate. They need to know they are at risk environmentally when living or working in overcrowded, hazardous places; when traveling on highways; when heat, air pollution, or water pollution is excessive. They are at risk behaviorally when they smoke or drink excessively, overeat, abuse medications, feel depressed for prolonged periods of time, or push themselves relentlessly toward high achievement.

Risk factors can be controlled and even though clients can manage only a few at a given point in time, these activities mark the beginning of movement toward positive states of health. It is a sad fact that "normal" behavior practiced in current society is risky behavior. A major initial task of the community health nurse is to secure the attention of a client who regards an activity as ok, but which in reality is self-destructive

---

[1] Dunn, op. cit., pp. 4–5.
[2] O. Carl Simonton, Stephanie Matthews-Simonton, and James Creighton, *Getting Well Again*, Bantam Books, Inc., New York, 1978, p. 3. Copyright 1978 O. Carl Simonton. Reprinted by permission of Bantam Books, Inc. All rights reserved.
[3] Ibid., p. 27.

(such as drinking excessively, eating junk foods exclusively, or ignoring environmental hazards in the workplace). The nurse can start teaching at a beginning level of health promotion. This "health improvement" will entail persuading the client to become aware of a selected risk factor (affective learning), and informing the client about the risky behavior by giving convincing data about its long-term consequences (cognitive learning). Utilizing the teaching-learning principle that the best learning will occur if it is perceived as useful by the learner, the nurse can direct the client toward other resources which will verify the data already given and serve to broaden and deepen the perspective of the client regarding the specific risk factor. When the client participates in her or his own learning, motivation to change is more easily set in motion.

COMMON RISK FACTORS

Risk factors that seem to increase a person's chances for developing a chronic degenerative disease are identified as follows:

1 Slightly obese body mass
2 Elevated blood pressure (systolic and diastolic)
3 Smoking
4 Alcohol—more than 2 oz/day
5 Low level of exercise
6 High serum blood fats (triglycerides and cholesterol)
7 Hazardous agents in the environment
8 Glucose tolerance—higher insulin sensitivity

Each risk factor represents symptoms or behaviors which are so familiar and/or acceptable to American consumers that they almost escape notice.

In 1974 the Government of Canada published *New Perspective on the Health of Canadians.*[4] It introduced a useful concept which views all causes of death and disease as having four contributing elements:

1 Inadequacies in the existing health care system
2 Behavioral factors or unhealthy lifestyles
3 Environmental hazards
4 Human biological factors

Using that framework, a group of American experts developed a method for assessing the relative contributions of each of the elements to many health problems. Analysis in which the method was applied to the ten leading causes of death in the United States in 1976 suggests that perhaps as much as *one-half* of mortality in 1976 was due to unhealthy behavior or lifestyle; 20 percent to environmental factors; 20 percent to human biological factors; and only 10 percent to inadequacies in health care.[5]

[4] Marc Lalonde, *A New Perspective on the Health of Canadians,* Government of Canada, Ottawa, 1974.
[5] The Surgeon General's Report on Health Promotion and Disease Prevention, *Healthy People,* U.S. Department of Health, Education, and Welfare Publication 79-55071, Washington, D.C., 1979, pp. 8–9.

These data direct attention toward the necessity for health promotion programs. The American consumer must be made aware of symptoms and risky behaviors and possible consequences manifesting from each symptom or behavior. It is true that some individuals seem to be impervious to the consequences of selected unhealthy behaviors or lifestyles; however, this fact must not dilute the efforts of health professionals toward promoting and improving the health status of persons at risk. The diseases and/or health problems that commonly are associated with the identified risk factors are reported in *Disease Prevention and Health Promotion,* a report of the Departmental Task Force on Prevention,[6] as follows:

Obesity is an extremely common health problem which is based on nutritional imbalance. Obesity is frequently associated with hypertension, coronary heart disease, and adult-onset diabetes.

Hypertension is associated strongly with cerebrovascular accident. Professional and public awareness of hypertension as a risk factor has increased treatment of hypertensive individuals, thus reducing the blood pressure to normal for millions of people.

Cigarette smoking accounts for an estimated 25 percent of coronary heart disease deaths. It also is responsible for one in every five cancer deaths. Cigarette smoking interacts with certain occupational exposures (such as asbestos and uranium) to greatly enhance the risk from either occupational exposure or smoking alone. Smoking is also associated with the disabling disease, chronic obstructive pulmonary disease.

Alcohol abuse is a risk factor for certain cancers such as upper gastrointestinal cancers. Alcohol abuse can begin in adolescence, young adulthood or middle age, remain a lifelong problem, and lead to premature death.

Substantial evidence from studies suggests that vigorous activity lowers cholesterol and triglycerides and lowers risk of fatal heart attack. Regular exercise is physiologically sound, of value in weight control, possibly preventive with respect to heart disease, and contributes to general well-being.

Reduced daily cholesterol intake, saturated fat intake, and caloric intake have been recommended as a prudent diet for primary prevention of cardiovascular disease. Current research suggests high density lipoprotein (HDL) protects against heart attacks. The concentration of HDL, taken in conjunction with that of total blood cholesterol, gives a more accurate prediction of an individual's risk of heart attack than the total cholesterol value alone.

The occupational setting is a primary environmental source of exposure to carcinogens. These sources of carcinogens, mutagens, and teratogens can be controlled by either preventing release of the agents into the environment or removing them from the environment. Other available methods for controlling hazardous agents include:

1 Substitution of the hazardous material with a safer one
2 Change in the manufacturing process to prevent escape or release of the offending agent
3 Isolation of the agent in some type of enclosure

[6] Report of the Departmental Task Force on Prevention, *Disease Prevention & Health Promotion: Federal Programs and Prospects,* U.S. Department of Health, Education, and Welfare Publication 79-55071B, Washington, D.C., 1978, pp. 23–54.

4 Control of the source by engineering techniques such as exhaust methods

5 Personal protective devices such as special clothing

6 Education and motivation of workers and managers to comply with safety procedures

Air pollution and environments containing irritant particulate matter contribute seriously to chronic respiratory diseases.

Diabetes mellitus and impaired glucose tolerance are associated with atherosclerosis and may be genetically related.

LIVING LONGER AND HEALTHIER

Efforts to improve the health of the American people lies in examining what "the people do or don't do to and for themselves. Individual decisions about diet, exercise, and smoking are of critical importance and collective decisions affecting pollution and other aspects of the environment are also relevant.[7]

A well-known study of nearly 7000 adults who were followed for 5½ years by Belloc and Breslow showed that simple basic health habits contributed toward longer life and better health.[8] The health habits included:

1 Eat between meals once in a while, rarely, or never

2 Breakfast almost every day

3 Moderate exercise (active sports, long walks, bike riding, swimming, gardening) often or sometimes

4 Seven or eight hours sleep a night

5 No smoking

6 Moderate weight

7 No alcohol or in moderation

Additional findings stated that

1 A 45-year-old adult who practices three or less of these habits has a life expectancy of 21.6 years and can expect to live to about 67. An adult with six or seven of these habits can look forward to 33.1 years, to 78.

2 The physical health status of those reported following all seven good health practices was consistently about the same as those 30 years younger who followed few or none of these practices.[9]

For clients interested in becoming more fit, feeling better, and reducing illness potential, the practice of prospective medicine, wellness clinics, and holistic health centers are to be found in any major metropolis. Books, articles, periodicals, newspaper items describing how to feel better, how to heal self, becoming well, relieving stress,

[7]Victor R. Fuchs, *Who Shall Live?*, Basic Books, Inc., Publishers, New York, 1974, p. 55.

[8]Nedra B. Belloc, Lester Breslow, "Relationship of Physical Health Status and Health Practices," *Preventive Medicine*, 1:409–421, August 1972.

[9]Nedra B. Belloc, "Relationship of Health Practices and Mortality," *Preventive Medicine*, 2: 67–81, March 1973.

etc., are proliferating as consumers become more responsive and eager to improve their sense of well-being.

HEALTH PROMOTION AS A PART OF PREVENTION

All health professionals are familiar with the three levels of prevention as classified by Leavell and Clark. In brief, primary prevention connotes health promotion, which involves activities directed toward promoting general well-being and is not focused on a particular disease. Primary prevention also includes specific protection for selected diseases such as immunizations for diphtheria, whooping cough, tetanus, and smallpox. Secondary prevention focuses on early diagnosis and instigating measures to stop progression of disease processes or handicapping disabilities. Tertiary prevention deals with rehabilitation activities for disabled patients in an effort to return the person to a level of maximum usefulness.[10]

Community health nurses deal with all three levels of prevention but give emphasis to the level requiring greatest attention in their particular setting. For example, nurses working in home health agencies tend to focus on the tertiary level. For nurses who are concentrating on teaching wellness in group work and health promotion classes, the focus is on the first level of primary prevention. A precise definition of prevention can be elusive when one contemplates the activities encompassed in the first level of prevention. Shamansky and Clausen clarified the first level, *primary prevention,* as meaning

> prevention in the true sense of the word; it precedes disease or dysfunction and is applied to a generally healthy population. The targets are those individuals considered physically or emotionally healthy, exhibiting normal or maximum functioning. Primary prevention is not therapeutic; it does not consist of symptom identification and use of therapeutic skills.
>
> Primary prevention includes generalized health promotion as well as specific protection against disease. The purpose is to decrease the vulnerability of the individual to illness or dysfunction. Health promotion encourages optimum health and personality development to strengthen the individual's capacity to withstand physical and emotional stressors.[11]

However, close examination of the word *prevent* reveals its meaning as "to come before or precede" or "to act in anticipation of." In reality, the implication presumes anticipation of a potential illness or recognition of the prepathogenesis period. *Promote* means "to further the growth or establishment of (something)." The word *promotion* synthesizes more closely with movement toward improved health and seems to more accurately portray the process of assisting clients toward increasingly positive states of health. In other words, prevention recognizes the negative possibility of disease states occurring (which they very well may); whereas promotion assumes a posi-

---

[10] Hugh R. Leavell and R. Gurney Clark, *Preventive Medicine for the Doctor in His Community: An Epidemiologic Approach,* 3d ed., McGraw-Hill Book Company, New York, 1965, pp. 19-28.

[11] Sherry L. Shamansky and Cherie L. Clausen, "Levels of Prevention: Examination of the Concept," *Nursing Outlook,* 20(2):104-108, February 1980, p. 106.

tive view of greater wellness states. Even though health promotion is generally accepted as subsumed within primary prevention, it is and can be regarded as projecting different expectations of future events affecting health status.

PREPARING FOR HEALTH PROMOTION

"Good health can be experienced positively or negatively, as something tangible or as an absence of health-related problems."[12] Whether health is promoted from a positive or negative frame of reference, the goal of health promotion and enhancement of the well-being of clients and/or the public is of utmost concern. When considering health promotion strategies for groups, give thought to the selection of problems according to the following criteria:

1 Number of persons affected (or at risk)
2 Severity of the problem
3 Duration of the effect
4 Number of potential life-years lost
5 Cost to society (if pertinent)[13]
6 Present state of knowledge of consumers about the problem
7 Acceptability of intervention measures to consumers
8 Determination of what behaviors to modify
9 Potential benefits accruing for consumers

Integrate the community health nursing process with the selection of the most feasible problem, then write goals and objectives as a blueprint for the health promotion strategy. For help in writing objectives, see Objective Evaluation of Outcomes at the end of Chap. 3.

Intervention strategies with clients and groups which are helpful to keep in mind regarding their usefulness to health promotion programs include:

1 *Reminders* Reminders prompt or cue the occurrence of a desired behavior.[14] When nursing students remind prospective consumers of an impending proposed health program by means of a personal invitation or personal telephone call, this action ensures greater attendance than public posters or letters delivered through the mail.

2 *Tailoring* Tailoring refers to the process of fitting the prescribed regimen and intervention strategies to specific consumer characteristics.[15] This can be handled by a careful assessment of the target population. For example, if an exercise program is proposed for elderly citizens, aerobics and exercises designed specifically for geriatric clients will be much more appealing than a general vigorous calisthenic class. One

[12] Paul Brearley, et al.: *The Social Context of Health Care*, Basil Blackwell & Mott Ltd., 1978, p. 7.

[13] Report of the Departmental Task Force on Prevention, *Disease Prevention & Health Promotion: Federal Programs and Prospects*, U.S. Department of Health, Education, and Welfare, Washington, D.C., 1978, p. 166.

[14] P. Bryan Haynes, D. Wayne Taylor, and David L. Sackett, *Compliance in Health Care*, The Johns Hopkins University Press, Baltimore, Md., 1979, p. 176.

[15] Ibid., p. 179.

group of senior students tailored a class on strokes for residents of a retirement home in the following way.

> We decided that many times the elderly are too respectful of the health personnel they deal with in that they do not question their doctor's instructions or ask for further explanations. This is due in a large part to the way most of them were brought up—the opinion of the doctor was not to be questioned. In this way they are missing valuable information concerning their health because their doctors are either too busy to explain or they feel their clients are not interested in explanations. We feel every person has a right to know about the illness she or he may have and is entitled to full explanations. So we wanted to offer ourselves as resource persons to the residents to enable them to ask questions they might have concerning strokes.

3 *Contracting* Contracting refers to the process of specifying a set of rules regarding some behavior of interest and formalizing a commitment to adhere to them.[16] In these rules, a positive consequence occurs after the desired behavior and does not occur if the desired behavior does not occur. For groups of people who are not convinced that walking a mile per day will increase their sense of well-being, a contract can be proposed whereas the individuals will be persuaded to walk 1 mile 3 times a week for a period of 2 months. Skinfold measurements of arms, thighs, and abdomen taken before and after the 2-month period can be compared in addition to a subjective evaluation of one's own sense of well-being before and after the contracted period for walking. For individuals wanting to feel better, a positive outcome resulting from this contract will be sufficient as a starting point for engaging in more concentrated fitness programs.

4 *Self-monitoring* Self-monitoring is a process of observing and recording one's own behavior.[17] Self-monitoring can be used effectively if the client is motivated to change. Of importance is checking the self-monitored report for accuracy and providing feedback to the client. For the client who is willing to monitor and record intake of soft drinks for 1 week (rather than recording weight gain or loss) the behavior has the possibility of being regulated as a consequence. The self-regulation will follow the client's perception of the actual frequency of the action. Self-monitored records provide data for further examination and study. For example, the client and nurse may want to explore the relationship of numbers of soft drinks consumed per week with weight gain or loss per week. Or, examination of the cost of soft drinks per week may be compared with alternative low-calorie choices.

5 *Reinforcement* Reinforcement refers to any consequence that increases the probability of the behavior being repeated.[18] Many groups use the reinforcement strategy to reward members' behavior. Weight loss groups, for example, give praise or public acclaim to members losing the most pounds. Verbal support and encouragement from community health nurses regarding any desired behavior of clients is extremely essential for promoting health strategies.

Evaluation of health promotion strategies establishes the appropriateness of criteria used in the selection of the health problem and the success or failure of outcomes,

---

[16] Ibid., p. 181.
[17] Ibid., pp. 184–185.
[18] Ibid., p. 185.

objectives, and interventions used. Evaluation of strategies, whether verbal or written, provide useful feedback for modification of future health promotion programs.

PROGRAMS FOR PROMOTING HEALTH

An overview of health promotion activities is offered for the purpose of stimulating nursing students with ideas that can be used in health promotion projects for consumers and groups. Additional content for each subject area will have to be gained from explicit sources such as specialty books, articles, voluntary community agencies, governmental agencies, and resource persons and disciplines within each community. Much valuable knowledge is gained when nursing students pursue a self-directed course of action. Not only is their health promotion project potentially destined to be a good one, but many key persons of allied disciplines with whom they have consultation, become involved and provide invaluable contributions leading to a more attractive comprehensive presentation.

Exercise

Former U.S. Surgeon General Dr. Jesse L. Steinfel has said, "It will make you more effective in your work and at the same time bring personal compensations, one of which is that exercise appears to retard the aging process."[18a] Exercise is the means to an alert, vigorous, and lengthy life. Inactivity can kill you.[19] Physical activity can and should be fun, not a chore, and it should be done *daily*. Body tissues and functions are improved by physical activity.[20]

Many citizens are responsive to the idea of exercise and enjoy participating in a program of active sports such as tennis, golf, swimming, bicycling, regular visits to a spa, jogging, attending yoga or body conditioning classes, and similar activities. For citizens who are generally inactive, depressed, listless, and bored, and such people can be found, the challenge for the community health nurse is to entice or persuade these people to start exercising daily—a little at a time, yet increasing the tempo and complexity of movements as their physical fitness progresses. What are some specific benefits of exercise?

Increased strength and endurance (leads to more efficient use of energy even in mental tasks)
Maintains proper circulation
Increased poise and grace
Improved muscle tone and posture
Reduction of chronic tiredness
Reduction of chronic tension
Improved control of weight

[18a]Philip Goldberg, *Executive Health,* McGraw-Hill Book Company, New York, 1978, pp. 130–131.
[19]Laurence E. Morehouse and Leonard Gross, *Total Fitness in 30 Minutes a Week,* Simon & Schuster, Inc., New York, 1975, p. 20.
[20]Ibid., p. 75.

Reduced aches, pains, stiffness
Fewer serious accidents
Improved appearance
Reduction of degenerative disease risk factors[21]

Clients of any age may of their own volition increase their habitual levels of physical activity. For the sedentary client, however, there is no assurance that there are not contraindications for a vigorous exercise program. For this reason nurses should take a health history, do a health assessment, and based on the findings recommend an examination by a physician preliminary to starting a regular exercise program.

For nurses proposing to start an exercise program for a selected group of consumers, the word "exercise" may elicit an "alarm reaction" from some physicians. For this reason, less threatening terms such as conditioning, range of motion, movement, or walking programs might be considered. When planning exercise programs, some general guidelines need to be considered.

1 Exercises for warming up and cooling down are necessary preceding and following every regular session. The purpose of the light warm-up exercises is to gradually increase respiration, heart rate, and body temperature, and to stretch ligaments. The warm-up exercises should include stretching routines and should be done slowly to prepare the body for more vigorous exercise. A 5-minute cool-down period helps to avoid problems such as cramps or nausea.

2 Comfortable loose clothing and properly fitting shoes are recommended.

3 Exercise should be adapted to the client's exercise tolerance level. This means the client should be able to execute a given exercise without undue discomfort or fatigue.

4 Exercise "overloading" should be applied to induce a higher level of performance. In overloading, the individual's exercise is increased in intensity or is extended for a longer time than normally.

5 The exercise plan should provide for progression. Progression is applied by increasing the exercise incrementally in intensity and duration.

6 Individuals must desire to improve. Motivation to become more fit is essential.

7 Advance the unfit client's psychological limits of effort. Frequently, the client's psychological tolerance for exercise is reached before physiological limits are attained. Careful assessment of the client's psychological and physiological reactions assists in determining the best approach to use for persuading the client to accept gradually increasing exercise dosages.[22]

8 Watch for signs of competition. Clients should be enjoying the exercise, not competing with another member of the group. If possible, set up exercise routines that lessen the possibility of competition occurring.

Exercise programs can consist of a wide variety of movements, including simple to complex, specific to general, limited to diverse. Aerobic dancing, yoga exercises,

---

[21]Philip Goldberg, *Executive Health,* McGraw-Hill Book Company, New York, 1978, p. 131.

[22]H. Harrison Clarke, "Exercise and Aging," in Geral Dene Marr Burdman and Ruth M. Brewer (eds.), *Health Aspects of Aging,* A Continuing Education Book, Portland, Oreg., 1978, p. 137.

running, swimming, simple movements, karate, and bicycling are some of the options. The world's oldest exercise is walking. It is the cheapest, easiest, most accessible, least conspicuous, and may be the best.[23]

Relaxation

"Attitudes toward relaxation are the most naive of all. Most individuals assume that collapsing in front of the TV, working in the garden, spending a quiet afternoon with a book, and working out on the tennis court are effective means of relaxing and reducing stress."[24] However, if these individuals maintain a mental anxiety and neurophysiological functioning characteristic of prolonged unabated stress while engaged in their "relaxing" pursuits, the purpose they are seeking is not being accomplished. The amount of muscle activity that takes place at rest, or during relaxation, can vary enormously from person to person. To reduce significant wear and tear occurring in everyday life, deep relaxation measures must be learned and practiced.

What is true relaxation? Relaxation means the complete absence of holding any part of your body rigid. By relaxation of muscles is meant the complete absence of all contractions. Limp and motionless, the muscle offers no resistance to stretching. It is physically impossible to be nervous in any part of your body which is completely relaxed.[25]

Rest is nature's remedy for tension. Learning to relax or control tensions leads to more efficient living through conservation of human energy. By conserving human energy, freedom to accomplish those things a person wants to do is increased because fatigue states are avoided.

Abdominal Breathing Learning to breathe deeply and completely is useful for reducing tension. Abdominal breathing is practiced in yoga and is an activity that can be done inconspicuously when under stress or preceding a stressful event. It can be utilized habitually and with calming results. It is best done while seated in an upright position.

Abdominal Breathing Method[26] For practice place your hands on your abdomen right below the navel. The fingertips of each hand should touch one another.

Breathe through your nose. Many people habitually breathe through their mouths, an almost sure sign of stress overload, and not nearly as healthy.

Inhale very slowly. As you inhale, push the abdomen out as though it were a balloon expanding. Your fingers should separate.

As the abdomen expands, your diaphragm will move downward, allowing fresh air to enter the bottom part of the lungs. Keeping your back straight will aid the process of maximizing inhalation.

---

[23]Goldberg, op. cit., p. 140.

[24]Kenneth R. Pelletier, *Mind As Healer, Mind As Slayer: A Holistic Approach to Preventing Stress Disorders,* Delacorte Press, New York, 1977, p. 23. Copyright 1977 Kenneth R. Pelletier. Reprinted by permission of Delacorte Press and Seymour Lawrence.

[25]Edmund Jacobson, *You Must Relax,* McGraw-Hill Book Company, New York, 1962, pp. 84–85.

[26]Goldberg, op. cit., pp. 201-202.

As the breath continues, expand the chest. More air should now enter, filling the middle part of the lungs.

While slightly contracting the abdomen, raise your shoulders and collarbones. This should fill the upper part of the lungs.

At this point, the entire respiratory mechanism has been employed and no portion of the lungs is left unfilled. Hold the breath for about 5 seconds.

Exhalation is as important as inhalation. Proper exhalation not only expels all used air, it opens space for fresh air to enter. After holding the breath, begin slowly to exhale through the nose. As you do so, draw in the abdomen. This will lift the diaphragm. The expanded rib cage will return to its normal position, and the lungs will empty.

Remember to exhale slowly, and let all the air empty out. If comfortable, hold it a second or two before beginning the inhalation again. When you resume, remember to inhale slowly and completely.

Your first few practice sessions may leave you with a slightly dizzy feeling. That is normal. Teaching clients to do abdominal breathing is appropriate in many diverse settings. Nurses can suggest this procedure frequently, particularly when they sense that the client is tense. The procedure can be described as a helpful exercise that the nurse and client can do together. In this way, both client and nurse receive the benefit of an immediate stress reduction technique.

Visualization For persons deeply desiring a particular goal (a car, home, educational degree, etc.) it is common practice to create a mental image of the desired event. By forming the image, the person makes a clear mental statement of what is wanted. By repeating the statement or imagery, the person soon expects the desired event to occur. As a result of the positive expectation, the individual begins acting in ways consistent with achieving the desired result, and in reality helps to bring it about.[27] A hypothesis for the effectiveness of visualization practices is the principle that psychological energy follows patterns of thought.[28] Nurses can encourage clients to use their imagination creatively and visualize healing processes and improved health status. "Where the mind tends to focus, the emotions and the physiology are likely to follow."[29] Simonton has described his use of relaxation and visualization measures to promote healing of cancer successfully with clients willing to follow this treatment regimen. Anderson corroborated the effectiveness of visualization by reporting about clients with diagnoses of neurodermatitis, obesity, and asthma who responded with positive results following the regular practice of relaxation and visualization.[30] As explained by Anderson, the "thought process involved in visualizations, images, and words precedes activity."[31]

Nurses can teach clients who want a change in their health status to practice the

[27] Simonton, op. cit., p. 118.
[28] Pelletier, op. cit., p. 250.
[29] Ibid., p. 251.
[30] Robert A. Anderson, *Stress Power! How to Turn Tension into Energy*, Human Sciences Press, New York, 1978, pp. 211-213.
[31] Ibid., p. 206.

basic relaxation visualization procedure regularly as follows:

1 Go to a quiet room. Shut the door, sit in a comfortable chair, feet flat on the floor, eyes closed.

2 Become aware of your breathing.

3 Take in a few deep breaths, and as you let out each breath, mentally say the word, "relax."

4 Concentrate on your face and feel any tension in the muscles of your face and around your eyes. Make a mental picture of this tension—it might be a rope tied in a knot or a clenched fist—and then mentally picture it relaxing and becoming comfortable, like a limp rubber band.

5 Experience the muscles of your face and eyes becoming relaxed. As they relax, feel a wave of relaxation spreading through your body.

6 Tense the muscles of your face and around your eyes, squeezing tightly, then relax them and feel the relaxation spreading through your body.

7 Move slowly down your body—jaw, neck, shoulders, back, upper and lower arms, hands, chest, abdomen, thighs, calves, ankles, feet—until every part of your body is more relaxed. For each part of the body, mentally picture the tension, then picture the tension melting away, allowing relaxation.

8 Now picture yourself in pleasant, natural surroundings—wherever feels comfortable for you. Mentally fill in the details of color, sound, texture.

9 Continue to picture yourself in a very relaxed state in this natural place for 2 to 3 minutes.

10 Create a mental picture of any ailment or pain that you have now, visualizing it in a form that makes sense to you.

11 Picture any treatment you are receiving and see it either eliminating the source of the ailment or pain or strengthening your body's ability to heal itself.

12 Picture your body's natural defenses and natural processes eliminating the source of the ailment or pain.

13 Imagine yourself healthy and free of the ailment or pain.

14 See yourself proceeding successfully toward meeting your goals in life.

15 Give yourself a mental pat on the back for participating in your recovery. See yourself doing this relaxation and mental imagery exercise 3 times a day, staying awake and alert as you do it.

16 Let the muscles in your eyelids lighten up, become ready to open your eyes, and become aware of the room.

17 Now let your eyes open and you are ready to resume your usual activities.[32]

Progressive Relaxation Progressive relaxation is a learned program for retraining muscles to obtain complete relaxation with minimal signs of residual tension. Jacobson states that a course in scientific relaxation or tension control teaches an individual to run her or his own organism successfully. Advantages concurrent with this accomplishment may be increased job productivity, longer daily working ability, clearer thinking, lessened self-consciousness, harmonious staff meetings and relations, diminished sensitivity to criticism, lessened friction, lessened anxiety, decreased fatigue, decreased

[32] Simonton, op. cit., pp. 120-123.

absenteeism, and better working attitudes.[33] In a course of scientific relaxation, students are taught to become familiar with the sensation, location, and degree of tensions, to note the control sensation which is the sensation from muscular contraction. As students progressively learn tension control, they utilize a self-discipline which leads to relaxation, self-operation, and improved general health.

Bernstein and Borkovec have written an informative training manual which describes progressive relaxation training in terms of its history, current status, research findings, clientele who can benefit, the rationale for relaxation training, basic procedures, and possible problems with suggested solutions. The manual is concise, is in paperback, and is available for health professionals who wish to teach relaxation training to prospective clients. As cautioned by Bernstein and Borkovec, relaxation training is not a panacea for all clients; it is a technique which must be used with discrimination and judgment. It has been found to have considerable value for persons with high tension levels[34] and can be initiated with clients who are responsive and consenting to preventive measures as suggested by health professionals.

In an article written for business executives, Benson described the "relaxation response" as a simple way for individuals to alleviate stress and thus moderate or control many of its undesirable effects—effects which may range from simple anxiety to heart disease. The "relaxation response" is an innate integrated set of physiologic changes which appear to counteract the harmful physiologic effects of stress.[35] The relaxation response elicits changes similar to those described by persons promoting the regular practice of meditation. It cannot be denied that conscious relaxation, meditation, or temporary withdrawal from the busy activities of the day, when done regularly and for brief time periods, will have beneficial effects for all individuals engaged in the practice. However, for persons with high tension levels and showing physiological damage, such as elevated blood pressure, learning progressive relaxation and practicing it daily diminishes the amount of work required of the heart; and general health, a sense of well-being and renewal, is the result.

As explained by Jacobson, taking a rest or nap each day is beneficial, yet it is not as effective in lowering blood pressure as the employment of scientific relaxation. Until an individual has acquired habits of muscular relaxation when resting, the arms and other parts of the body can continue to be in a tense state. Training to relax is an easy treatment and produces lasting results.[36]

Persons of all occupational levels and ages exhibit varying degrees of tension levels and are potential candidates for progressive relaxation training. A project of four relaxation classes was conducted by two senior nursing students with a population of elderly citizens living in a retirement facility. Preceding each class, blood pressure readings were taken, then a 30-minute tape was played giving instructions for eliciting the relaxation response. Following the tape, blood pressure readings were taken again.

[33] Edmund Jacobson, *How to Teach Scientific Relaxation: Instructor's Text*, Auspices, Foundation for Scientific Relaxation, Inc., Chicago, 1958, p. 17.

[34] Douglas A. Bernstein and Thomas D. Borkovec, *Progressive Relaxation Training*, Research Press, Champaign, Ill., 1973, p. 11.

[35] Herbert Benson, "Your Innate Asset for Combating Stress," *Harvard Business Review*, 52(4):49–60, July–August 1974.

[36] Jacobson, *You Must Relax*, op. cit., p. 231.

Since the attendance of the class was voluntary, participation of the residents dropped gradually, possibly due to a variety of extraneous factors. However, the data collected at each session showed a reduction in blood pressure following the elicitation of the relaxation response. The average drop in blood pressure per session for each group varied from 3.9 to 16.6 mmHg drop. It was found that the particular individuals who attended the four classes regularly had a consistent progressive decline in blood pressure readings which implied the benefits of regularly applying the technique.

For community health nurses who wish to teach progressive relaxation training, thorough knowledge of the technique, personal experience with it, attention to the physical setting, knowledge of muscle groups and familiarity with the sequence for training, and evaluative forms and devices are all requisite before initiating any teaching sessions. Training classes can be utilized in a variety of settings with a diverse range of citizens who consent to participate. Information can be given about stress, consequences of stress, process of relaxation, tension control, physiologic changes, body awareness, significance of breathing, and related subjects. The need for citizens to learn techniques of relaxation and its benefits is an opportunity which is a "natural" for community health nurses and should not be overlooked, particularly when practicing primary prevention.

Other Relaxation Measures Autogenic training, biofeedback, transcendental meditation (TM) are some of the techniques being practiced by health professionals to relax clients and promote a sense of calm, peacefulness, and control. All of the techniques require a relaxed posture and/or state of mind to begin with, concentration, and openness to new feelings and experiences. All of the techniques require extensive study and training by health professionals before putting them into practice.

Autogenic Training *Autogenic training* is a deep relaxation technique developed by a German psychiatrist, Johannes Schultz, in 1932. It is a method of rational physiologic exercises designed to induce distinct physical sensations and lead to deep relaxation of a purely physical nature. Through this process, individuals learn to abandon themselves to an ongoing organismic process rather than exercising conscious will. It is a technique that depends to a great extent on autosuggestion.[37] It is used by health professionals to induce deep relaxation, normalize body functions, and promote healing physiological changes.

Biofeedback *Biofeedback* "is simply the feedback of biological information to the person whose biology it is." As described by Brown, "the real biological feedback drama unfolded when it was discovered that we could tap the hidden secrets of the completely internal, life-governing functions of the body, that we could capture the internal signals and transform them into externalized information-bearing signals that could be sensed, perceived, recognized, and acted upon by our brain's control system."[38] Biofeedback equipment can monitor events such as brain waves, heartbeat, muscular tension, or skin temperature. These events are then transformed into

[37]Pelletier, op. cit., pp. 229–231.
[38]Barbara B. Brown, *New Mind, New Body* Bantam Books, Inc., New York, 1974, pp. 4–5.

readily observable signals—lights, tones, wavy lines on a monitor. As individuals perceive their own internal world of psychologic functioning, they are able to regulate the body's physiologic and subjective processes. Biofeedback is being used in a variety of ways by many health professionals. Brown projected the possibility that biofeedback can be one of the most potent and practical tools for explorations of the power and the energy of the mind. The principle that the mind and body can use information about themselves to gain new awareness and greater vitality creates exciting options for revealing inner well-being.[39] Biofeedback has excellent potential for use in self-care and promotion of greater states of health.

Transcendental Meditation The *TM Technique* is a simple mental practice derived from ancient Indian tradition and adapted for modern use by Maharishi Mahesh Yogi. Practicing TM involves the use of a mantra, a meaningless sound individually assigned to the learner by a trained instructor. Correct use of the mantra is said to automatically reduce the level of excitation and disorderly activity of the nervous system, quieting the mind while maintaining alertness. Simultaneously, metabolic changes occur which point toward a deep state of rest, which enables the body to normalize the damage of stress and strengthen the system to ward off excessive strain in the future.[40] Many benefits derived from the use of TM have been validated by studies and reported in professional and business journals.

Use of Humor As a Stress Reduction Technique Since stress comes in all varieties, not just physical, a person's emotional and psychological strength goes a long way in determining resistance and vulnerability.[41] Clients have the opportunity to choose from a variety of stress reduction techniques advocated by health professionals. The attractiveness and potential effectiveness of a given technique, the distinction of the health professional offering the technique, and the public acclaim and popularity regarding the effectiveness of the technique all influence clients' decisions regarding which technique to put into practice. A tip suggested by Selye is "to try to keep your mind constantly on the pleasant aspects of life and on actions which can improve your situation. . . . Nothing paralyzes your efficiency more than frustration; nothing helps it more than success."[42]

Humor has been said to facilitate the release of energy accompanying excessive tension. Cousins described his use of laughter to reduce pain he was experiencing. He called this part of his recovery program an "exercise of affirmative emotions as a factor in enhancing body chemistry."[43] Cousins watched "Candid Camera" films and some old Marx Brothers films and found that 10 minutes of genuine belly laughter had an anesthetic effect and gave him at least 2 hours of pain-free sleep. Laughter provides internal exercise for a person and it creates a mood in which other positive emotions can be put to work.[44] Laughter is a means for facilitating pleasant optimistic

---

[39] Ibid., p. 371.
[40] Goldberg, op. cit., pp. 212–213.
[41] Ibid., p. 30.
[42] Hans Selye, *Stress without Distress,* J. B. Lippincott Co., New York, 1974, p. 142.
[43] Norman Cousins, *Anatomy of an Illness As Perceived by the Patient,* W. W. Norton & Company, New York, 1979, p. 39.
[44] Ibid., p. 146.

thoughts and redirecting energy toward positive health states. Finding books, films, jokes that are genuinely funny to the client can be a prescriptive activity assigned to the client by the nurse. It is a therapeutic activity worth trying with clients to reduce stress, alleviate pain, or redirect mental energies into a positive vein.

Nutrition and Health

Obesity is one of the serious nutritional health problems in the United States. Contributing to the problem is the sedentary nature of our culture which indulges in excessive TV watching and eating junk foods. Income is not necessarily a single important factor that contributes to obesity, as much as eating high-calorie foods, junk foods, sweets, habitually eating as a conditioned response, having a daily cocktail, inactivity, eating at all social gatherings or coffee breaks, snacking at all hours of the day or night, eating too fast, and cleaning up the plate. Affluent and poor alike have problems with nutrition. Selected groups of consumers are demonstrating an avid interest in nutrition as evidenced by the proliferation of natural food and health food stores, soup and salad restaurants, recipe and diet books.

Studies are showing that nutrition has a great deal to do with our daily capacity to perform. Findings of a study done by Viteri demonstrated that when a group of respondents received a diet supplemented with high quality protein and calories, they spent 33 percent of their time in rest or sleep and 67 percent of their time being active during or after work. In comparison, a nonsupplemented group of subjects who were studied at the same time spent 49 percent of their time at rest or sleep and 51 percent of their time being active at work or after work. The study stated that the nonsupplemented subjects were extremely tired and almost exhausted during the work period whereas the supplemented respondents were not.[45] This study suggests that people who are receiving inadequate nutrition (by scarcity, lack of income, ignorance, or choice) are being robbed of a percentage of their potential active life, their vitality, their sense of well-being, and their freedom from excess fatigue.

In another study done by Cabak and Najdanvic, it was reported that children who were hospitalized for severe malnutrition at less than 12 months of age had a reduced IQ in the later school years as compared to children who had not been malnourished.[46] This study suggests that nutrition not only affects physical energy and vitality, but also intellectual development. In view of the suggested associations which these studies bring out regarding the effect of nutrition on physical and mental performance, it seems imperative for community health nurses to evince a deep interest and curiosity about the diet patterns of the families they visit.

Even though nutrition is included in all nursing curricula, nurses' knowledge of recommended nutritional practices is not always up-to-date and specialized. Frequently, there is little agreement on precisely what we should and should not eat. Articles can be found in reputable journals supporting or disclaiming any of the current nutritional recommendations. It is important for nurses to know about nutri-

[45] Milton Terris, "Approaches to an Epidemiology of Health," *American Journal of Public Health,* **65**(10):1037–1045, October 1975.
[46] Herbert G. Birch, "Malnutrition, Learning, and Intelligence," *American Journal of Public Health,* **62**(6):733–784, June 1972.

tional disputes and be able to recommend studies or professional journals which will broaden clients' knowledge about controversial issues. Ultimately, it is up to every client and nurse to determine their own stands regarding a given controversial issue.

The Changing American Diet As stated by Bland, 25 percent of Americans are seriously overweight due to the overingestion of nutrient-poor foods.[47] This happens partly because of our eating habits which can be popularly described as "bolting down" foods within our grasp, and our selection of junk foods (processed foods which are often purchased at fast food establishments).

Brewster and Jacobson express concern about the increase of dietary fat, refined sugars, and the decrease of less complex carbohydrates that Americans consume today.[48] The consumption of carbohydrates as represented by rye, barley, buckwheat, corn flour, and corn meal has dropped drastically in recent years, whereas sweeteners have increased markedly. Sweeteners contribute virtually no nutrients—only calories—to our diet. The "empty" calories can cause obesity, which in turn raises the risk of heart disease, diabetes, and other health problems. According to the authors, the most alarming change in our diet is the increased intake of fat which they associate as having a linkage with cardiovascular diseases and some cancers. They implicate fast food restaurants as having greatly influenced the American diet, leading to an increase in the consumption of ice milk, french fries, fish, chicken, beef, cheese (particularly pizza cheese), chili sauce, tomato products (catsup, paste, sauce), pickles, and soft drinks.

Dietary Goals for the United States Dietary goals for the United States[49] as reported by the Senate Select Committee on Nutrition and Human Needs in 1977 were written with the objective of improved health through informed diet selection by every American. The recommendations are listed below.

1 *Increase the consumption of complex carbohydrates* (whole grains) *and "naturally occurring" sugars* (fruits and vegetables). Whole grains are identified as the complex carbohydrates, or starches which include brans, whole wheat, millet, bulgur, brown rice, dried beans, etc. The complex carbohydrates are high in fiber and contain a great variety of vitamins, minerals, and sometimes generous amounts of protein. In a study of the intake of crude fiber in the American diet for selected time periods between 1909 and 1975, it was found that trends showing the decline of crude fiber consumption in the United States supported the hypothesis that fiber intake has decreased coincidentally with increases in degenerative diseases.[50]

Increased consumption of fruits, vegetables, and whole grains is important with respect to supplying adequate amounts of micronutrients, vitamins, and minerals.

[47]Jeffrey Bland, *Nutrition and the Health Practitioner: A Reference Source in Clinical Nutrition,* 1979, p. 2. Copyright Jeffrey Bland, Ph.D., 1979, Tacoma, Wash.

[48]Letitia Brewster and Michael F. Jacobson, *The Changing American Diet,* Center for Science in the Public Interest, Washington D.C., 1978.

[49]Select Committee on Nutrition and Human Needs, U.S. Senate, *Dietary Goals for the United States,* 2d ed., Government Printing Office, Washington, D.C., 1977.

[50]Steven N. Heller and L. Ross Hackler, "Changes in the Crude Fiber Content of the American Diet," *The American Journal of Clinical Nutrition,* 31(9):1510–1514, September 1978.

This is particularly important for those clients who are limiting their food intake to control weight or save money.

2 *Reduce the consumption of refined and processed sugars.* Sugar is needed to generate the energy necessary for the complex processes within our cells. However, we do not need as much sugar as we actually eat. The problem with voluntarily cutting down on obvious sugar intake is that the consumer can affect only approximately 25 percent of the sugar and other sweeteners ingested. An informed approach for consciously reducing the intake of refined and processed sugars requires careful reading of food labels and voluntarily eliminating the consumption of soft drinks and processed foods from the diet. Clients also must be watchful for refined starches (white bread, noodles, spaghetti, rice, pastry) which are examples of hidden sources of sugar.

3 *Reduce overall fat consumption.* Or, decrease meat consumption and use more poultry and fish. Red meat is a prime source of fat in the diet. To reduce fat intake, eat meat less often, buy leaner cuts, broil meat so fat drips off, and use more poultry, fish, and low-fat dairy products.

4 *Reduce saturated fat consumption to account for 10 percent of total energy intake* and *balance that with monounsaturated and polyunsaturated fats so that equal proportions are represented in the fat intake.* Saturated fats are the main kind of fatty acid made by the animal body. Monounsaturated fats are usually made by plants, but some can be made by animals. Polyunsaturated fats, which are often called essential fatty acids, can only be made by plants and are needed for normal cell function. Saturated fats elevate serum cholesterol, monounsaturated fats have little or no effect on serum cholesterol, and polyunsaturated fats lower serum cholesterol.

A high-fat diet is counterproductive to weight loss and thus to the prevention of many chronic diseases. Cholesterol and triglycerides are the two principal fats in the bloodstream which when abnormally high, act as an irritant to artery walls and contribute to the formation of plaques which obstruct blood flow. Plaques are not entirely made of cholesterol—they also contain fibrin, collagen protein, minerals, triglycerides, and phospholipids. Lipid substances (cholesterol, triglycerides, and phospholipids) are dispersed in the blood stream by linking up to a protein called *lipoproteins.* Lipoproteins are divided according to their volume and density. The four groups are named (1) *Chylomicron* (the largest and least dense), (2) very low density lipoproteins (VLDL), or *Prebeta-lipoproteins,* (3) low density lipoproteins (LDL), or *beta-lipoproteins,* and (4) high density lipoproteins (HDL), or *alpha-lipo-proteins* (the smallest and most dense). Recent evidence indicates that the ratio of HDL to LDL is now considered the key risk factor for coronary artery disease. HDL contains more protein and smaller amounts of cholesterol and triglycerides. Large field trials have demonstrated that a high blood level of HDL is associated with a lowered incidence of coronary artery disease.

5 *Reduce cholesterol consumption to about 300 mg/day.* Cholesterol is a vital substance found in every body cell. A nutritional controversy exists regarding the association of the amount of cholesterol in the diet and the level of cholesterol in the blood. The body produces cholesterol according to its needs and how the intake of cholesterol through diet affects cholesterol production is a controversial issue. Until more concrete evidence is gained, it is recommended that cholesterol intake be limited in the diet.

6 *Limit the intake of sodium by reducing the intake of salt to about 5 g/day.* For the consumer voluntarily cutting his sodium intake, more vigilance is required than merely using less salt in cooking and eliminating the salt shaker at the table.

Deliberate effort should be made to avoid salty snack foods and salty processed foods. When reading labels, look for salt, monosodium glutamate (MSG), sodium nitrite, and a variety of other additives. For clients willing to forego their preference for the taste of salt and accept "bland tastes" of food, the natural unsalted taste of food *can* become enjoyed if given sufficient time for the taste buds to adjust.

Nutritional Assessment Program Since diet is an integral part of every person's life, an informed nutritional screening program is a recommended procedure which should be implemented by all health professionals as an educational health promotion activity. As advocated by Bland, a nutritional assessment program generally has four components.[51]

1 *Anthropometric measurements* These measurements include height and weight, skin-fold measurements (triceps, subscapular, or midaxillary), arm circumference, upper arm muscle diameter, and head circumference (especially in infants and children).

2 *Clinical assessment* This assessment consists of the client's history and physical examination. Certain physical signs such as easily plucked hair or pale conjunctivae are indicative or suggestive of malnutrition.

3 *Biochemical assessment* This assessment encompasses common laboratory tests, such as serum albumin and a complete blood count, and/or functional laboratory tests such as fecal fat and D-xylose tolerance test.

4 *Dietary methodologies* These are used to determine an individual's dietary or nutritional intake and to assess the need for intervention or correction. These determinations may be obtained through 24-hour recall, dietary records, history of foods eaten over a long period of time, or self-administered questionnaire for general dietary data or information on specific foods.

Every person responds to foods differently. One family member may be able to eat lots of fat, sugar, and salt with no apparent ill effects, but that does not mean that all members of the family can do likewise. For this reason each individual can profit from a nutritional assessment. There is no single diet suitable for every individual. Tastes, habits, and needs are individualized and an intelligent nutritional program takes this into account.

For nurses seeking more information about nutrition, workshops, books, and study programs are available for updating knowledge. For nurses having minimal interest in the field of nutrition, it is imperative that they are able to assess the client's need for a nutritional assessment program and refer the client to appropriate resources.

Counseling about Nutrition

It is extremely difficult to persuade people to change food habits and can rarely be done based on a "It's good for you" approach. It is always advisable to elicit the family's opinions about food before introducing any of your own ideas. However, before the nurse engages a family in discussion about nutritional ideas and habits,

---

[51] Bland, op. cit., pp. 3–4.

it is good preparation for the nurse to browse through local grocery stores and look at food displays and prices in the neighborhood. In view of what is found, the nurse may want to help low-income families set up buying clubs or food cooperatives or at least inform them where food cooperative stores are located. The nurse may want to try cooking some recipes which avoid preprocessed preprepared foods and see if the end result is tasty or not. A good recipe book to experiment with is *Diet for a Small Planet* by Lappé.[52]

The purposes of adequate nutrition are to provide for body growth and development, to maintain general health and resistance to disease, to provide for activity, and to maintain a desirable weight. Margaret Mead has said, "Food affects not only man's dignity, but the capacity of children to reach their full potential, and the capacity of adults to act from day to day."[53]

Every nurse learns that a normal, adequate diet includes a balance of proteins, carbohydrates, and fats in combination with vitamins, especially vitamins A, B-complex, C, and D; minerals, especially calcium and iron; and an adequate amount of fluids. The problem, and at the same time the challenge, in teaching is to interpret to the homemaker in the family or the person living alone what this means in terms of economics, availability of food, attractive food combinations, preferences of family members, and what contributes to growth and development and to general health and well-being.

In nutrition teaching and working for change in dietary habits, the nurse should help the homemaker or person living alone to build whenever possible on the accustomed diet. A "meat and potato" diet meets many nutritional requirements and with the addition of such leafy vegetables as spinach, broccoli, or a salad and some fruit could be made a satisfactory one. Low-income families tend to use a diet high in "starchy" foods, because it is less expensive, is temporarily filling, and gives quick energy. However, it does not meet the body's requirements for growth and development of muscles, bones, and teeth or for general well-being.

There are many approaches to teaching nutrition that will enable the alert nurse to help the homemaker or the person living alone. There are times when a visit is made before the remains of breakfast or lunch have been cleared away and by observing unobtrusively, the nurse can learn something about the family's eating patterns. In discussing diet and foods, the nurse needs to ask questions that will provide more information than just a "yes" or "no" response.

A review of a record of the family's menus for 2 or 3 days will provide insight into some of the nutrition problems. In one instance, the sixth-grade daughter of a family had a severe problem of overweight. By reviewing the family menus, including snacks the girl had at school, for 3 days, it was discovered that the snacks alone—candy bars, ice cream, and doughnuts—came to more than 600 cal/day. This brought out several psychological problems of which the family was not aware.

The nurse needs to be nonthreatening in teaching, recognizing that the home-

[52] Frances Moore Lappé, *Diet for a Small Planet,* Friends of the Earth, Ballantine Books, New York, 1971.
[53] Margaret Mead, "Changing Significance of Food," *Journal of Nutrition,* 2(1):17–18, Summer 1970.

maker may be doing the best possible under the circumstances and in the face of such problems as meal preparation on a low income and meal planning with foods available from "surplus foods" and "food stamps." Some nurses have recipes they can share or exchange with homemakers for casseroles, the cooking of cheap cuts of meat, and simple desserts. On occasion, a productive way to teach is to accompany the homemaker to the market to give assistance in economy buying and to show how to read the labels and compare sizes and prices of cans and packages.

Not only are the nutritionists in health centers, health departments, and hospitals available to the nurse for consultation, but also many private health organizations, such as the local heart association, employ nutritionists who can be most helpful. Nutritionists associated with some of the commercial businesses such as food processing plants and dairies often help. They are interested in the nutrition problems the nurse encounters in work with families. In one "company" town suffering from a severe economic depression, the nutritionist from the local gas and electric company worked with the nurse to present some cooking demonstrations of low-cost menus and provided copies of the recipes demonstrated.

When certain dietary restrictions conform to religious beliefs or cultural practices regarding the eating of meat or other foods, substitutions can be worked out. Assistance for this can be secured from a local nutritionist.

Nutritional Supplements Nutritional supplements play an important role in reinforcing the body's biochemical needs and helping to avoid disease states resulting from stress factors, toxic materials in the environment, and decreased value of certain prepared foods. As explained by Bland, each person has specific biochemical needs for maintaining a proper nutritive balance. This balance is unique for each person as dictated by biochemical individuality or specific physiological strengths and weaknesses. Weak spots can occur in any one of three general areas where nutrition is important:

1 Energy production and maintenance through breakdown of foods
2 Building of the body's defense systems or immunity
3 Building replacement tissue and cellular material to combat tissue degeneration

Current eating habits of Americans have led them to consume many refined foods to which chemicals have been added such as humectants, antioxidants, emulsifiers, flavorings, stabilizers, etc. Most of these compounds place unknown amounts of stress upon our physiology after entering the food chain. Proper nutritive supplements help augment the body's defense against the pathology resulting from these chemical and physical stress factors. The more we expose ourselves to toxicants, air pollution, and empty-calorie foods, the more the need for selective supplementation.

Since every person has specific biochemical needs, supplementation has to be approached on an individual basis. However, the following suggestions are offered by Bland for supplementation.[54]

[54] Jeffrey S. Bland, "The Sense and Nonsense of Nutritional Supplements," *Pharmacy West*, May 1976, p. 28.

Table 8-1 Suggested Vitamin B-Complex Supplementation

Vitamin	Requirement
Vitamin B_1	15–20 mg
Vitamin B_2	15–20 mg
Vitamin B_3	20–30 mg
Vitamin B_6	10–30 mg
Vitamin B_{12}	10–20 μg
Biotin	0.3–0.6 mg
Choline	50–100 mg
Folic acid	400–1000 μg
Inositol	250–500 mg
P-aminobenzoic acid	50 mg
Pantothenic acid	100–200 mg

1 Increase intake of vitamin C to 500 to 1000 mg/day and vitamin E to 100 to 400 IU/day. These vitamins have an effect upon reducing the cell destructive process and resulting cellular aging processes.

2 The vitamin B-complex family increases the efficiency of cellular energy production and metabolism. Suggested B-complex supplementation is shown in Table 8-1. Excess amounts of these water soluble agents which are not used by the body will be excreted, and not yield to accumulation contributing to toxicity.

3 Vitamin A is important in night vision and proper mucous tissue and epidermal tissue support. The supplementation should not exceed 20,000 IU/day.

4 Vitamin D is essential for proper bone structure and aiding in the prevention of bone resorption in middle age. It is also fat soluble and excesses should be avoided. A starting supplementary level is 100 IU/day.

5 The minerals, zinc, magnesium, iron, potassium, and iodine should be present in a biochemically supportive diet. These minerals are essential for proper nervous system, adrenal system, circulatory system, and immunological system functions.

6 Certain essential amino acids such as lysine, methionine, tryptophan, and phenylalanine are necessary to supply proper protein precursors and building blocks for brain transmitting substances. These are particularly helpful in cases where people have untoward dietary habits or protein assimilation problems.

Nutritional supplementation requires an informed approach. For nurses interested in promoting the health status of clients through nutritional means, referral to recognized nutritional experts is recommended.

Folk Medicine: Use of Herbs Folk medicine practice is the curative and maintenance behavior used by individuals to solve health problems. The response of many consumers to the ideas of folk medicine and herbalism (the knowledge and study of herbs) is growing. Visits to health food stores, natural or organic food stores, spice or herbal shops will reveal a wide selection of foods, supplements, and herbs. Consumer advocates can always be found in these stores who are knowledgeable, firm, and persuasive about particular products recommended for purchasing. Some people buy herbs for medicinal reasons, some like to try different herbal teas experimentally, and some buy for healing purposes. An intellectual curiosity and a willingness to listen to persuasive arguments about the use of herbs and folk remedies is enlightening. Many of the folk remedies and the folklore of different ethnic groups have merit and bear investigation before discrediting them altogether. It is good practice never to laugh at or ridicule a belief no matter how weird it sounds. The wise nurse will listen and learn about home remedies and practices the family is carrying out and will suggest complementary health measures as necessary or advisable.

Losing Weight   For clients who want to lose weight, much discussion is necessary before a specific weight loss program can be specified. Assessment of the client's past efforts toward losing weight, current eating habits, amount of existing stress in daily life, habitual responses to increased stress, beliefs regarding efficacy of diet methodologies, current level of motivation, current food or drink addictions, enjoyment of eating and drinking—are just some of the factors requiring thorough investigation.

When the nurse and client agree that the client is ready, a nutritional assessment is advised preliminary to instituting a planned program. Diet programs must be individualized and geared toward activities most easily fulfilled by the client. A written contract with the client or a prescriptive activity which the client has agreed is reasonable and attainable should be given a prominent location in the client's home to serve as a daily reminder. Weight loss should be approached in a positive manner, rather than negative. For example, the client should be encouraged to think about acquiring a new exquisite taste for crunchy beautiful salads as opposed to "giving up" icky-sweet cheesecakes for dessert. Whatever the contract or prescriptive activity, the goal should be perceived in a positive way and the encouragement and expectation should be focused positively. For example, the prescriptive activity might be stated: "Goal. Demonstrates the strength and ability to eliminate sweet desserts and glasses of wine from regular diet for 1 week."

The client should be reinforced verbally for all positive behaviors at the same time that measurement of skin folds or weighing on the scale is done. Losing weight effectively is best done slowly and steadily. Minute evidences of success in losing weight must be acknowledged as positive indicators of ultimate success. A basic factor underlying weight loss is the client's motivation and perseverance. It is essential for the nurse to provide regular and consistent support to the client, through whatever means seems to appeal to the client's ego and sense of accomplishment.

Smoking Cessation

Of all the risk factors contributing to a chronic degenerative disease, smoking is one of the most difficult to change. For clients who want to stop smoking, exploration of the variety of smoking cessation programs available in the community must be done to determine methods used for quitting. Clients can be encouraged to enroll in the program which they believe to be most suitable and likely for them to achieve success. Many clients may choose to stop smoking "cold turkey" whereas others may need support and assistance to learn skills that promote self-control and self-directed change. Farquhar suggests a four-step plan that nurses may wish to utilize with clients.[55]

[55] John W. Farquhar, *The American Way of Life Need Not Be Hazardous to Your Health,* W. W. Norton & Company, Inc., New York, 1979.

1 *Identifying the problem*   Since smoking rates vary with each client, it is a good idea to determine exactly the number of cigarettes smoked each day. A simple tally sheet which is marked conscientiously for a period of 1 week will give a fairly accurate count of cigarettes smoked.

2 *Determining commitment to quit smoking*   Eliciting the client's beliefs about her or his capacity to quit smoking must be investigated thoroughly. Identifying potential resistances to change is one of the most important steps in promoting the cessation of smoking. Counterbalancing negative belief barriers with convincing positive alternatives must be thoroughly examined. Discovering a specific antidote for each client to use when faced with the urge to smoke will arm the client with a substitute activity which may provide distraction from the need for a cigarette. Encourage the client to seek a buddy (preferably an ex-smoker) who can give the client social support.

3 *Increasing awareness of smoking patterns*   The first level of awareness is knowing how many cigarettes are smoked a day. The second level of awareness gauges how strong the desire is for each cigarette smoked. The third level reveals the circumstances or cues that trigger the smoking urge (i.e., finishing a meal, feeling tense, drinking coffee or a cocktail, etc.). All three levels can be monitored in a smoking diary by the client who responds to an investigative approach. The important lesson of the diary is to learn which cues trigger the desire to smoke and which carry the strongest urge. Every cigarette is preceded by an urge that can be rated. By learning the circumstances and cues that trigger the most intense urge, experimentation with alternative activities can be practiced until a satisfactory substitute is found.

4 *Building an action plan to quit smoking*   Self-help skills for quitting as suggested by Farquhar are (a) tapering, (b) quitting, and (c) maintenance.

Tapering is a suggested plan for clients who smoke more than 15 cigarettes a day. If the client is able to taper the number of cigarettes smoked to 12 or 15 a day, the experience of learning to suppress the urge to smoke combined with the satisfaction in being able to do so brings subjective rewards which will assist the client to quit altogether. The process of tapering successfully requires that the client learn how to suppress the urge to smoke, enlist social support from family or friends, and develop alternative actions incompatible with smoking. Suppression of the urge to smoke is facilitated by means of imagery and relaxation skills. Have the client think of both positive and negative images of smoking, practice both positive and negative images until the best ones are found for each individual client. Testing for the best images is accomplished by eliciting from the client if she or he can actually *see* and *feel* the positive and negative emotions in the imagery. When this happens, encourage the client to practice the imagery sequence, starting with negative images, relaxing, and shifting to positive images. If the urge-suppression imagery practice can be accomplished in a period of 1 minute, it can be evoked during work or social occasions as frequently as needed. Discuss who the client would like to assist in bolstering her or his effort to taper smoking. Talk about constructive ways the social support person can interact with the client to ensure the best results. Explore with the client smoking substitute activities. Which activity will be the best substitute? Suggested alternatives for smoking include relaxation skills, physical activity such as exercise, eating low-calorie foods, chewing sugarless gum, or other ideas originating from the client. Encouraging the client to write a self-contract for tapering smoking will help to clarify goals and the specific strategies decided upon for the plan of action. The written contract with set deadlines assists the client to carry out the plan.

To strengthen the client for quitting and maintaining the new status as a non-smoker, discussion of potential temptations and ways of resisting them will arm the client with needed behaviors. Encourage the client to write a list of strengths which enabled her or him to quit smoking. Support the client to reward self for completing a successful stop-smoking program. Engage in rehearsals with the client on how to turn down a persuasive offer of a cigarette. Concentrate on the positive behaviors the client used in quitting smoking.

It is not easy to quit smoking and success comes with persistent effort. The nurse can be a constructive supportive person for the client who truly wishes to stop smoking. For clients who are not ready to stop, the nurse can offer a few objective facts about the consequences of smoking, then cease talking about the subject. Assessing client behaviors and being sensitive to and accepting their decisions about smoking has more positive effects in the long run than building client resistance by repeatedly talking about the deleterious effects of smoking. For some clients, the promotion of their health turns out to be a long-term goal for the nurse and requires patience and persistence. The nurse must be watchful for minute indications of readiness to change and capitalize upon these moments whenever they occur.

Dealing with Alcohol-Related Problems

Many families with an alcoholism problem are not immediately detected by community health nurses as having this particular problem because all overt evidences of drinking are disguised in any number of interesting ways. Sometimes nurses will be aware that a family member drinks to excess but do not offer their services because of a feeling of inability to cope with the problem, a preset conviction that nothing constructive can be effected, or an attitude of disapproval based on their own feelings regarding the use of alcohol.

Knowledge about alcohol, how it affects the body physically, behaviorally and socially, indicators of alcohol-related problems, resources for information and treatment should be known by community health nurses.

Ethyl alcohol, or *ethanol*, is the absolute alcohol content in a drink. The ethanol varies from 40 to 50 percent in American distilled spirits, 10 to 14 percent in table wines, and 4 percent in most American beers. The concentration of ethanol in a 12 oz can of beer, a 4 oz glass of table wine, and an 1 oz shot of distilled spirits is relatively equal: ½ oz. The amount of ethanol consumed and the length of time before intoxication varies with each individual. Ethanol is classified as a simple incomplete food with limited nutritional value. It contains calories but lacks vitamins, amino acids, and minerals. Ethanol (above very low blood-alcohol levels) is a depressant which anesthetizes control areas in the central nervous system. If alcohol is consumed regularly at intoxicating levels, pathophysiological effects occur.

Can alcohol be beneficial? A moderate intake of alcohol can:

1 Lessen feelings of tiredness and fatigue
2 Lessen feelings of tension, anxiety, and pressure

   3   Lessen feelings of self-consciousness
   4   Increase feelings of relaxation
   5   Increase a sense of euphoria
   6   Increase feelings of self-esteem
   7   Facilitate a feeling of solidarity among a group of drinkers in a social environment
   8   Facilitate greater honesty and openness
   9   Facilitate talking and laughing
 10   Release inhibitions
 11   Bring about changes in the body's physical functioning (i.e., arouse the appetite, dilate peripheral blood vessels and cause a feeling of warmth, act as a mild sedative, reduce the acuity of the senses)

All of the above responses as associated with a moderate intake of alcohol essentially means a consumption of no more than 2 oz of alcohol a day.[56]

Pathophysiological Effects of Alcohol According to Abernathy, the following pathophysiological effects occur when excess amounts of alcohol are consumed over a long period of time.

Emotions Alcohol decreases cognitive functions and allows the emotions to predominate. With the release of inhibitions, the behavioral manifestations of the emotions are more noticeable and sudden variations in mood may occur. Anger or rage, sadness, and euphoria are commonly experienced during heavy drinking and often displayed in an exaggerated manner.

Personality Alcohol, when long misused, alters the personality. The particular changes caused by alcohol misuse are related to the individual's basic personality structure and individual response to the long-term effects of alcohol.

Sleep While low doses of alcohol induce relaxation and sleepiness, large doses produce sleep disturbances. These are experienced as restlessness and early awakening with difficulty returning to sleep. Results include fatigue, irritability, impairment of concentration and memory, and a variety of physical discomforts.

Sexual Functioning While alcohol may assist in overcoming guilt and lack of self-confidence, promote a feeling of sexiness or amorousness, and release inhibitions, actual performance is impaired. Chronic heavy use of alcohol can result in sexual frigidity or impotency.

Central Nervous System (CNS) Effects Long-term excessive use of alcohol can result in premature aging of the brain. This alcohol-related organic brain syndrome is permanent and irreversible.

---

[56] "The Effects of Alcohol on Body Functions," in The National Center for Alcohol Education, *The Community Health Nurse and Alcohol-Related Problems,* U.S. Department of Health, Education, and Welfare, June 1978, pp. 137–141.

One well-known, but not universal, CNS effect of excessive alcohol use is the blackout. Unlike fainting or "passing out," an individual experiencing a blackout walks, talks, and acts normally, and appears to be aware of what is happening. Yet later, he or she has no recollection of events during the blackout. Reactions to finding out that a blackout has occurred include passive indifference, disbelief, intrigue, and marked fright. Not all persons with alcohol problems experience blackouts.

Pathological Alcohol Reaction   Some people, after drinking only a small amount of alcohol, lose contact with reality, get out of control, violent, and physically destructive. The episode may last several hours. The victim usually collapses in a state of exhaustion and awakens with no memory of what occurred. Pathological alcohol reaction is differentiated from blackout because of the extremely violent behavior that is its prominent feature.

Nutritional Deficiencies   A common nutritional deficiency disorder, *peripheral polyneuropathy,* is characterized by weakness, numbness, partial paralysis of extremities, pain in the legs, and impaired sensory reaction and motor reflexes. This condition is reversible with adequate diet and supplemental thiamine and other B vitamins. If the polyneuropathy is left untreated, it may progress to *Wernicke's encephalopathy.* It is characterized by opththalmoplegia, nystagmus, ataxia, apathy, drowsiness, confusion, and inability to concentrate. Without treatment, it can be fatal.

Gastrointestinal Disorders   Alcohol is an irritating chemical and in strong solution can damage the mucosa and result in esophagitis and gastritis. Increased capillary fragility can result in gastric bleeding. Erosion and ulceration of the mucosa can occur, and gastric or duodenal ulcers are a frequent result.

Cardiovascular Problems   Alcohol affects the cardiovascular system extensively. It causes vasodilation of the peripheral vessels, producing flushing, heat loss, and a sense of warmth, and simultaneously it causes vasoconstriction of the great vessels, producing resistance, thus increasing the work load on the heart.

Hepatic Problems   Enlargement of the liver occurs with prolonged heavy alcohol use, probably as a result of accumulation of triglycerides in the hepatic cells. Alcohol-induced hepatitis and cirrhosis are more serious disease processes.

Pancreatitis   Acute pancreatitis exhibits symptoms ranging in severity from a gastritis-like sensation to severe pain with nausea and vomiting and rigidity of the abdominal musculature. The most serious consequences of this condition include necrosis and hemorrhaging of the organ.

Decreased Immunity and Complications of Other Conditions   Alcohol-dependent persons frequently have a lowered resistance to infections of all types because of the depressing effect of alcohol on the immunological system, especially white blood cells. Upper respiratory infections and pneumonia are common. Injuries, including surgical wounds, require longer to heal.

Effects on the Fetus Alcohol crosses the placental barrier and can have significant adverse effects on the fetus. A particular recurring pattern of fetal abnormalities, called *fetal alcohol syndrome* (FAS) can happen. Most common in the FAS are prenatal growth deficiencies and postnatal growth deficiencies persisting through early childhood. Mental deficiency or developmental delay are almost always present. Fine motor dysfunction including tremulousness, weak grasp, and poor eye-hand coordination are present in most children with FAS.[57]

Indicators of Alcohol-Related Problems and Nursing Intervention Alcoholism should be suspected as an existing problem when the community health nurse is appraised of family disruptions, recurring financial problems, behavior problems exhibited by children, violent arguments, child abuse, wife battering, absenteeism from work or school, serious disruptions in social relationships, and recurring neglect of professional, occupational, or household responsibilities. It is possible that alcoholism will not necessarily be associated with the above indicators; however, the nurse must always rule out the existence of alcohol abuse in the assessment of family situations. When the nurse believes that alcoholism is a factor associated with the family situation, careful preparation must be planned toward the most appropriate intervention method. First of all, the nurse must determine the best person to intervene with the individual or family. Nurses who work best with clients with alcohol-related problems have an open mind, can speak directly and positively, can be practical, patient, realistic, and empathic.

For nurses who choose to intervene directly with the client, the following information must be elicited before determining the best treatment alternative.

1 What is the extent of the client's involvement with alcohol?
2 Has general functioning been affected?
3 What seems to be the client's greatest problem?
4 What is the client's treatment history?
5 How does the client perceive his or her problem?
6 How does the client's family perceive the problem?
7 What are the client's financial resources?[58]

Deciding on the best approach to use with a specific client takes ingenuity, knowledge of the client, persistence, and patience. Initially, education of the client and family about the facts of alcoholism must be carried out. Surprisingly, not all individuals realize the chronicity, progression, and pathological effects of alcohol. Developing a working relationship with the client, family members, or significant others ensures the utilization of appropriate support measures when needed. Communicating with members of allied disciplines (physicians, ministers, friends) enlarges

[57]Mari Wirfs Abernathy, "Alcohol-Related Problems: A Perspective," in the National Center for Alcohol Education, *The Community Health Nurse and Alcohol-Related Problems,* U.S. Department of Health, Education, and Welfare, Washington, D.C., June 1978, pp. 5–13.
[58]Joanne M. Pedersen, "Guidance and Referral of People with Alcohol-Related Problems," in The National Center for Alcohol Education, *The Community Health Nurse and Alcohol-Related Problems.* U.S. Department of Health, Education, and Welfare, Washington, D.C., June 1978, pp. 65–68.

the support network available for the client. Sometimes, a group confrontation between the client and persons caring about the client is necessary for the client to realize that the problem is a serious one. Treatment alternatives can be explored and discussed.

Many community resources are available for information, referral, and treatment. Becoming acquainted with the services of all agencies dealing with alcohol-related problems, philosophy of treatment, methodologies used, incorporation of supportive members (families, friends) assists the nurse in advising the client about alternatives for corrective action.

Working with clients with alcohol-related problems is a difficult assignment for any nurse. Because of the various settings in which the community health nurse works, she or he must be alert and observant for problems associated with alcohol use. Recognizing the prevalent consumption of alcohol in American society, the community health nurse must assume responsibility for teaching about the effects of alcohol to all consumers willing to listen. The average American lacks essential basic information or possesses an abundance of misinformation about the effects of alcohol as a chemical in the body system. Attempting to prevent alcohol misuse or minimize the consumption of alcohol of the average American constitutes a challenge for the nurse committed to health promotion activities.

Ecology and Environment

A person's involvement with the natural environment is inescapable. How you live and what you do has an impact, either directly or indirectly, on the world around you. Whether you are overtly concerned or not, social actions related to pollution (air, noise, water), recycling, disposables, solid wastes, conservation of energy and natural resources, and population control affect *you.*

Historically, as humanity has evolved, the sociocultural system has been able to protect and insulate us increasingly from certain injurious effects of our environments. In other words, over time the human population has adapted to its native environment and maintained a dynamic equilibrium with processes of environmental change.[59]

In our current era, there is a great deal of concern about the encroachment of undesirable problems such as pollution, overcrowding, and limited natural resources due to technology and carelessness. Where there is high population density (urban environment), there is increasing worry about the environmental problems of noise, accumulating garbage, occasional power outages, smog, traffic congestion, high crime rates, etc. In addition, metropolitan areas tend to manifest disordered relationships due to crowding, stress, deprivation, and lack of territorial control.[60] Many existing environments are unhealthy places in which to live, work, play, or visit. Many citizens of the United States live and work, whether cognizant of it or not, under a variety of

---

[59] Solomon H. Katz and Anthony F. C. Wallace, "An Anthropological Perspective on Behavior and Disease," *American Journal of Public Health,* **64**(11):1050–1052, November 1974.

[60] John Cassel, "An Epidemiological Perspective of Psychosocial Factors in Disease Etiology," *American Journal of Public Health,* **64**(11):1040–1043, November 1974.

stresses and potentially hazardous conditions that are likely to affect their state of health.

For residents living in urban areas, the city is a human-constructed environment with little evidence of plant life. The rural areas contain a very low density of erected structures dominated by a rural landscape of woods and fields. The suburban areas represent a blend of both city and town with a more equal balance of plant life and structures.[61]

Each community has its distinctive history, geography, neighborhoods, climate, and flavor. Each community and its residents must be assessed individually in terms of the variety of factors affecting the health of the population.

According to Cassel, Hinkle, and Kasl it is the social environment and not the physical environment which is the primary determinant of the health and well-being of people who live in cities. In other words, within wide limits, it is not the physical condition of the house, neighborhood, or human settlement that determines a person's health so much as the individual's social background, perception of environment, and relation to other people and to her or his social group.[62] As an example of this hypothesis, it is pointed out that the well-to-do who live in Manhattan are healthier than the poor residents in that city, even though they share the same dirty air, the same noise, and the same density of people per acre of land or even per dwelling unit. The correlates of social position are not limited to education, occupation, income, and type of dwelling; they include maternal health, infant mortality, child care, family size, frequency of family disruption and of major family problems, and all of the habits, attitudes, and behavior that a person learns from the social milieu in which she or he grows up. These, it seems, are more important determinants of health and behavior than the physical characteristics of the buildings lived and worked in, of the surrounding neighborhood, or of the cities.

It is true that major improvements in health have occurred in the past through better housing, cleaner water supplies, adequate sanitation, and higher standards of education. However, it is also recognized that not all persons who harbor organisms, such as the tubercle bacillus, or pneumococcus, contract those respective diseases. The organism is a necessary factor for the development of a disease, but it is rarely a sufficient factor. As pointed out by White, data must be collected about the circumstances under which the disease occurred, the interactions between the client and the environment, the noxious agents involved, and the social, cultural, biological factors influencing the vulnerability of the client for the disease.[63] As stated by Kennedy, illness is both a social and biological phenomenon. A person's health and well-being depend in a significant way upon perceptions, attitudes, and expectations

[61] Donald A. Kennedy, "Community Health and the Urban Environment," in Lawrence E. Hinkle, Jr. and William C. Loring (eds.), *The Effect of the Man-Made Environment on Health and Behavior,* Department of Health, Education, and Welfare Publication CDC-77-8318, Washington, D.C., 1977, p. 10.

[62] Lawrence E. Hinkle, Jr., "Some Implications of These Papers," in Lawrence E. Hinkle, Jr., and William C. Loring (eds.), *The Effect of the Man-Made Environment on Health and Behavior,* Department of Health, Education, and Welfare Publication CDC-77-8318, Washington, D.C., 1977, p. 301.

[63] Kerr L. White, "Health Problems and Priorities and the Health Professions," *Preventive Medicine,* 6:560–566, 1977.

about the world in which she or he operates. Health also depends upon the individual's pattern of participation in the activities and needs of various groups, organizations, communities, and societies that compose the sociosphere.[64]

If the above premises are accepted as true, community health nurses can contribute significantly toward wellness of individuals by eliciting data that is comprehensive and sensitive to social, cultural, physiological, mental, emotional, and environmental factors influencing clients' well-being. Not all histories taken by health professionals cover all facets influencing the health of individuals. Valuable and significant data can be assembled by community health nurses and used creatively to educate clients regarding the benefits of health promotion measures.

To have an effect on environmental problems, the community health nurse must be cognizant of community action procedures as a means for changing pathological behavior patterns of individuals or social groups or introducing protective health patterns. A familiarity with social epidemiology leads one to investigate cultural situations, social situations, and personality situations as they interrelate with the host and agent, so as to provide knowledge about intervention points toward which prevention can be directed. As stated by Graham, there is much epidemiological knowledge about the agent, vector, and host, and what should be done to effect prevention; however, behavioral changes that are necessary and the sociological knowledge regarding how this behavior can be successfully altered to effect prevention is lacking.[65] Scientific studies can be initiated by community health nurses which study social factors influencing the behavior of individuals in specific environments, and findings may instigate new directions for health promotion activities.

On a local scale, nurses should be knowledgeable of current environmental and ecological issues. By practicing energy conservation measures such as reducing the amount of electric energy used daily; riding buses, car pooling, bicycling, or walking to work; saving recycled materials; planting a garden; reducing the amount of water used daily, the nurse can command respect as a role model who offers concrete, explicit, workable methods based on practical experiences.

SUMMARY

The American population is becoming better acquainted with the concept of wellness and the variety of ideas promoting health, improved lifestyles, adoption of health practices that lower risk of disease, and knowledge of noxious agents in everyone's environment. Community health nurses must be ready to prescribe activities which will help clients specifically to move toward improved states of health. Activities receiving an overview in this chapter include exercise, relaxation, visualization, humor, and nutritional assessments. Noxious agents about which all individuals need more education are smoking, the consumption of excessive amounts of alcohol, and environmental hazards. The health promotion activities and discussion of selected health problems in this chapter represent only a few of the wide variety of health promotional programs and methodologies advocated by health professionals and lay persons alike. Community health nurses must be alert to the emergence of new methodologies

[64] Kennedy, op. cit., p. 24.
[65] Saxon Graham, "The Sociological Approach to Epidemiology," *American Journal of Public Health,* **64**(11):1046–1049, November 1974.

and make informed decisions regarding the adequacies of proposed programs before recommending and prescribing them specifically for their clients.

SUGGESTED READING

Anderson, Robert: "The Perfect Pre-Run Stretching Routine," *Runner's World,* May 1978, pp. 56–61.

Anderson, Robert A.: *Stress Power! How to Turn Tension into Energy,* Human Sciences Press, New York, 1978.

American College of Sports Medicine: *Guidelines for Graded Exercise Testing and Exercise Prescription,* Lea & Febiger, Philadelphia, 1976.

American Medical Association: *Fit for Fun,* American Medical Association, Chicago, Illinois, 1978.

Ardell, Donald B.: *High Level Wellness,* Bantam Books, Inc., New York, 1977.

Ashford, Nicholas: *Crisis in the Workplace,* Massachusetts Institute of Technology Press, Cambridge, Mass., 1976.

Barksdale, L. S.: *Building Self-Esteem,* Barksdale Foundation, Idyllwide, Calif., 1974.

Belloc, Nedra B.: "Relationship of Health Practices and Mortality," *Preventive Medicine,* 2:67–81, March 1973.

Belloc, Nedra B., and Lester Breslow: "Relationship of Physical Health Status and Health Practices," *Preventive Medicine,* 1:409–421, August 1972.

Benson, Herbert: *The Relaxation Response,* William Morrow & Company, Inc., New York, 1975.

Berry, Carol, and Tom Ferguson: "How to Stay Healthy in a Polluted World," *Medical Self-Care,* No. 8, Spring 1980, pp. 3–12.

Bland, Jeffrey S.: *Your Health under Siege: Using Nutrition to Fight Back,* The Stephen Greene Press, Brattleboro, Vt., 1981.

Boston Women's Health Book Collective: *Our Bodies, Ourselves,* Simon & Schuster, Inc., New York, 1973.

Breslow, Lester, and Anne R. Somers: "The Lifetime Health-Monitoring Program," *The New England Journal of Medicine,* 296(11):601–608, March 17, 1977.

Brown, Barbara B.: *New Mind, New Body: Bio-Feedback: New Directions for the Mind,* Harper & Row, Publishers, Inc., New York, 1974.

Cooper, Kenneth H.: *The Aerobics Way,* Bantam Books, Inc., 1977.

Carlton, Bill: "A Study of the Health and Sickness Behavior of Selected Adults in Southeast Kentucky," *Public Health Reports,* 93(4):356–361, July–August 1978.

Cousins, Norman: *Anatomy of an Illness as Perceived by the Patient,* W. V. Norton & Company, Inc., New York, 1979.

Davis, Louis E. et al.: *The Quality of Working Life,* The Free Press, New York, 1975.

Deutsch, Ronald: *The New Nuts among the Berries,* Bull Publishing, Palo Alto, Calif., 1979.

Doyle, Rodger, and James Redding: *The Complete Food Handbook,* Grove Press, Inc., New York, 1976.

Eckholm, Erik P.: *The Picture of Health,* W. W. Norton & Company, Inc., New York, 1977.

Estes, Nada J.: *Nursing Diagnosis of the Alcoholic Person,* The C. V. Mosby Company, St. Louis, 1980.

Elting, L. Melvin, and Seymour Isenberg: *You Can Be Fat-Free Forever,* Penguin Books, Inc., New York, 1974.

Farquhar, John W.: *The American Way of Life Need Not Be Hazardous to Your Health,* W. W. Norton & Company, Inc., New York, 1979.

Ford, Loretta C.: "Influencing Health Values," *Health Values: Achieving High Level Wellness,* **1**(1):17–21, January–February 1977.

Fuchs, Victor R.: *Who Shall Live?* Basic Books, Inc., New York, 1974.

Gartner, Alan, and Frank Riessman: *Self-Help in the Human Services,* Jossey-Bass Publishers, San Francisco, 1977.

Goldberg, Philip: *Executive Health,* McGraw-Hill Book Company, New York, 1978.

Hamburg, David A.: "Disease Prevention: The Challenge of the Future," *American Journal of Public Health,* **69**(10):1026–1033, October 1979.

Haynes, R. Brian, D. Wayne Taylor, and David L. Sackett: *Compliance in Health Care,* The Johns Hopkins University Press, Baltimore, Md., 1979.

Hinkle, Lawrence E., Jr., and William C. Loring (eds.): *The Effect of the Man-Made Environment on Health and Behavior,* U.S. Department of Health, Education, and Welfare, Publication CDC-77-8318, Washington, D.C., 1977.

Hittleman, Richard: *Be Young with Yoga,* Warner Paperback Library, New York, 1962.

Hochbaum, Godfrey M.: *Health Behavior,* Wadsworth Publishing Company, Inc., Belmont, Calif., 1970.

Jacobson, Edmund: *How to Teach Scientific Relaxation,* Instructor's Text, Auspices, Foundation for Scientific Relaxation, Inc., Chicago, 1958.

Jacobson, Edmund: *You Must Relax,* McGraw-Hill Book Company, Inc., New York, 1962.

Jarvis, D. C.: *Folk Medicine,* Fawcett Publications, Inc., Greenwich, Conn., 1958.

Jospe, Michael: *The Placebo Effect in Healing,* Lexington Books, D. C. Heath and Company, Lexington, Mass., 1978.

Knowles, John H.: *Doing Better and Feeling Worse,* W. W. Norton & Company, Inc., New York, 1977.

Krieger, Dolores: *The Therapeutic Touch,* Prentice-Hall, Inc., Englewood Cliffs, N.J., 1979.

Lappé, Frances Moore: *Diet for a Small Planet,* Friends of the Earth, Ballantine Books, 1971.

Lazes, Peter M. (ed.): *The Handbook of Health Education,* Aspen Systems Corporation, Germantown, Md., 1979.

Lust, John B.: *The Herb Book,* Bantam Books, Inc., New York, 1974.

"Making Health Education Work," *American Journal of Public Health,* supplement, **65**:1–44, October 1975.

McCamy, John C., and James Presley: *Human Life Styling,* Harper & Row, Publishers, Inc., New York, 1975.

Milio, Nancy: "A Framework for Prevention: Changing Health-Damaging to Health-Generating Life Patterns," *American Journal of Public Health,* **66**(5):435–439, May 1976.

Morehouse, Laurence E., and Leonard Gross: *Total Fitness in 30 Minutes a Week,* Simon & Schuster, Inc., New York, 1975.

National Center for Alcohol Education: *The Community Health Nurse and Alcohol-Related Problems,* A Book of Readings, U.S. Department of Health, Education, and Welfare Publication ADM-281-75-0013, Washington, D.C., June 1978.

National Institute on Drug Abuse: *A Woman's Choice—Deciding About Drugs,* U.S. Department of Health, Education, and Welfare Publication ADM-79-820, Washington, D.C., 1979.

Pantell, Robert H., James F. Fries, and Donald M. Vickery: *Taking Care of Your Child: A Parent's Guide to Medical Care,* Addison-Wesley Publishing Company, Reading, Mass., 1977.

Pelletier, Kenneth R.: *Mind as Healer, Mind as Slayer,* Delacorte Press, New York, 1977.

Pender, Nola J.: "A Conceptual Model for Preventive Health Behavior," *Nursing Out-Look,* 23(6):385–390, June 1975.

Pritikin, Nathan, and Patrick M. McGrady, Jr.,: *The Pritikin Program for Diet & Exercise,* Bantam Books, Inc., New York, 1979.

Report of the Departmental Task Force on Prevention: *Disease Prevention and Health Promotion: Federal Programs and Prospects,* U.S. Department of Health, Education, and Welfare Publication 79-550718, Washington, D.C., September, 1978.

Roberts, Toni M., Kathleen McIntosh Tinker, and Donald W. Kemper: *Healthwise Handbook,* A Dolphin Book, Garden City, New York, 1979.

Roemer, Milton: *Rural Health Care,* The C. V. Mosby Company, St. Louis, 1976.

Royal Canadian Air Force: *Exercise Plans for Physical Fitness,* Pocket Books, New York, 1962.

Samuels, Mike, and Hal Bennett: *The Well-Body Book,* Random House, Inc., New York, 1973.

Sehnert, Keith, and Howard Eisenberg: *How To Be Your Own Doctor (Sometimes),* Grosset and Dunlap, New York, 1975.

Select Committee on Nutrition and Human Needs, U.S. Senate: *Dietary Goals for the United States,* 2nd Ed., Government Printing Office, Washington, D.C., 1977.

Selye, Hans: *Stress without Distress,* New America Library, New York, 1974.

Simonds, Scott K.: "Toward a Nonsmoking Society," *Health Values: Achieving High Level Wellness,* 2(1):22–30, January–February 1978.

Simonton, O. Carl, Stephanie Matthews-Simonton, and James Creighton: *Getting Well Again,* Bantam Books, Inc., New York, 1978.

Sheehy, Gail: *Passages,* Bantam Books, Inc., E. P. Dutton & Company, Inc., 1976.

Sobell, David S.: *Ways of Health,* Harcourt-Brace-Jovanovich, New York, 1979.

Stellman, Seanne, and Susan Daum: *Work is Dangerous to Your Health,* Vintage Books, New York, 1973.

"Stress, A Special Feature," *American Journal of Nursing,* 79(10):1953–1964, November 1979.

Surgeon General's Report on Health Promotion and Disease Prevention: *Healthy People,* U.S. Department of Health, Education, and Welfare Publication 79-55071, 1979.

Tager, Mark and Charles Jennings: *Whole Person Health Care,* 2d ed., Victoria House, Inc., Portland, Oreg., 1978.

Terris, Milton: "Approaches to an Epidemiology of Health," *American Journal of Public Health,* 65(10):1037–1045, October 1975.

Toffler, Alvin: *The Eco-Spasm Report,* Bantam Books, Inc., New York, 1975.

Vickery, Donald, and James F. Fries: *Take Care of Yourself, A Consumers' Guide to Medical Care,* Addison-Wesley, Reading, Mass., 1977.

Watts, Alan W.: *This Is It,* The Macmillan Company, New York, 1969.

Waldbott, George L.: *The Health Effects of Environmental Pollutants,* The C. V. Mosby Company, St. Louis, 1973.

White, Leon S.: "How to Improve the Public's Health," *The New England Journal of Medicine,* 293(15):773–774, October 9, 1975.

Chapter 9

Valuing the Aged

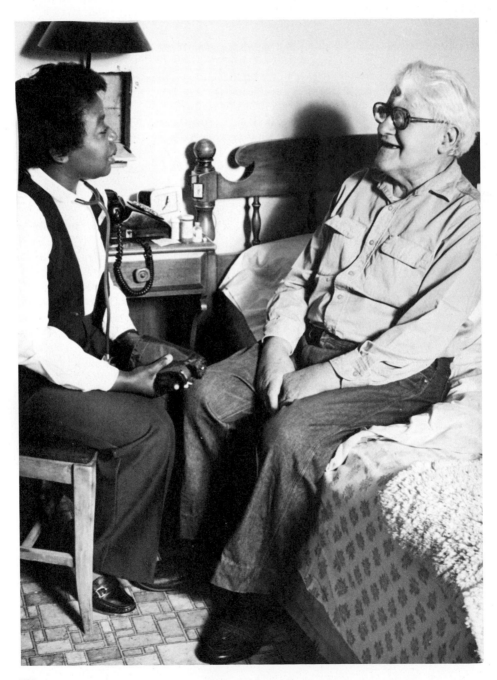

Aging is a process that can be viewed from several perspectives. The positive view is analogous to the aging of wine—the more years that it ages, the more priceless and exquisite it becomes—a veritable treasure to possess! The natural view accepts the normal sequence of aging as when the hardy crocus withers; the beautiful rose loses its bloom and gradually drops its petals; the apple becomes dry, wizened, or wrinkled; the leaves of the vine maple become brillant before fading and becoming brown and dry. The negative view is analogous to fashion. When an item is no longer in style, it is considered old, useless, and generally discarded. All these views of the aging process are existent in our society, and are transferred to our aging citizens for assimilation as they see fit.

Gerontological and geriatric nursing has emerged as a popular, special field and has provided valuable content for community health nurses. Insights relative to the processes of aging and how it affects persons in our society have provided nurses with a basis for understanding physical and behavioral changes. With this increased understanding, nurses are able to support healthful living practices among the aging and to more readily identify symptoms and signs of incipient disease. Interpretations by nurses enable elderly clients and their families to better utilize medical, social, and personal resources in planning for more healthful and satisfying living in the later years.[1]

DESCRIPTIVE DATA ABOUT THE AGED

As defined by the lawmakers, 65 years of age is the legal time for people to retire with social security benefits, and this influences the attitudes and expectations of many citizens regarding the transition to becoming old. Most older people live in a family setting, usually in their own households. Of every 100 older people, 28 live alone or with nonrelatives. Only 5 percent of old people live in institutions. Most elderly people live in the central city; approximately 35 percent live in small towns, and 5 percent live on farms.[2]

Ninety percent of senior citizens have some income from retirement payments; others work, but a great majority are categorized as poor economically. The elderly have chronic diseases and have medical expenditures 3½ times those of people under 65 years of age.[3] In personality and behavior, senior citizens are people as various and as individual as any younger group; possibly, they are more so.[4]

In a longitudinal study done by Maas and Kuypers, the lifestyles and personality orientation of 142 respondents were examined over a 40-year time period.[5] Most of the subjects were economically well-off and very few had below average incomes. All the respondents were parents of children when originally selected for study.

---

[1] Myrtle Irene Brown, "Nursing of the Aging and Aged," in Austin B. Chinn (ed.), *Working with Older People: Clinical Aspects of Aging,* vol. 4, U.S. Department of Health, Education and Welfare, July 1971, p. 354.

[2] Jack Botwinick, "Who Are the Aged?" *Geriatrics.* 29(7):124–129, July 1974.

[3] Ibid., p. 126.

[4] Ibid., p. 129.

[5] Henry S. Maas and Joseph A. Kuypers, *From Thirty to Seventy,* Jossey-Bass Publishers, San Francisco, 1974, pp. 1–215.

A conclusion of this study, based on the accumulated data, shows that there are innumerable potentials for variety in lifestyle in old age. The findings brought out that fathers characteristically had a continuity of lifestyle from young adulthood into old age, due to relatively few changes in their environment, other than retirement. For mothers, lifestyle changes were more apparent, sometimes radical, due to pressures of marital, parental, occupational, and environmental factors that forced adaptation to a greater or lesser degree. It was found that qualities of life in old age are highly associated, in complex ways, to qualities of life 40 years earlier. Mothers revealed continuities in personality, from early adulthood to old age, more so than fathers, and this finding was most evident for those mothers whose late-adult personality was characterized by anxiety and ego disorganization. The only suggested explanation for this finding was the presence, both in old age and in early adulthood, of depressive tendencies, low self-worth, tension, and high self-doubt.

Conclusions from these findings suggest that old age, to be properly understood, should be viewed as an integral part of the life cycle and not as a terminal period apart from the earlier years of life. Wives and mothers should expand their interests and involvement beyond the circle of the family if their later years are not to become problematic ones. Health is a crucial correlate of total personal functioning in old age. Health problems in old age are likely to be clearly foreshadowed in the early-adult years.[6]

For community health nurses, whether talking about housing, retirement, economic factors, leisure-time experiences, or health services, it must be remembered that aging persons have a wide diversity of interests, capacities, and needs and should be provided with a wide diversity of opportunities and provisions. As pointed out in the Maas and Kuypers study, most parents in their old age are not traveling a downhill course; they are involved in rewarding and diversely patterned lives. They demonstrated that different ways of living can be developed as social environments change with time. For some, old age provided a second and better chance at life.[7]

PROBLEMS OF THE AGED

Some of the crises which must be met by the elderly include the following: completion of the parental role; withdrawal from active community and organizational leadership; termination of marriage through death of one's mate; loss of an independent household; loss of interest in distant goals and plans; the necessity of depending on others or on society for support, advice, and management of funds; physical disabilities, such as arthritis and cataracts; assumption of a subordinate position to adult persons; taking up membership in groups made up largely of old people.[8] Other crises which are often unanticipated are loss of mobility due to failing sight or inability to walk any distances, the potential for robberies or muggings, nutritional

---

[6] Ibid., p. 1–215.
[7] Ibid., p. 215.
[8] Paul L. Niebanck, *The Elderly in Older Urban Areas,* Institute for Environemntal Studies, University of Pennsylvania, Philadelphia, 1965, pp. 96–97.

deficiencies due to limited mobility, depressed affect, inadequate funds, change in living situation, and possibility of falls, fractures, and fires.[9] The manner in which the elderly person copes with and adjusts to these crises as they occur in life depends on the individual's personality, attitude, and past experiences, which may have been negative or positive. In order for aging to occur satisfactorily, it is essential that flexibility in adjustment to new situations be developed. Frequently, clients are not aware of crisis potential and may need to be alerted to preventive practices or improved coping mechanisms which will serve as precautionary measures.

Community health nurses can play an important role in assisting the elderly to strengthen their coping abilities, as the nurses interact with the aged in their home situations. In some cases, clients do not seek help actively because of a variety of factors, such as pride of independence, a stoic acceptance of difficulties, a sense of helplessness, a fear of the unknown, or unawareness of available resources.[10] When these particular clients come to the attention of the nurse, she or he must take the initiative to become thoroughly aware of the home situation, assess the health status and capabilities of the client, elicit the concerns of the client, and introduce preventive measures which will support optimal, satisfying living conditions. In so doing, the nurse must have a relationship with the client which is trusting and understanding of the basis for all actions taken.

Retirement

Retirement has a definite effect on the elderly, because it forces them to change many of their basic relationships and habits. Some of the expectations directed toward retired persons is that they will assume responsibility for managing their own lives; they will live within their income regardless of its adequacy; they will avoid becoming dependent on their families or on the community; they will engage in leisure time or volunteer roles.[11] Whether retirement is anticipated as desirable, inevitable, or dreadful, the complexity of this social role becomes gradually apparent as specific privileges, expectations, and relationships evolve. A new framework of activity and interests have to be developed. Since a basic psychological hunger of people is for time structure, the retired person must find new purposeful and satisfactory ways of structuring the day. A variety of tasks, activities, or hobbies can be undertaken, dependent upon the energy, enthusiasm, and interest of the person. Sometimes a reduction of income affects the manner in which the retired person lives. Or the income may be ample but a decline in health changes the living pattern so that some former activities can no longer be enjoyed. When widowhood occurs, this often means a severance of a fundamental relationship that has given stability and meaning to life. The process of readjustment is a lengthy one, and often important decisions have to be made during this critical period which affect the remainder of the person's life.[12]

[9] Priscilla Pierre Ebersole, "Crisis Intervention with the Aged," in Irene Mortenson Burnside (ed.), *Nursing and the Aged,* McGraw-Hill Book Company, New York, 1976, pp. 272–273.
[10] Ibid., p. 280.
[11] Robert C. Atchley, "Retirement," in Irene Mortenson Burnside (ed.), *Nursing and the Aged,* McGraw-Hill Book Company, New York, 1976, p. 532.
[12] Niebanck, op. cit., pp. 97–102.

Loneliness

The elderly often experience a deep sense of loneliness and isolation as they try to reaffirm meaning to their lives. Conti described several elderly persons who had individually adapted to lifestyles that were unsatisfactory because of their loneliness. She described how the community health nurse visited these persons who initially denied their loneliness, but consented to receiving the attention of a "caring" person and eventually made adjustments to more satisfactory coping patterns. For some, this meant attendance of senior citizen groups for socialization or participation in a range of activities. The work of the nurse with these elderly people meant communicating her value of them as human beings and showing acceptance, understanding, and patience with them before they were ready to reveal their feelings or willingness to make a change in adjustment.[13] Pets are very important to some elderly persons. For those clients who have difficulty with the English language, bringing persons to visit who speak their native tongue gives pleasure. Certain times of the day or night are lonely periods for some clients. By arranging a telephone call or social visit at these particular times, the loneliness may be assuaged.[14]

Nurses should be particularly observant of symptoms of depression in the elderly. Because the aged have difficulty tolerating the loss of physical health, special attention should be focused on impairments of vision, hearing, or ambulation. When a client complains of anxiety, nervousness, insomnia, loss of energy, loss of appetite, the nurse should become alerted to feelings of depression. The therapy of hope is one of the best strategies to use as opportunities are devised for social contacts and the strengthening of self-esteem. In as many creative ways as the nurse can discover, efforts should be directed toward increasing the sense of usefulness of the client. Simple rewards are satisfying and appreciated when given in recognition of even a small gain.[15] By caring and being sensitively supportive of the client's concerns, the nurse strengthens the client to face each day.

Elderly persons sometimes move slowly and think slowly, but they are very responsive to the enthusiasm and warmth of young people and delight in any kind of exchange with young people. They also are very responsive to sensory stimulation and should be touched or stroked whenever a practical opportunity arises. Sensory experiences are important for psychological well-being. For example, the nurse should always feel the pulse, whether it needs to be known or not, comb the hair, press the ankle for edema, or give a reassuring body squeeze whenever wanting to communicate approval or acceptance. In many ways, elderly persons are like little children and do not mind being treated with warmth, fun, or simple games. If encouraged to attend small group discussions where a subject of interest is being explored, participants can find this to be a stimulating way of sharing ideas or receiving recognition, particularly when they have an able nurse leader or facilitator.

[13] Mary Louise Conti, "The Loneliness of Old Age," *Nursing Outlook,* 18(8):28–30, August 1970.

[14] Irene Mortenson Burnside, "Mental Health in the Aged," in Irene Mortenson Burnside (ed.), *Nursing and the Aged,* McGraw-Hill Book Company, New York, 1976, p. 143.

[15] Irene Mortenson Burnside, "Depression and Suicide in the Aged," in Irene Mortenson Burnside (ed.), Nursing and the Aged, *McGraw-Hill Book* Company, New York 1976, p. 172.

MYTHS ABOUT AGING

Some myths about the elderly which must be checked out in terms of the acquaintance of the nurse with any aged client include the following:

1 The expected passive behavior pattern of the person in retirement. The right to "take it easy" has been earned, and the client now can rest. Does the client conform to this myth? Is the client content? What is her or his philosophy of life? Is satisfaction with resting evident?

2 Dependence on others for advice and assistance is a natural and inevitable consequence of advancing age. Does the client accept dependence graciously or seem to be fiercely independent? Who are the acceptable persons from whom advice and assistance will be taken?

3 Custodial care in institutions is the answer to chronic illness, invalidity, and mental disturbances. How does the client feel about institutional care? Has she or he personally visited any nursing or retirement homes? If custodial care is needed, what does this mean to the individual?

4 Withdrawal from social participation tends to accompany departure from employment. Is the client active socially? Has the client withdrawn from former social groups voluntarily? Is she or he lonely? Is encouragement needed to join new groups, such as a senior activity center?

5 No preparation for retirement is required or expected. How is the client adjusting to retirement? Were most of the changes anticipated? How would she or he advise others to prepare for retirement?

6 Older persons are unable to learn new skills.[16] Since cognitive processes do not decline with age, what generally happens in learning a new skill is the necessity for unlearning a well-established way of doing things. This means willingness to change. For most individuals, the initial response to a new idea is resistance which is more a function of intelligence, cultural, and experiential factors than one of age.[17] Will the client be willing to try out a new skill? Is the client a *possibility* thinker—a person who perceptively probes every problem proposal, and opportunity to discover the positive aspects present in almost every human situation? Or is the client an *impossibility* thinker—a person who makes swift, sweeping passes over a proposed idea, scanning it with a sharp, negative eye, looking only for reasons why something will not work instead for visualizing ways in which it could work?[18]

WORKING WITH THE AGED

For nurses visiting the elderly in their homes, it is a delight to witness the uncovering of each personality as the history of each person is evoked. The pictures, belongings, and other memorabilia in the home provide the nurse with clues regarding the client's interests and sources of comfort. Elderly persons love to talk with animated nurses

[16] Ernest W. Burgess, *Aging in Western Society,* The University of Chicago Press, Chicago, 1960, p. 20.

[17] Kathy Gribbin, "Cognitive Processes in Aging," in Irene Mortenson Burnside (ed.), *Nursing and the Aged,* McGraw-Hill Book Company, New York, 1976, p. 49.

[18] Robert H. Schuller, *Move Ahead with Possibility Thinking,* Doubleday & Company, Inc., Garden City, N.Y., 1967, pp. 2–3.

who are client-centered and willing to draw out their thoughts about past events, present concerns, and future desires. Whenever special interests, skills, and hobbies are discovered that had meaning for them in the past, they might respond to persuasion to resume the favored activities, if feasible. Sometimes a modification of procedures must be devised because of physical impairments or economic factors.

A firm, persistent, persuasive, encouraging approach works well with elderly clients. The "laying on of hands" is advisable whenever an opportunity presents itself, i.e., taking a pulse, checking for edema of extremities, or reaching out with a friendly touch.

As pointed out by a nursing student:

> . . . even if health care is readily accessible to the elderly client, the formal technological care they receive is not the care they want. Frequently they are lonely. A client may dutifully take medications for hypertension, cardiac or respiratory diseases every day and have monthly checkups, but may not be healthy if she or he does not feel someone is definitely concerned—not blood pressure or urine, but the total human being. Affection is a primary element in caring for the elderly, and many of our older citizens are environmentally isolated in our modern life. If an older person lives alone, she or he may not see or talk with another person for a week or more. As isolation develops, the elderly person may not bother with reading a paper or using other communication media. With the decrease in sensory stimulation, apathy and/or mental deterioration becomes an inevitable eventuality.

The Advocate Role with Elderly

Nurses are well acquainted with the term "advocacy" and most believe that they participate as client advocates. However, when a situation arises that involves a choice in favor of the physician versus the client, or the employing agency versus the client, nurses frequently choose the route safest for their own survival. Often, that means the client loses a needed advocate. Being an advocate means taking a risk in behalf of the client. As stated by Kohnke, advocacy is the "act of defending or pleading" the case of another. Or, as it is used in nursing, *advocacy* is the act of informing and supporting a person so that the best decisions possible for the self can be made.[19] Acting as an advocate according to Kohnke's definition means (1) informing clients of what their rights are in a particular situation and then making sure they have all the necessary information to make an informed decision, and (2) supporting clients in the decisions they make. If the client makes a decision which the nurse judges to be a poor one, it is still the client's right to make such a decision. It is even more difficult for the nurse if the client's decision is in opposition to his physician's wishes or institutional policy. However, it must be remembered that individuals who make decisions also bear responsibility for the consequences of that decision. A true nurse advocate who does not want to be labeled as a "rescuer" avoids making decisions *for* clients. That nurse focuses on giving all necessary information to the client so that the client makes her or his own best and informed decision.

[19] Mary F. Kohnke, "The Nurse as Advocate," *American Journal of Nursing,* 80(11):2038–2040, November 1980.

Many elderly clients need advocates. When working with and educating clients about their particular life situations, nurses can act as advocates but they must also inquire about supporting family members, friends, and neighbors. The person closest to and most supportive of the client's needs must be counseled about the client's rights, informed of all aspects of the client's situation, and encouraged to act as the client's advocate or in behalf of the client's interests, depending on the situation. Elderly persons often need reassurances that they can make right and responsible decisions. When the nurse and significant supportive persons in the client's environment reinforce the ability of clients to decide for themselves according to their innate wishes, a respect and dignity is accorded them which they have earned.

For elderly clients who are unable to make informed decisions because of confusion, memory loss, or related reasons, family members or significant supportive persons acting in behalf of the client must be informed of all alternatives available in the client's situation and must bear responsibility for making correct decisions. Nurses can serve these clients best by encouraging, educating, and supporting family members and/or authorized representatives how to act in the role of client advocates.

Health Assessment   To maintain the health status of elderly citizens, community health nurses must function as warm, caring, person-centered nurses and as client advocates. *Advocacy* is action designed to help the powerless (or aged) acquire and use power to make social systems (health organizations) more responsive to recipient needs.[20] When acting as a client advocate, the nurse has the opportunity and responsibility to teach relevant health information concurrently with the health assessment of the client. As the client perceives and understands the meaning of the health information and realizes the availability of goals and options for responsible action, the health decisions can be made purposefully and with a sense of control over outcomes that are realistic and feasible for her or his life situation. When searching for ways to clarify health information more explicitly for elderly clients, nurses can make use of visual tools (see Chap. 3), provide sufficient time for decisions, and accentuate the options with fewest risks.

A complete assessment of elderly clients include:

1   A health assessment of each referred client.
   a   A health history which includes historical information, past health history, family history, occupational history, sexual history, and current health complaints.
   b   A review of systems inclusive of vital signs, blood pressure, height, weight, heart sounds, lung sounds, inspection of feet and nails. Has the client had a recent physical examination? If using a corrective device (hearing aid, glasses, dentures), is it in good working order?
   c   Examination of all medications taken, frequency, method of administration, purpose of medications, client's understanding about the importance of each medication and possible side effects, reminder system for taking medications as

---

[20] Joan C. Rogers, "Advocacy: The Key to Assessing the Older Client," *Journal of Gerontological Nursing,* 6(1):33–36, January 1980.

prescribed by the physician. Elderly clients "frequently have multiple chronic disease states that require long-term multiple drug therapy."[21] Errors of omission, erratic dosage, and overdosage when medications are self-administered are not uncommon.

d A nutritional assessment of diet history. Determine the adequacy of nutrients (minerals, vitamins) in the diet, assess the client's knowledge about essential foods, foods to avoid, regularity of meals, practice of snacking, recommended supplemental foods, food likes and dislikes, fluid intake. "The person who eats alone should be suspected of marginal nutrition and this fact should lead to observation and inspection for further signs."[22]

e Assessment of activity of daily living (ADL) of each client, ability to give self-care, mobility, housekeeping ability, amount of exercise done on a daily basis, client's receptivity to learning simple exercises, avocational interests.

f Determination of client's ability to relax or method of reducing stress, client's receptivity to learning relaxation measures.

2 Examination of the home for environmental hazards, need for minor repairs, recommended safety measures.

3 Determination of the significant family members or neighbors in case of emergency.

4 Exploration of client's knowledge of available community resources according to personal needs, such as senior citizen centers, meals on wheels, transportation resources, recreational facilities, volunteer opportunities, mobile library, home health services, and educational facilities.

5 Assessment of client's lifestyle, friends, frequency of socialization with others, recreational interests, hobbies, crafts, ability to reach out and join others, client's willingness to learn new occupational skills.

6 Assessment of characteristics of client's neighborhood and the residents in that neighborhood. The accessibility of services such as food, drugs, banks, post offices, church, welfare office, etc.; the safety of the neighborhood during daylight and night hours.

While interviewing elderly clients, the nurse must clarify the purpose for each question asked and the relevancy of each question to the client's current health status. Practice patience, persistence, and rephrasing of questions until satisfactory responses are obtained. For the most part, nurses customarily ask questions eliciting past health history, family history, and current health complaints. Data which are frequently overlooked comprise historical information, the occupational history and the sexual history of the client.

Questions encouraging a life review by the client draw forth past events and the client's perception of these life events. The process of *life review* is a naturally occurring and universal mental process in which past experiences progressively return to consciousness. It is not synonymous with, but includes, reminiscence.[23] As the client engages in reexamining her or his whole life, the nurse can be an excellent listener,

[21] Ronald C. Kayne, "Drugs and the Aged," in Irene Mortenson Burnside (ed.), *Nursing and the Aged,* McGraw-Hill Book Company, New York, p. 438.

[22] Mary Opal Wolanin, "Nursing Assessment," in Irene Mortenson Burnside (ed.), *Nursing and the Aged,* McGraw-Hill Book Company, New York, p. 406.

[23] Sandra Chubon, "A Novel Approach to the Process of Life Review," *Journal of Gerontological Nursing,* 6(9):543–546, September 1980.

can point out client strengths and positive accomplishments, can assist with looking anew at unresolved conflicts and reorganizing the meaning of such events toward improved quality of life for the client. A life review shared with the nurse for therapeutic reasons is inclusive of significant reminiscences and will enable the client to see special meanings and purpose in life. Chubon described a case study in which she encouraged an elderly woman to read a novel simulating the client's own life. Analogies apparent in the novel assisted the client to view a past unresolved conflict differently.[24] Methods initiated for resolving and focusing on significant events that emerge during a life review are varied and depend on the creativity of the nurse. Pleasurable memories and events that portray positive skills, talents, and accomplishments of the client can have therapeutic outcomes reflecting the innate strengths of the client.

Occupational histories elicit the occupations and various work settings with which the client has been familiar. Sometimes, this history gives clues which can be associated with the current health status of the client. The long-term effects of many environmental hazards in work settings are insidious and do not emerge for many years. A careful appraisal of past occupational histories, hazards commonly associated with each work environment, and current health problems and/or lifestyle habits of the client can lead to nursing diagnoses which are accurate and conducive toward the adoption of strategic nursing interventions.

Very little is known regarding how the elderly perceive and understand sexual changes brought about by aging and illness. Even though the capability and capacity for sexual response in the later years is well-substantiated in the literature, societal belief tends to stress that human sexual response cannot be retained and that sexual desire just fades away with age and/or illness. For nurses who sense that a sexual history will be beneficial for clients in terms of their health status, concerns, lifestyle, and life situations, an inquiry about sex and sexual activity as a natural physiological function can be introduced. If clients are not responsive to the inquiry, it must be remembered that sexual attitudes for many elderly persons were formed in an era when sex was not discussed openly. If clients show an interest in the inquiry, opportunity is granted to exchange information about the physical, psychological, and social aspects of sexuality, counsel about human sexual responses as normal functions, and explore and interpret recent studies about sexuality and aging. Recommendations and/or individualized suggestions can be offered which will enhance the client's quality of life. Correcting misinformation, listening to needs expressed by clients, and reinforcing behavior acceptable to clients are possible teaching functions originating from an inquiry about sexuality.

When requesting a nutritional history, it helps to remember that faulty diets in the aged are commonly results of loneliness and financial worry, which can lead to a malnutrition so severe that life cannot be enjoyed. Loneliness tends to increase poor eating habits, such as overeating of starchy, unbalanced meals and nibbling sweets, eating too little food at irregular times, or foods that contain slight nutritional value, at times a "tea and toast" diet. Some elderly people excuse themselves for this by a "what's the use?" attitude.

[24] Ibid.

The nurse's challenge is to encourage an interest in all aspects of the meal: the planning, shopping, cooking, and eating. People should be encouraged to have their meals in as pleasant a situation as possible, to eat slowly and savor the food. For some, listening to the radio, watching television, or reading while eating can contribute to the pleasure of the meal.

Many retired men and women living alone have never learned to plan, buy, or cook a meal, and they need help to undertake such a program for themselves. There are some community resources to help them, such as senior citizens center classes and clubs. They particularly need help with shopping when the food budget is limited, for it may be a problem in relation to small buying and cooking. Emphasis should be on the importance of a varied diet selected from the four major food groups. A home economist has offered the following suggestions for planning and shopping under these situations for this group.

1   Keep up-to-date on food prices by watching advertisements.
2   Buy no more food at one time than can be used easily; a big economy-sized package is not a bargain if it grows stale or spoils or the person tires of it.
3   Buy dry mixes for breads, cakes, and puddings; a portion can be used and the remainder will keep in a cool place.
4   Cook small amounts when possible; half a cup of shelled peas or cut string beans make a normal serving.

Chronic diseases requiring diet restrictions occur frequently in this age group, including diabetes and cardiac disturbances, also degenerative diseases such as cancer and paralysis agitans. The physician will prescribe diets for these conditions, but the nurse will need to explain—more than once—why it is important to avoid salt or sugar and why soft foods may sometimes be necessary. Salt and sugar substitutes are available at pharmacies and grocery stores; they can make meals more palatable. Often clients must experiment with them to find the one they like best, as their flavors differ.

It is important to point out to the elderly, especially those living alone, the close relationship of nourishing food to good health and a sense of well-being in order to enjoy life.

When all essential data have been gathered, the nurse has knowledge of most of the client's needs, and can make a contract with the client which fulfills the need with highest priority. Often, the need as determined by the nurse is not the one having highest priority with the client. When this happens, it is generally advisable to work with the need the client has identified.

For example, a nursing student described the home of an elderly male client as being a "tumbled down, dark, damp hovel." She went on to say "When I first saw the conditions in which Mr. C. was living, my first thought was to get him out of there and tear down the house. I then assumed that if he would not leave the place, he would *certainly* want to clean it up. But Mr. C.'s perspective of his needs differed greatly from mine. His greatest concerns were to ensure the continued satisfaction of his physical needs; mine were for his safety needs. His need priority included refilling needed prescriptions, getting new glasses so he could read again, and cleaning out the driveway so that 'you and the meal lady can get in.'"

For another student working with an arthritic, hypertensive elderly lady who had been advised by family and friends to move into a retirement facility and who had numerous reasons for delaying such a move, discussion of the client's situation led to the realization that the elderly lady hoped to die in her home. So, as a temporary but necessary and immediate measure, the student negotiated with the client to fulfill two goals: (1) order a bedside telephone to replace the telephone on the wall in case of emergency and (2) visit her physician whom she had not seen for a year and secure a current assessment of her physical condition. By working with the client to fulfill immediate needs, compliance with future advisable medical and nursing measures become more assured as changes in health status occur.

While actively engaged in working with elderly clients, the community health nurse may be calling and coordinating with professionals of many related disciplines, such as the physician, nurse practitioner, physical therapist, occupational therapist, nutritionist, social worker, consumer advocate for senior citizens, homemaker, housekeeper, or environmental health specialist. By freely consulting with members of the related disciplines, services are individualized, clarified, and facilitated for elderly clients. At all times, family members and significant others should be kept informed and approving of all developments and decisions.

GROUP WORK WITH THE ELDERLY

For nursing students wanting to work with the elderly, many opportunities exist for small group discussions and/or educational programs describing specific characteristics of illness care, health care, self-care, health promotion, and related subjects. The elderly like to learn how aging processes affect their body. Many are interested in health promotion activities which have the potential for improving chronic disease states. For example, an elderly 74-year-old woman who has been practicing tai chi daily for the last 4 years explained that this Chinese meditative exercise improved her arthritis dramatically. Her commitment to tai chi on a daily basis has not only relieved her of the symptoms of arthritis but has accentuated a vigor and zest for living which is infectious.

Evidence is strong that by keeping active and fit, an elderly person can minimize the losses that accompany aging.[25] Encouraging groups of elderly citizens to join a walking group or swimming group, explaining the benefits of aerobic exercises, providing incentives to participate in such groups are "fun" projects that nursing students can initiate. Cooking classes exploring the implications of vegetarian diets, junk food withdrawal, shopping at the supermarket, eliminating or reducing salt and sugar in the diet, cooking for one, are nutritional projects stimulating for elderly citizens and enterprising nurse teachers. The field of health promotion offers many opportunities for expanding the knowledge and skills of elderly citizens toward improved states of wellness.

[25] James H. Price and Stephen L. Luther, "Physical Fitness: Its Role in Health for the Elderly," *Journal of Gerontological Nursing,* 6(9):517–523, September 1980.

In view of congregate living represented by the many forms of public and private housing such as low-income apartments for the elderly, retirement homes, condominiums, retirement villages, and similar collective housing experiments, there are usually individuals who will be responsive to learning how to help neighbors in times of crisis or need. When classes are offered for the purpose of teaching elderly persons how to care for self or their neighbor in need, the classes increase a sense of self-sufficiency and promote a "helping" environment in geriatric communities where loneliness and isolation tend to prevail. The content of the classes can focus on health services available in the community, accessibility of these services, what to do in times of crisis, and preventive strategies for maintenance of health. Efforts to promote community spirit and camaraderie among elderly populations can be hard work, yet have rewarding results. If community organization principles are used conscientiously (see Chap. 4), success in these enterprises is almost assured.

RESOURCES FOR THE ELDERLY

In every community, resources for the elderly are multiplying and services are available which provide a wide variety of programs designed to meet the physical, emotional, social, recreational, economic, and environmental needs of senior citizens. To become knowledgeable about the services in each local community, the nurse or citizen must locate the information and referral center for senior citizens. This can be done by securing a people's yellow pages book, or looking in the yellow pages of the local telephone book for the headings: aging, senior citizen services, social service organizations, or social and health services. The mayor's office in every community, the welfare department, or social security office should also be able to direct telephone inquiries to the proper local resources.

Services that are available through senior service centers or departments of aging cover a gamut of needs. A visit to these agencies is very illuminating and frequently engenders enthusiasm to reach out and inform more aging citizens about the opportunities they might be missing. Questions are answered or directions given about the many resources available, such as health care facilities, medicare, medicaid, housing, employment, transportation, volunteer opportunities, social security, supplemental security income, food stamps, leisure-time activities, educational opportunities, and senior services activities and events.

Volunteer Opportunities

A program with which to be familiar is RSVP (Retired Senior Volunteer Program) which is sponsored by ACTION, Washington, D.C. It offers senior citizens, 60 years of age and older, the opportunity to volunteer for a variety of interesting and vital jobs. The volunteer chooses the activity in which she or he has expertise or an interest and, subsequently, gives real services or teaches important skills needed by the clientele with whom she or he is working (school children, disadvantaged persons, handicapped individuals, other senior citizens, etc.). Activities from which the volunteer can select are inclusive of occupations, such as recreational and craft interests, newspaper or newsletter abilities, employment services, office or food preparation skills, handyperson skills, musical or entertainment abilities, or friendly visiting. In-service, on-the-job training sometimes is given in community agencies receiving volunteer aid if it seems necessary. While giving service, volunteers are covered by an insurance plan which gives protection for accidents on the job or travel to and from a station. Sometimes, mileage compensation is given, if desired. Periodically, social events are planned to provide recognition, honor, and awards to volunteers. RSVP not only gives senior citizens the opportunity to volunteer services, it also serves as an excellent resource for the disabled and homebound elderly who need some kind of assistance in the home.

Health Care

Health care facilities, such as local health departments, visiting nurse associations, and home-care agencies, are cognizant of the needs of the elderly and occasionally offer free programs screening citizens for early symptoms of diabetes, glaucoma, tuberculosis, and hypertension. Or, foot-care clinics are maintained on a regular basis so that senior citizens can have their nails clipped, corns and calluses examined for infection, receive preventive protective remedies, counseling, and referral.

Many home-care agencies provide health care and supportive services to sick and disabled persons in their places of residence. This includes medical, nursing, dental, physical therapy, occupational therapy, homemaking, and housekeeping services as recommended. Day-care centers provide supervision for elderly persons who cannot be left alone for extended periods of time. The goal of the day-care center is to keep citizens residing in their own homes as long as possible yet provide them with a protective daytime therapeutic environment according to their needs. Day-care centers are particularly valuable resources for family members who want their aging member to be in a protective environment while they work during the day.

On an increasing scale, nurse practitioners are making their services available in retirement homes, low-income housing projects, and senior citizen centers. They do health assessments, foot care, screen for hypertension, diabetes, glaucoma, counsel about preventive health measures, refer special problems to physicians or to appropriate community resources as necessary. When residents become acquainted and familiar with the services of the nurse practitioner, they respond very positively to the ministrations and suggestions for improved daily living.

Protective and Advocacy Services

Familiarity with legal services for citizens is becoming essential for nurses to know. In every community there are legal resources which will advise or give information about what to do when a problem is causing concern. People's yellow pages maintains a list of legal resources, and local telephone books have listings of numbers to call for information, such as the mayor's office or community information and referral services. Legal knowledge and direction frequently needed by nurses and family members are ways for securing common legal protection of persons and property, such as power of attorney, guardianship, trusts. Explanations and requirements for acquiring specific protection can be secured from any legal aid or legal referral agency.

Helping elderly citizens or family members to protect their money and property is a preventive measure that can always be encouraged by nurses. Making a will, the appointment of an executor of the will, joint ownership of bank accounts and trusts, and after-death arrangements should be suggested as important preventive functions to have clarified among family members.[26]

The Gray Panther Movement suggests that people in their later years need not remain passive and impotent when faced with unacceptable conditions. With increasing assertiveness and organization, the senior citizens are mandating appropriate responses from all sectors of society as to appropriate provision of their needs. Elderly citizens should be encouraged to request that their names be put on the mailing list of state and local committees for aging. In this way, they are kept informed of all legislation pertaining to their interests.[27] Through organizations which present a united front, senior citizens secure publicity, public concern, and remedial action for many problems which are of particular concern to them.

Financial Resource

Supplemental security income (SSI) is a minimum income for older people with limited financial resources who are 65 years or older and people under 65 who are blind or severely disabled. The monthly checks take the place of basic cash payments which were once paid by state and local public assistance offices to the aged, blind, and disabled. People who are eligible for SSI may be earning a small amount of money or have no income, or have minimal assets which can be turned into cash. To determine if qualifications of senior citizens meet expected criteria, it is advisable to call a social security office to obtain the most recent essentialities for eligibility. The amount of payment to each citizen is variable according to the income and assets each individual or couple has. Even though the Social Security Administration runs the program, supplemental security income is not the same as social security. People who get social security can get supplemental security income also if they are eligible for both sources of payment.

Aged, blind, and disabled people receiving SSI checks also are eligible for medical assistance and social services from the state public assistance office. To determine the extent of specific services available for these clients, the local welfare office should be contacted.

Nutrition Resources

The food stamp program is funded by the United States Department of Agriculture and enables low-income households to buy more food of greater variety to improve their diets. Food stamps are coupons that can be used as cash at authorized food stores to buy food, seeds, and plants for growing food. They cannot be used to buy tobacco, alcoholic beverages, paper products, soap, or anything inedible. To purchase food stamps, participants pay a sum of money based on their family size and net monthly income. Households with a low net income are eligible for food stamps. A *household* is a group of people living together who buy and cook their food together. They pool

[26] Bernita M. Steffl, "Prevention Measures and Safety Factors for the Aged," in Irene Mortenson Burnside (ed.), *Nursing and the Aged,* McGraw-Hill Book Company, New York, 1976, pp. 483–485.

[27] Marie A. Fasano, "Community Resources," in Irene Mortenson Burnside (ed.), *Nursing and the Aged,* McGraw-Hill Book Company, New York, 1976, pp. 504–517.

their income and share expenses. While most households are families, other groups of people who are not related to each other can also be a household.

Application for the food stamp program is made by requesting an interview with a representative of the state agency (welfare office). It is advisable for all applicants to have documents showing: where the household is; how many are in the family; the proof of income; paid bills and receipts showing expenses, such as rent, medical bills, child care, education; a savings account passbook; and the most recent checking account statement. If a household is eligible, an authorization to purchase (ATP) card is issued. The amount each household is required to pay for food stamps each month is determined in the eligibility interview.

A requirement of the program is that all able-bodied individuals in the household between 18 and 65 years of age must register for work and accept suitable employment. When registered, they report to the state employment service, and are referred to employers when suitable employment is found. For food stamp recipients who are over 60 years of age, are physically handicapped, feeble, or cannot prepare all their meals, meals on wheels will accept food stamps. In the event of a disaster, such as a fire, hurricane, tornado, flood, storm, or other severe catastrophes, the food stamp program can be converted into an emergency plan which issues free food stamps to all adversely affected households. To apply for emergency assistance, disaster relief agencies or the welfare office must be contacted. It is the responsibility of each household to report an increase or decrease of household size, change of income, or other alterations of household status within 10 days of the change. Misuse of food stamps and ATP cards is illegal and subject to penalty.

Other Resources

Senior citizen centers or information and referral centers are the best sources of knowledge about all available services provided in the community. They can answer inquiries about transportation resources, bus schedules, and services. They know if mobile libraries are available for individuals who are homebound. They can provide information about meals on wheels or locations of hot meals in neighborhood settings. They have a listing of all adult education classes held in local community settings and dealing with a variety of subjects—theoretical, vocational, or recreational. For citizens who want to focus on pure enjoyment, information is available about dances, bingo games, card games, field trips, and other activities that represent some of the amusements planned for senior citizens. A wide variety of special services are constantly in the process of development, so inquiries regarding special needs should always be made in the event that services are obtainable or that ideas for new services will culminate into special projects.

Avocational counseling is a free professional service which helps disabled and retired citizens to discover their interests and potentials and then finds activities in their communities best suited to their needs. Avocational activities include a range of interests, such as games, sports, nature, collecting, art, music, education and culture, volunteer work, and organizations.[28] When a citizen is desirous of learning more about a

[28] "Health Professionals Told of Avocational Counseling," *Geriatrics,* **29**(5):43, May 1974.

special interest, inquiries should be directed toward senior citizen centers or information and referral centers.

For community health nurses who have never visited local community facilities giving special services to specific clientele, it is advisable to become acquainted with these resources. Many community facilities give service to all ages of clientele; however, when a certain portion of senior citizens are actively interested in a particular service, it is helpful to study the basis for the magnetism of the service, the facility, or the promised results. Suggested places to visit with an open mind, observe, and make use of all the senses are health food stores, nutrition and vitamin centers in supermarkets, low-income housing authority offices, missions on skid road, centers serving hot lunches, herb stores, natural food stores, and health clinics in inner cities.

CHRONIC DISEASE STATES AND DEATH

For those individuals and family members who must learn to adjust to the changes evoked by the symptoms of chronic and degenerative diseases, such as multiple sclerosis, arthritis, emphysema, terminal carcinoma, cerebral vascular accident (stroke), and similar debilitating diseases, special attention must be given. Not only the client but all family members are affected in some way or other by the required adaptation to the existence and concurrent dependencies produced by chronic diseases. All clients and families adjust in their own individualistic ways and many need assistance in learning to accommodate with essential changes necessitated by the disruption of roles and tasks in the home. Many professional references deal with the stages of adaptation or coping mechanisms undergone by clients when chronic diseases are diagnosed or terminal prognoses are given. However, few authors as yet take heed of the distinct adjustments expected of family members who are directly affected by the change of status of the client, a family member with a one-time vital role in the family structure. Kubler-Ross discussed the physical and emotional adjustments undergone by family members of clients who were dying and recognized that family members also went through emotional stages of adjustment very similar to those described for dying clients. She pointed out the importance of someone to befriend family members, allow them to work through their rational or irrational feelings about a pending death, and ease the movement of feelings toward acceptance without guilt.[29] The family-centered community health nurse is the qualified person for the role of comforting and assisting family members when chronic degenerative diseases are diagnosed and terminal prognoses are anticipated.

The stages of adaptation or coping mechanisms undergone by clients and family members when they realize the necessity for accepting a change in their lives have been identified by various authors as sequential and progressive in nature for most people. According to Crate, who studied stages of adaptation for the diagnosis of multiple sclerosis, the first stage is one of *denial* and *disbelief*, which is manifested in a variety of ways, depending upon the individual's lifestyle of coping with crisis or conflict. Denial can be exhibited for a short period or it can be long-lasting. The nurse should listen to

---

[29]Elisabeth Kubler-Ross, *On Death and Dying,* The Macmillan Company, New York, 1969, pp. 157–180.

all expressions of feeling noncritically and help the individual to articulate with clarity. By drawing out existing feelings of resentment and bitterness, the nurse facilitates the adjustment process. The second stage consists of a *developing awareness,* which is commonly manifested as anger. By being empathic, the nurse can listen to arguments, criticisms, and attacks without responding as a singled-out target. The nurse must be aware that anger is a realistic defense when a person's life is capriciously changed without consent. The nurse must consciously not argue with the client or moralize about any issue. The third stage is one of *reorganization,* in which relationships with family members are adjusted and accommodations are made in the activities of daily living. At this time the nurse must continue to listen to the expressions of feelings of the client and family members, suggest suitable practical rehabilitative methods for readjusting their household routines, encourage the use of appropriate self-help devices, and give verbal support for accomplishments successfully attained by the persons assuming new roles and duties. The fourth stage consists of *resolution* or *identity change,* in which the client acknowledges the reality changes seen in self. The client begins to identify that she or he is similar to other clients with the same diagnosis. Dependent upon the diagnosis and the home situation, the nurse at this point must consider releasing the client, encouraging her or him to become self-directive within limits, and to seek out relationships with others.[30]

For clients and families who are concerned about the time when admission to an institution becomes imminent, the nurse must elicit the perceptions of the client regarding the meaning of institutionalization. Acute care hospitals are generally viewed differently from nursing homes, convalescent homes, or retirement homes. Family members must be alerted to the advantages and disadvantages of particular institutions in terms of the client's viewpoint, physical condition, recommended treatments, and home situation. A problem-solving approach can be used with the client and family members as all alternatives for care are carefully considered. Visits to the institutions to view their assets and limitations can be encouraged. An assessment and recommendation from the attending physician always is valuable at this critical moment of decision making for clients and families. For the most part, if the client voluntarily decides to enter a selected facility, the transition from home to institution is greatly eased for all concerned.

When the diagnosis is a terminal one, the early stages of denial and anger precede the latter stages of adaptation, which are aptly described by Kubler-Ross as those of bargaining, depression, and acceptance. *Bargaining* is a period when the client makes a bargain with God in the hope that death will be postponed. *Depression* is the natural state during which a client is filled with sorrow that she or he will soon lose everything and everyone. If allowed to express sorrow, the client becomes emotionally prepared for the final stage of *acceptance.* During the final stage, effective communications are predominantly nonverbal rather than verbal.[31] For an ordinarily talkative nursing student who did not know how to say what he wanted to say to a young mother dying of

[30] Marjorie Crate, "Nursing Functions in Adaptation to Chronic Illness," *American Journal of Nursing,* 65:72–76, October 1965.

[31] Elisabeth Kubler-Ross, *On Death and Dying,* The Macmillan Company, New York, 1969, pp. 82–136.

cancer, he chose to sit with the client for a period of time in quietness and empathy. This nonverbal expression seemed to give comfort and peace to the client.

The concept of hope was graphically described by Kubler-Ross as an essential ingredient in all people. They are nourished by it and appreciate any small fragment of hope that is offered on a realistic basis. The hope may not necessarily be directed toward total cure, but a remission of the illness or an anticipation about the next life.[32] Until the client gives some cue that she or he is ready to talk, the nurse is in a position where asking direct questions may seem awkward. If the nurse has a knowledge of the client's religion, values, and beliefs, she or he is better able to speak words of comfort and strength that prepare the client for the final task. Communicating a genuine individualized concern to the client, accepting the health status realistically in a verbal or nonverbal manner, and incorporating hope in such a way that the client finds it believable is the most supportive behavior the nurse can give.

Hospice An emerging resource that is effectively meeting the needs of dying clients and their families is hospice. *Hospice* is characterized as a caring community. It is a program for the terminally ill and their families. The goal of a hospice service is not the endless prolongation of life, but ensuring that what remains of life is free from pain, and is comfortable and satisfying to the client, whether receiving care at a special hospice facility or at home. Family members are considered an integral part of the service given to the client and receive the comfort and help they need to live with the dying client until death as well as to cope with bereavement following the death.[33] Hospice may be a home care program, a free-standing institution, a separate hospital department or an interdisciplinary team. Various models of hospice offer outpatient services or day care, home care in conjunction with institutional settings, or a combination of models.[34]

Health personnel giving hospice services often represent a team effort, inclusive of nurses, social workers, physicians, chaplains, physiotherapists, nutritionists, pharmacists, legal counselors, volunteers, and allied disciplines. Twenty-four-hour service seven days a week frequently is available. Health professionals giving hospice services are special people who demonstrate expertise in the management of pain—social, psychological, spiritual, and physical.[35] They have knowledge of symptom control in the physical management of dying clients and give expert counsel to clients and family members psychologically, spiritually, and socially. The health team members work closely together and maintain a sense of purpose and accomplishment through regular meetings providing necessary support for each other, the opportunity to share experiences and receive sustenance as needed when undergoing particularly stressful periods.

The success of hospice services is apparent in most communities as increasing numbers of clients exhibit an attitude of acceptance or improved "quality of life" pre-

[32] Ibid., pp. 138–156.

[33] Barbara J. Ward, "Hospice Home Care Program," *Nursing Outlook,* 26(10):646–649, October 1978.

[34] Kenneth P. Cohen, *Hospice: Prescription for Terminal Care,* Aspen Systems Corporation, Germantown, Md., 1979, p. 68.

[35] Ibid., p. 89.

ceding a peaceful death. Hospice services represent a health resource with which all nursing students should be acquainted.

SUMMARY

An overview of some of the problems, concerns and resources for aging as commonly encountered by community health nurses was given. Nurses can be supportive of aging as a process which leads to more healthful and satisfying living in the later years. In working with the aged, the nurse must be a warm, caring, person-centered individual who carefully applies and individualizes the nursing process with each client. Knowledge and familiarity with the ever-growing community resources and services available for all senior citizens is essential, as well as illuminating.

SUGGESTED READING

Baer, L. S.: *Let the Patient Decide: A Doctor's Advice to Older Persons,* The Westminster Press, Philadelphia, 1978.

Becker, Ernest: *The Denial of Death,* The Free Press, New York, 1973.

Binstock, Robert H., and Ethel Shanas (eds.): *Aging and the Social Sciences,* Van Nostrand Reinhold Company, New York, 1976.

Botwinick, Jack: *Aging and Behavior: A Comprehensive Integration of Research Findings,* 2d ed., Springer Publishing Co., Inc., New York, 1978.

Burnside, Irene Mortenson et al.: *Psychosocial Nursing Care of the Aged,* McGraw-Hill Book Company, New York, 1980.

Busse, E. W., and E. Pfeiffer, (eds.): *Behavior and Adaptation in Later Life,* Little, Brown and Company, Boston, 1977.

Burdman, Geral Dene Marr and Ruth M. Brewer: *Health Aspects of Aging,* A Continuing Education Book, Continuing Education Publications, Portland, Oreg., 1978.

Butler, Robert N., and Myrna I. Lewis: *Sex after Sixty. A Guide for Men and Women for Their Later Years,* Harper & Row Publishers, Inc., New York, 1976.

Carnevali, Doris L., and Maxine Patrick (eds.): *Nursing Management for the Elderly,* J. B. Lippincott, Philadelphia, 1979.

Chubon, Sandra: "A Novel Approach to the Process of Life Review," *Journal of Gerontological Nursing,* 6(9):543–546, September 1980.

Dickinson, Peter A.: *The Fires of Autumn: Sexual Activity in the Middle and Later Years,* Drake Publishing, Inc., New York, 1974.

Finch, Caleb E., and Leonard Hayflick (eds.): *Handbook of the Biology of Aging,* Van Nostrand Reinhold Company, New York, 1977.

Goldman, Ralph and Morris Rockstein (eds.): *The Physiology and Pathology of Human Aging,* Academic Press, New York, 1975.

Hess, Beth B. (ed.): *Growing Old in America,* Transaction Books, New Brunswick, N.J., 1976.

"Hypertension: A Special Feature," *American Journal of Nursing,* 76(5):765–780, May 1976.

Kiernat, Jean M.: "Adaptive Living and Accident Prevention for the Aged," *Allied Health and Behavioral Sciences,* 2(1):61–75, 1979.

Mishara, Brian L.: *Alcohol and Old Age,* Grune & Stratton, Inc., New York, 1980.

Pearson, Linda Joan, and M. Ernestine Kotthoff: *Geriatric Clinical Protocols,* J. B. Lippincott Company, Philadelphia, 1979.

Poe, William D., and D. A. Holloway: *Drugs and the Aged,* McGraw-Hill Book Company, New York, 1980.

Price, James H., and Stephen L. Luther: "Physical Fitness: Its Role in Health for the Elderly," *Journal of Gerontological Nursing,* 6(9):517–523, September 1980.

Riggs, Richard, "Perceived Health Needs, Problems, and Interests of the Aged," *Health Education,* March–April 1978, p. 3.

Rockstein, Morris and Marvin L. Sussman (eds.): *Nutrition, Longevity, and Aging,* Academic Press, New York, 1976.

Saxon, Sue V.: *Physical Change and Aging: A Guide for the Helping Professions,* Tiresias Press, New York, 1978.

Schutz, Howard G.: *Lifestyles and Consumer Behavior of Older Americans,* Praeger Publishers, Inc., New York, 1979.

Spencer, Marion G., and Caroline J. Dorr: *Understanding Aging: A Multidisciplinary Approach,* Appleton-Century-Croft, New York, 1975.

Stokes, Shirlee Ann, Louise M. Rauckhorst, and Mathy D. Mezey: "Health Assessment—Considerations for the Older Individual," *Journal of Gerontological Nursing,* 6(6):328–337, June 1980.

Ward, Barbara J., "Hospice Home Care Program," *Nursing Outlook,* 26(10):646–649, October 1978.

Weg, Ruth B.: *Nutrition in Later Years,* University of Southern California Andrus Center, Los Angeles, 1978.

Woodruff, Diana S., and James E. Birren (eds.): *Aging: Scientific Perspectives and Social Issues,* D. Van Nostrand Company, Inc., New York, 1975.

Wolff, Ilse S.: "Retirement: A Different Season," *Nursing Outlook,* 21(12):763–765, December 1973.

Yurick, Ann G. et al.: *The Aged Person and the Nursing Process,* Appleton-Century-Crofts, New York, 1980.

Chapter 10

Applying Epidemiology, Statistics, and Research

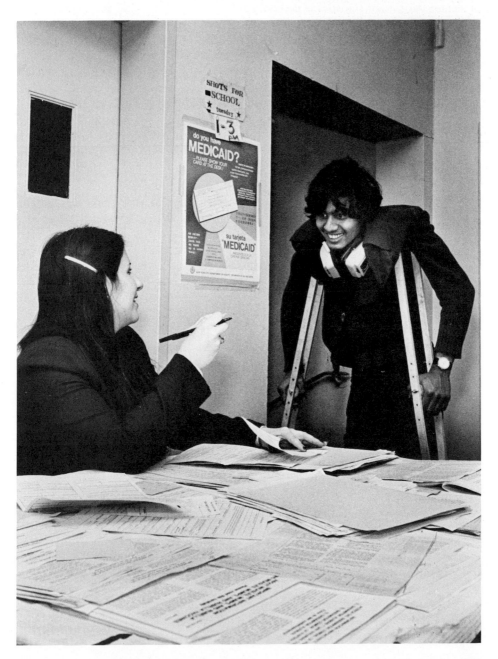

The emphasis on clinical, laboratory, and epidemiologic research in the past decade dictates that the nurse have an understanding and appreciation of research methods and statistics. The Community Health Nursing Section of the American Nurses' Association requires the nurse to have knowledge of the research method within the broad categories of evaluating, studying, and research. Also, an understanding of epidemiology and statistics is necessary for continuing appraisal and evaluation of health situations which concern clients, families, and communities.

STUDY AND RESEARCH

Searching for increased knowledge in a systematic way requires curiosity, self-discipline, and familiarity with research methods. Nursing students who wish to promote the advancement of improved client care must have a beginning acquaintance with basic principles and methods in order to study any aspect of the health-illness continuum which concerns them. For the nurse who is sufficiently curious about an intriguing health problem, a beginning step into research activities can be initiated by doing a ministudy. By investigating the variety of methods for doing studies, getting an idea from readings whether any other nurse has done a similar study, and determining exactly what is to be found out, the neophyte nurse can start investigative activities which may bring exciting discoveries to light. Some problems that might be interesting to study include identification of consumers' attitudes and opinions regarding specific health issues or advertised products, the coexistence of specific stress factors with specific chronic diseases, and the investigation of factors that promote wellness in families—why some families rarely if ever have upper respiratory illnesses while others seem to have them constantly. Other areas of interest are only limited by the concerns of the nurse, and the demands of her or his position. They could include learning about the skin care routines followed by adolescents with acne, or how families react if one of the children has enuresis. What factors influence the utilization of health care facilities in the community?

Nurses working in the community, wanting to improve the health status of its residents, need to become better acquainted with research methods, evaluation, and interpretation of results. They need knowledge of the principles and methods of epidemiology because their client is the community. *Epidemiology,* and its research techniques, describes and explains the distribution and determinants of disease in population groups, with the ultimate goal of promoting health and furthering preventive measures. This is in contrast to clinical research, which pertains to the individual client who usually already has sought health care, and the efficacy of diagnostic tests or therapeutic regimens. The community health nurse often is trying to prevent the need to seek curative health services.

The purpose of presenting an elementary discussion of epidemiologic and statistical concepts is to enable the nurse to participate in or to conduct studies. Familiarity with these concepts will be of value in presenting and analyzing quantitative data, such as showing how great a problem hypertension is in the community. Also, it will help the nurse be more critical of the validity of the proliferating new knowledge in the health sciences area. Terms such as variation, population, sample, data, observations, and central tendency, which may be familiar to the nurse in other contexts, are explained from the point of view of epidemiology and statistics. The authors present this limited discussion knowing that the material is too elementary for some readers, that it will be a review for others, and that it will be helpful for some; it is in no way intended to bring about mastery in the sciences of epidemiology and statistics. (The student is directed to references in the bibliography at the end of the chapter for a detailed discussion of both subjects.)

DEFINITIONS

Epidemiology has been defined above. Basically, its purpose is to learn why some people get sick and others do not and then apply the knowledge to prevent other people from getting sick. Another way of saying this is that epidemiology tries to identify "risk factors"—those elements or variables in an individual's life or environment which give her or him a greater than average risk of developing a particular disease—and then developing a strategy to counteract those facts and thus reduce the risk.

The term *statistics* is defined in various ways. For the purpose of this presentation, statistics refers to a systematic approach for obtaining, organizing, and analyzing numerical facts so that scientific conclusions can be drawn from them. Statistics allow for description and for inferences. The rather specialized techniques that are used for biological data are often called biostatistics. They present fact rather than an assumption or hunch.

Vital statistics in the broad sense refers to births, deaths, populations, illnesses, marriages, and divorces. In the narrow sense the term refers to births, deaths, and populations. Illnesses in the population are classified as *morbidity statistics,* deaths as *mortality statistics.* Generally marriage and divorce statistics are used more frequently by social agencies than by health agencies. Since the disciplines of public health and community health nursing are concerned with people, vital statistics are an important tool in their fields.

SOURCES OF DATA

The family record is an excellent source for such statistical information as age, sex, ethnic background, and specific disease or condition. Information from the records facilitates program planning and is useful in evaluating the services given to the family. Study of the records should also give the interested and curious nurse ideas as to some of the problems that need to be researched in order to learn more about them. Roberts and Hudson developed a method of studying the client's progress through the record. Their study method gives direction for collecting, presenting, and analyzing data concerning the following:

1   The scope of needs identified in clients and families by the community health nurse (Does the client or family also recognize these needs?)
2   The progress made by families in meeting their own needs for nursing care (What factors seem to influence how successfully this is done?)

3 The proportion of persons who obtain needed immunizations and diagnostic tests (Which families do, and which do not, get their children immunized, and why?)

4 The number and kinds of conditions which are brought to medical attention for diagnosis, periodic medical evaluation, and treatment (Are the preventive programs in the community really aimed at the most important targets?)

5 The extent to which clients with chronic illness and disability attain self-care[1] (Again, why are some successful in doing this, and others not?)

The questions in parentheses were added to indicate possible questions that an alert nurse might have and may wish to research for answers.

Information from records is used in compiling monthly and annual reports required by the agency. Such information is used by the local community health agency as well as by state and federal health agencies, grant-in-aid programs. voluntary and contracting agencies—insurance companies, schools, or industrial firms that pay for services—and by sponsoring or coordinating groups, such as the community chest or the united funds. The information is used to make comparisons with previous years, to predict and to determine needs for ensuing years, and to interpret to the community in order to obtain better understanding and support for community health nursing services.

The staff nurse rarely is responsible for compiling the agency's monthly or annual reports but is responsible for knowing the information contained in them. Such responsibility includes knowledge and understanding of the major accomplishments of the year, such as quantitative and qualitative attainments, concerns and plans for change, trends in activities and service needs, and the relation of service given to the estimated needs for such services.

Staff nurses may be involved in compiling statistics for special investigations of such topics as well-child care, child abuse, premature births, epidemiologic problems, home-care programs, school health, congenital defects, rehabilitation, mental retardation, migratory workers, and many more. The individual nurse may be interested in conducting a study within her or his district. The opportunities are unlimited and will vary according to the nurse's interest and the policies of the agency.

Technological advances in data processing, programming, and computers make for a much more efficient way of collecting, analyzing, and presenting data.

PRINCIPLES OF EPIDEMIOLOGY

Epidemiology, in the strict sense of the word, is a branch of medical science and centers on distribution and causation of disease in populations with the goal of discovering means of disease prevention. The methods used to determine disease causation can be adapted to many other areas of concern. At first it was concerned with the epidemic diseases, as the word indicates, but now it is being applied to all diseases, including trauma. It is more a system of methods than a body of knowledge, and uses knowledge from many areas such as biostatistics, microbiology, and clinical medicine.

---

[1] Doris E. Roberts and Helen H. Hudson, *How to Study Patient Progress,* Public Health Service Publication 1169, April 1964, p. 1.

One of the underlying principles is that no disease occurs by chance alone, because each follows its own recognizable pattern of occurrence. The pattern may not be seen when looking at one sick person, but when information is collected on many people with the same diseases, some common elements in their total life experience may begin to emerge. Compiling a list of these common elements helps to delineate the group in the community that has a high risk of developing that specific disease. Currently this is well-illustrated by the fact that cigarette smokers have a much higher risk of developing lung cancer than people who do not smoke. The "profile" of the group at high risk for coronary heart disease is fairly well known. It includes such risk factors as being male, over-weight, underactive, a smoker, high blood cholesterol level, high blood pressure, and certain personality characteristics. Knowledge of the risk factors provides a basis for preventive programs. Today, preventive efforts against the major diseases are not as simple as producing a vaccine and administering it. The efforts to prevent disease may affect a person's lifestyle.

Health is a state of equilibrium, a delicate balance of many factors. When this balance is lost, disease results. These factors can be grouped as those related to the host, the agent, and the environment. The host is the human being at risk of acquiring a disease. Some of the factors which determine whether or not the host will do so include age, sex, genetic background, general health status, immunologic status, personal health habits, and more. The agent is the factor which is essential to disease causation, such as microorganisms, physical forces, chemicals, or even food. Environmental factors are all those things external to the particular host, including other people. Disease prevention depends, in large part, on what we know about these factors and their interrelationships. As an example, we have learned how to prevent some infectious diseases by giving vaccine. We have protective clothing and heating devices to protect us from harm by extreme cold weather.

Disease causation is complex. Some diseases, such as coronary heart disease, may be the outcome of several interacting factors rather than of a single specific factor. Even when a specific infectious agent is known, there may be contributing factors that influence whether or not exposure to that agent will produce disease. Many common colds are caused by rhinoviruses, but a rhinovirus infection often fails to cause illness. Contributing factors here could include the person's general level of health or previous experience with that particular agent. When investigating the cause of a disease, it is necessary to pay attention to contributing causes as well as the primary agent.

Another important concept is that infection is not synonymous with disease. Sources of infection in a community are not limited to ill people. The term "infection" means that an infectious agent has invaded the host and started to multiply, in intimate relation to host tissues. There are at least four possible outcomes of this invasion. First, there may be overt clinical illness. Second, an inapparent, or subclinical, infection may occur in which the person shows no symptoms but is shedding the agent. In a study of family illnesses, rhinoviruses were recovered sometimes from healthy people. Another outcome is that the infected person may become a carrier. After recovery from clinical illness, the person may shed the agent, continuously or at intervals, for a long period of time. With typhoid fever, the ex-client sometimes excreted the agent at intervals for the rest of a lifetime, and so was still infected. Fourth, whether or not disease occurred, the agent may persist quietly in the host's tissue for long periods of time. Periodically it may produce symptoms. The best known example of this is probably herpes simplex, the cold sore. This is called a latent infection.

Knowledge of the distribution of disease over time is very valuable to the nurse in the community. Many diseases, such as hepatitis type A, are often present at a low level of incidence. This is the endemic, or background, level of incidence. When a significant increase in the number of new cases occurs, it is called an epidemic. That term originally referred to communicable diseases but more recently is being applied to chronic diseases as well, such as the "epidemic of coronary heart disease." Occasionally a disease occurs in large numbers in many countries, such as pandemics of influenza that affect most of the world.

An *epidemic curve* is merely a graphic display of disease onsets over time, be it hours, days, or weeks. It can give insight into the source of the disease. A school nurse who observes that several students develop hepatitis within a brief period (a few days to 2 weeks) and none after that will consider the possibility of common-source, or "point" outbreak. Figure 10-1 presents such an epidemic. A group of students drank water contaminated with hepatitis virus on only one day. Illness onsets began after a reasonable incubation period, and continued over a 2-week period, then stopped. The nurse would focus the investigation on events in the period consistent with the usual incubation period, i.e., 15 days before the first case to 35 days before the last one. This pattern of the epidemic curve strongly suggests that all the clients were exposed at the same time and probably at the same place.

If an unusual number of new cases keeps occurring over months, it indicates that the source of the infection is continuing in the community, and exposure is occurring intermittently. Figure 10-2 illustrates a typical continuing-source epidemic curve. It displays the onset dates of infectious hepatitis in a cottage-type institution over more

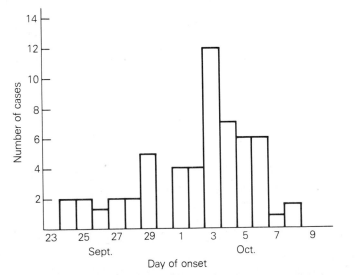

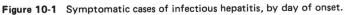

Figure 10-1 Symptomatic cases of infectious hepatitis, by day of onset.

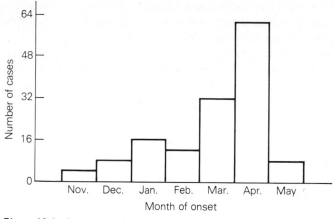

Figure 10-2 Symptomatic cases of infectious hepatitis, by month of onset.

than a 5-month period and indicates that exposure was occurring over a much longer time than the usual incubation period.

EPIDEMIOLOGIC INVESTIGATIONS

A nurse working with school children observed that some of them were having an unusual type of eye infection. In her concern for the health of her school, she learned how many students had this disease by observing those present and learning if any were absent because of it. She wanted to prevent a major epidemic. She phoned the family physicians of the sick children to learn if each one really had the same infection. Careful inspection of the list of children with the eye infection led her to recognize that they were all members of the swimming team. When she questioned them about this, she learned that they were on the team which practiced after school. Checking farther, she found that no members of the team that practiced early in the morning were sick. The school custodian told her that chlorine was added to the pool very early in the morning. Careful tests showed that by late afternoon the chlorine level in the well-used pool was low. From then on, chlorine was added at noon also. No new cases of eye infection occurred.

What had the nurse done? Most importantly, she had promoted the health of the pupils by stopping an epidemic. She had accomplished this by using two types of epidemiologic studies. First, she did a survey to find out precisely how many pupils in her "community" had the particular disease, and verified the diagnosis so that she knew it was indeed the same disease. It is necessary to learn how much disease occurs and who gets it before any efforts can be started to learn what causes it. The diagnosis must be reasonably accurate. The survey that determines this is a *descriptive observational study.*

Next, she had done a case-control study. She had gathered information about common exposures and experiences that the children with the infection had had—that all were members of the swimming team that practiced in the afternoon. This led her to the hypothesis that it could be caused by faulty chlorination, and the fact that no one on the morning-practice team (the control group) had an eye infection strengthened the possibility. The cooperation of the custodian and proper tests proved the hypothesis and resulted in preventing more eye infections.

The example illustrates some important features of case-control studies. They are designed to discover what possible causative factor is more often associated with people with infection than in otherwise similar healthy people. Factors to be studied may have been suggested by careful observation, extensive reading, or even by a hunch. Then to learn which factor(s) more frequently affects diseased people, the study must include a comparison or control group of unaffected people. They should be as much like the clients as possible except for presence of the disease. Selecting the right control group is one of the most important parts of the study. In conducting any study, the assistance of people with other areas of knowledge is usually needed. This the nurse got from the custodian. Probably the statistician is the one more frequently consulted in order to select the control group, analyze findings correctly, and draw proper conclusions.

Another type of epidemiologic investigation is called the *cohort study*. Once a factor has been shown to more often affect people with the disease, we need to estimate the risk associated with it. This type of investigation starts with a group of people, or cohort, exposed to the factor and observes them over a period of time to determine the frequency with which the disease develops. Again, a comparison group is needed, as similar as possible but not exposed to the factor. Studies of lung cancer used cigarette smoking as the suspect factor and observed smokers and nonsmokers over years for the development of lung cancer.

The major difference in study design is easy to recognize. The case-control study starts with the disease, while the cohort study starts with a possible causal factor. The former design will give you an estimate of relative risk or an answer to the question: How much greater are my chances of getting lung cancer if I smoke than if I do not? The cohort design will give you a direct estimate of risk: What are my chances of getting lung cancer if I smoke?

The study designs described so far are all observational designs, used to describe the pattern of disease occurrence in a community or to determine and analyze the importance of suspected causal factors. Another design is that of the *experimental study,* in which the investigator actually manipulates the experience of one group under study, but not that of the comparison group. For ethical reasons, these are usually limited to clinical trials or to evaluating the effectiveness of a vaccine.

STATISTICAL CONCEPTS AND TECHNIQUES

To aid the nurse in developing a systematic approach in classifying and analyzing data, certain statistical concepts and techniques are necessary. Those to be described are variation, qualitative and quantitative data, population and sample in collecting data, tables and graphs in presenting data, and analyzing the data.

First and foremost is the concept that any particular subject or subject area is characterized by variation. The field of nursing is an example, since nurses may work in a hospital, office, community health agency, clinic, school, or industry. Another example is provided by people. Some people are young, others are old; some are thin, others are obese; some are males, others are females; some have a specific disease, others do not. Human behavior differs, for no two persons are alike, and all respond to the environment in different ways. The variables or factors are the characteristics which have more than one value to be studied.

TYPES OF DATA

There are two types of data: qualitative and quantitative. *Qualitative data* refer to those variables that describe a quality or attribute observed in the people or subject being studied. The variables in qualitative data are referred to as enumerations, classifications, and discrete or counting data. Qualitative data are developed by counting the number of persons who possess or do not possess a quality or attribute, e.g., the number of persons who are male or not male, who wear dentures or do not wear dentures, who have chickenpox or do not have chickenpox. The number of children in a family or the number in a group is a discrete value, as one does not have a proportion or one-half of a child or person. Qualitative attributes are easy to classify since there is only a definite number of possibilities, such as sex, race, presence or absence of a disease. Caution must be taken in categorizing subjective judgments of such matters as severity of a disease, appearance, or behavior. Personal bias may affect the classification when it is made by other persons, even though specific criteria are set up. Also, counting data can be misleading when they are based on small numbers of cases.

Quantitative data or variables are those having measurable values, instead of counts or enumerations as in qualitative data. Quantitative variables allow for measurement by recording the amount of a variable possessed by each person (or thing) studied. Age in years is measured by subtracting the birth date from the present date. Incubation period for a disease is the time interval in hours or days between the infection of a susceptible person or animal and the appearance of signs or symptoms of the disease in question. Variables in quantitative data are called *continuous data*, in the sense that they are capable of assuming any value of measurement, as seen in measuring heights, weights, temperatures, and blood pressure.

Grouping of quantitative data in which the measurements are made in a continuous scale should be done with care to avoid loss of detail. For example, classifying 65 nursing students weighing 100 to 150 pounds would not tell how many students weighed 110, 120, 125, or up to 150 pounds. Generally, to determine groupings, one divides the range into equal size intervals from 5 to 20 and makes each group nonoverlapping with the succeeding one. The range is the difference between the largest and the smallest observations. For instance, if class intervals of 5 were used for weight, you would count the number of people falling into the class interval from 100 to 104.99; 105 to 109.99; or 110 to 149.99; and so on, through 149.99. The distribution is summarized in Table 10-1. Such characteristics as heights, temperatures, pulses, blood pressures, or specific laboratory findings also could be shown in a frequency distribution table.

Table 10-1 Frequency Distribution of Weight in Pounds of 65 Senior Nursing Students at School X

Weight, lb	Number of students
100–104.99	1
105–109.99	1
110–114.99	5
115–119.99	11
120–124.99	12
125–129.99	19
130–134.99	10
135–139.99	4
140–144.99	1
145–149.99	1
Total	65

COLLECTING THE DATA

The kind of data to be collected, the way in which they are collected and from whom or where, depend on the *hypothesis* or purpose of the study. Two concepts important to data collection are those of population and sample. *Population* refers to the full group, the universe, all the people in the community. In practice, access to the total population may be impossible or even undesirable. Epidemiologically, a population can be defined as all the people who meet a prescribed definition, such as the same sex, or age, or engaged in the same activity. Sometimes the word "population" is used in reference to the group on whom observations are to be made, e.g., the study population. The observations made are measurements of characteristics of people, such as cholesterol levels or height.

A *sample* is a portion or a fraction of the population or the universe which is to be investigated. *Sampling* is a method of selecting a smaller subgroup from the total population, which will be as representative of the entire group as possible. This helps you to generalize the results of your observations to the entire group. If you could assume that the 65 senior nursing students previously mentioned were truly representative of all such students you would generalize that the weight range for senior nursing students is from 100 to 150 pounds. It is impossible to select a truly representative subgroup or sample, so any generalizations to the larger group must be made with caution. However, samples are used—in part because of the tremendous saving of time and money that is accomplished by studying only a small portion of the whole population.

There are many types of samples, but only the *simple random sample* will be mentioned here. There is a sample selected from a population in some random way so that every individual in that population has the same probability of being included in the sample. This helps eliminate bias. Another advantage of the random sample is that there are mathematical techniques which allow for drawing conclusions about the population on the basis of the sample.

When dealing with small numbers, a way of selecting a sample would be to copy the name or measurement on a piece of paper, place the pieces of paper in a hat or box, mix them up, and draw without looking into the hat or box, so that the sample is drawn by chance alone. For larger samples, one technique is to assign consecutive numbers to the entire population and then use a table of random numbers to select the sample. Tables of random numbers are found in most statistics books.

The method of collecting data depends on the hypothesis, the size of the sample, and the variables being studied. A few sources of data are records from the community health nursing agency, clinic, school, or industry; employment records, birth and death certificates, United States census reports; and morbidity and mortality reports from local, state, national, or international agencies.

There are many ways of developing a form for recording the variables, or the information. The form may be a simple listing of facts, such as age and sex; a complex form may contain age, sex, race, housing, income, occupation, education, immunizations, behavior, attitudes and beliefs, and work history. The form may be a checklist used for entering a few items, or a punch card for many items, up to the limit of the card. Use of punch cards or large cards with a number of items makes tabulation more difficult unless mechanical means are employed.

TABULATING THE DATA

Tables are the most common way of presenting observations in a systematic arrangement, as they show the interrelationship among the variables. The simplest form of a table is a *two-column frequency table,* which may be used for quantitative or quali-

Table 10-2 Source of Referral for Nursing Service

Nursing service	Private physician	Patient or family	Hospital or out-patient department	Health department clinic	Community health nurse	School	Total
Newborn							
Infant							
Preschool							
School							
Adult							
Maternity							
Tuberculosis							
Communicable disease							
Noncommunicable disease							
Chronic disease							
Orthopedic disease							
Mental health							
Total							

tative data. The first column gives the classes into which data are grouped, and the second column lists the frequencies for each classification or group. Table 10–1 is an example of a two-column frequency table.

Since tables show the interrelationship between variables, the form may be arranged showing several variables. This type of table presents data in relation to the specific variable and in relation to any combination of the variables. For example, to determine the source of referrals to a district during a certain period of time, the data would be tabulated as shown in Table 10–2. In this example the total number of referrals from all sources can be determined. In addition, the table gives information concerning the interrelationship between the source of referral and the service given, as well as the combination of sources referring persons to a particular service.

A table should be self-explanatory, and the title should tell exactly what the table shows. All columns should be specifically labeled. Do not put more data in one table than the eye can readily comprehend. Lined columns can be distracting to the reader, so do not use them unless it is necessary to separate data.

GRAPHICAL PRESENTATION OF DATA

A *graph* is a pictorial way of showing quantitative data. It allows a rapid overview of the material presented. There are many types of graphs; a few of the most common, such as the bar graph, histogram, and polygon, will be presented. There are some guidelines that apply to all graphs. The simplest type that will show the data is the best to use. Any graph should be self-explanatory; the title should tell precisely what the graph shows; scales should be marked and labeled; and any symbols used should be explained. The data on a graph usually proceed from left to right, from bottom to top, with frequency of the event on the vertical scale and the method of classifying the data on the horizontal scale (see Fig. 10–3). Finally, when an arithmetic scale is used, the same distance on the scale must be allowed for equal numerical units.

The *bar graph* is the simplest type, with bars of uniform width usually arranged according to magnitude (Fig. 10–3). It is useful in comparing quantitative data or qualitative data of discrete type.

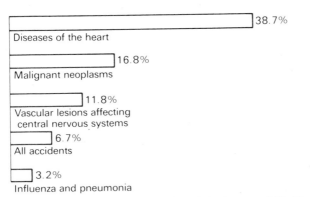

Figure 10-3 Five leading causes of death in the state of Washington in 1969.

Table 10-3 Relative Frequency Distribution of Weight in Pounds of 65 Senior Nursing Students at School X

Weight, lb	Frequency	Relative frequency, %
100–104.99	1	1.54
105–109.99	1	1.54
110–114.99	5	7.69
115–119.99	11	16.92
120–124.99	12	18.46
125–129.99	19	29.23
130–134.99	10	15.39
135–139.99	4	6.15
140–144.99	1	1.54
145–149.99	1	1.54
Total	65	100.00

The *histogram* is a bar chart showing frequency distributions of quantitative and continuous data. It is a series of adjacent rectangles, and the frequency of observations in the various bars, when added up, equal the total distribution of the variable being displayed. When the class intervals are of an unequal size, the relative frequency distribution may be used. The relative frequency is expressed in percent. It is calculated by taking the number of times a weight class occurred, dividing by the total observations in the entire group, and multiplying by 100. The relative frequency of the weight in pounds of the example in Table 10-1, is shown in Table 10-3 and in the histogram in Fig. 10-4.

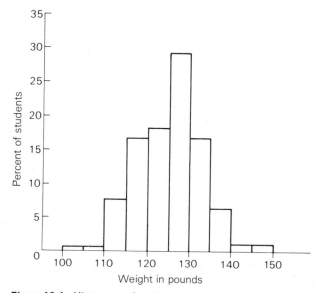

Figure 10-4 Histogram of weight in pounds of sixty-five students.

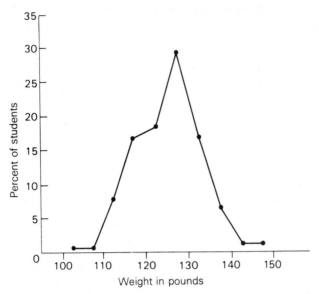

Figure 10-5   Frequency polygon of weights in pounds of sixty-five students.

The *frequency polygon* is essentially the same as the histogram; the data are computed in the same way. In the frequency polygon, the frequency is plotted at the midpoint of the class interval and each point is connected by a line. The rectangles of the histogram are replaced by the connecting lines at midpoint of the interval, resulting in a continuous line. Using the same data as in Fig. 10–4, a frequency polygon is plotted in Fig. 10–5. When the frequency polygon is superimposed on the

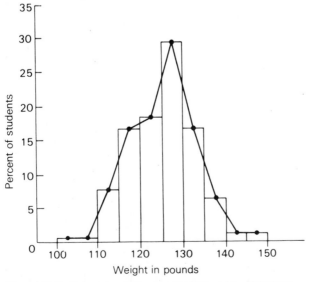

Figure 10-6   Frequency polygon superimposed on histogram.

histogram, it is evident that the frequency polygon is an approximation of the area of the histogram (see Fig. 10-6).

ANALYZING THE DATA

Analysis of data is a process for the purpose of drawing pertinent conclusions from them. The analysis of data is one of the most important parts of any study. The techniques used for drawing conclusions vary according to the hypothesis and the type and amount of data collected. This is why the problem must be clearly defined and the data carefully obtained and well organized.

Vital statistics furnish data on quantity, quality, and composition with respect to a population. The data give a picture of the population and allow for comparison, e.g., comparing the mortality of one group treated with a certain drug with that of another group not treated with the drug, or comparing the incidence or prevalence of disease in a given area with the incidence and prevalence in another area.

Data with qualitative characteristics usually are summarized in rates or ratios. A *rate* is really a proportion, and refers to the rapidity with which a specific event is occurring. The mortality rate tells at what speed people are dying. A ratio describes the relationship between two distinct, separate numerical quantities; neither is included in the other, e.g., the ratio of women to men. It is often used as an index or comparative summary.

Many different kinds of rates are used in studying the various factors involved in the causation and control of disease. Each rate serves a different purpose and is subject to different interpretation. In calculating a rate, the numerator and denominator must be from the same population, and the numerator is included in the denominator. The *numerator* is usually the number of events that have occurred over a specified period of time, and the *denominator* is the population at the middle of that time period. This is considered to be the *population at risk.* When the rate is an annual rate, the population as of July 1 of the specific year is used. The population is usually divided into units of 1000, and the rate expresses how rapidly a particular event is occurring in every 1000 people at risk. The denominator base unit is selected in order to give reasonable rates, neither too large nor in small figures of less than one. The unit selected for all deaths, the *crude mortality rate,* is 1000. The crude mortality rate can be expressed as 11.6 deaths per 1000 people in 1970, or 1160 per 100,000 or 1.16 per 100; they all show the same speed, but the 11.6 rate is more convenient to use. *Morbidity,* or disease incidence, rates are usually calculated for population units of 100,000. A *case fatality rate* is expressed as the number of deaths due to the specific disease per 100 cases of that disease, a percent. The crude death rate illustrates the principles involved; it is calculated according to the following formulation:

$$\text{Crude death rate} = \frac{\text{Number of deaths reported in a given year}}{\text{Estimated population July 1, same year}} \times 1000$$

The rate is easy to calculate. The numerator is found by adding up the number of deaths from all causes that occurred during a given period, usually 1 year. The denominator is the estimated population as of July 1 of same year, the base usually is 1000. The following example gives the calculation of the crude death rate for Seattle, Washington, in 1970:

$$\frac{\text{Total deaths in 1970}}{\text{Estimated population, 1970}} \times 1000 = \frac{6,092}{524,263} \times 1000 = 11.6$$

The findings are interpreted as indicating that, on the average, for every 1000 persons in the population of Seattle in 1970 there were 11.6 deaths from all causes.

Specific rates for deaths, diseases, age, sex, race, or any combination of these factors may be found as long as the numerator can be related to the same population. The following example gives the formula for the specific death rate from neoplasms in the state of Washington, 1969:

$$\frac{\text{Number of deaths caused by a particular disease}}{\text{Estimated population, 1969}} \times 100,000$$

$$\frac{4953 \text{ Deaths from neoplasms}}{3,203,218 \text{ Estimated population}} \times 100,000 = 154.6$$

The specific rate is interpreted as indicating that, on the average, 154.6 persons died from neoplasms per 100,000 population in the state of Washington in 1969.

Incidence and prevalence rates often are used to express the frequency with which a disease is occurring in a population. They have distinct meanings. The *incidence rate* refers to new cases of a disease which arise during a given time period, usually a year. The *prevalence rate* refers to the total number of cases of a disease in a population at a given point in time. For chronic diseases, such as tuberculosis, the prevalence rate is higher than the incidence; for acute diseases, such as the common cold, the incidence is greater than the prevalence. The formulas for the two rates are as follows:

Incidence rate =

$$\frac{\text{number of new cases of disease X}}{\text{occurring during a given time period}} \times 1000$$
$$\overline{\text{estimated population at risk at midpoint same time period}}$$

Prevalence rate =

$$\frac{\text{number of cases of disease X at a point in time}}{\text{estimated population at risk at that point in time}} \times 1000$$

It is important to distinguish between these two rates, and their names indicate their function.

Adjusted rates are often necessary when you want to compare rates of two or more geographic areas. Both the incidence and fatality of many diseases are influenced

Table 10-4 Morbidity from Disease K in Communities A and B

Sex	Community A			Community B		
	Cases	Population	Morbidity rate per 10,000	Cases	Population	Morbidity rate per 10,000
Males	50	10,000	50	50	15,000	33.3
Females	10	10,000	10	10	5,000	20.0
Total	60	20,000	30	60	20,000	30

by certain characteristics, such as age, sex, and race. Rates are adjusted in order to eliminate the influence of one or more of these factors, as the unequal sex distribution of the hypothetical populations illustrated in Table 10-4. The morbidity rate of 30 cases of disease K is the same for both communities, which would indicate that the experience with this disease was equal in them. Further examination shows the incidence of disease K is greater in males than in females, and the female/male ratio is not similar for community A and community B. To compare the true impact of disease K in the two communities, the rates must be adjusted for sex.

A simple method of adjustment of rates is to select a standard population and to apply the sex-specific rates of Communities A and B to this population. The last census can be used for the standard population, or the population of the two areas can be combined. The method for calculating these rates and the sex-adjusted rates for Table 10–4 is as follows:

1 Morbidity rate $= \dfrac{\text{cases of disease}}{\text{population}} \times \text{base}$

    a Community A:

$$\frac{60}{20,000} \times 10,000 = 30 \text{ cases per } 10,000 \text{ population}$$

    b Community B:

$$\frac{60}{20,000} \times 10,000 = 30 \text{ cases per } 10,000 \text{ population}$$

2 Sex-specific case rate $= \dfrac{\text{no. of cases per sex group}}{\text{population of sex group}} \times \text{base}$

    a Community A (males):

$$\frac{50}{10,000} \times 10,000 = 50 \text{ males}$$

b Community A (females):

$$\frac{10}{10,000} \times 10,000 = 10 \text{ females}$$

c Community B (males):

$$\frac{50}{15,000} \times 10,000 = 33 \text{ males}$$

d Community B (females):

$$\frac{10}{5,000} \times 10,000 = 20 \text{ females}$$

3 Specific sex population = Community A males

+Community B males

Specific sex population = Community A females

+Community B females

a Community A + B males = 10,000 + 15,000 = 25,000 males

b Community A + B females = 10,000 + 5,000 = 15,000 females

4 Expected cases = $\dfrac{\text{sex-specific rate}}{\text{base}} \times$ specific sex population

a Community A (males):

$$\frac{50}{10,000} \times 25,000 = 125$$

b Community A (females):

$$\frac{10}{10,000} \times 15,000 = 15$$

c Community B (males):

$$\frac{33}{10,000} \times 25,000 = 82$$

d Community B (females):

$$\frac{20}{10,000} \times 15,000 = 30$$

5 Sex-adjusted rate $= \dfrac{\text{total expected cases of each group}}{\text{total specific sex population}} \times \text{base}$

a Community A:

$$\frac{140}{40,000} \times 10,000 = 35$$

b Community B:

$$\frac{112}{40,000} \times 10,000 = 28$$

These sex-adjusted rates of 35 and 28 are now comparable. They reflect a higher rate for Community A than for Community B. For the sake of simplicity, race was considered to be similar in both communities. The age distribution for a disease or condition is often important, and it becomes necessary to adjust the rates according to age groups.

Age Groups

The age groups frequently used for all causes of morbidity and mortality are:

Under 1 year: infant
1 to 4 years: preschool
5 to 15 years: school
15 to 24 years: adolescent
25 to 44 years: young adults
45 to 65 years: middle age
66 plus: old age

However, computing the age-specific rates of two populations from the above groupings is difficult; therefore ages may be regrouped into a greater span of years. The important principle is that the groupings must be the same for the two populations.

Some of the formulas for computing rates and ratios commonly used in public health have been given. Others include:

Infant mortality rate =

$$\frac{\text{number of deaths under 1 year reported during given year}}{\text{number of live births reported during the same year}} \times 1000$$

Neonatal mortality rate =

$$\frac{\text{number of deaths under 28 days reported during given year}}{\text{number of live births reported during the same year}} \times 1000$$

Maternal mortality rate =

$$\frac{\text{number of deaths from causes of pregnancy during a given year}}{\text{number of live births reported during the same year}} \times 1000$$

Fetal death ratio =

$$\frac{\text{number of fetal deaths during a given year}}{\text{number of live births reported during same year}} \times 1000$$

Case fatality ratio =

$$\frac{\text{number of deaths from spec. disease during a given time period}}{\text{number of cases of the disease during the same period of time}} \times 100$$

Proportional mortality rate =

$$\frac{\text{number of deaths from a specific cause during a given year}}{\text{number of deaths reported from all causes during the same year}} \times 100$$

MEASUREMENT DATA

Data of all types, especially quantitative variables such as age or height, are summarized in terms of their distribution. Measures of central tendency describe this distribution, as measurements of variables tend to cluster around the highest point and will form a specific shape. The measures of central tendency are the mean, median, and mode.

The *mean* is the arithmetic average of a set of observations. It is calculated by adding up the value of each of the observations in a series and dividing by the total number of observations. Suppose that there is an outbreak of a waterborne disease in your district, and you want to determine the mean age at onset. To find the average of the sum of the ages in years, add the ages as follows: 12 + 15 + 16 + 16 + 17 + 18 + 18 + 19 + 20 + 20 + 20 + 22 + 24 + 25 + 28 + 30 = 320; then divide the sum by the total number of observations (16), i.e., 320 divided by 16, which equals 20 years. Each of these numbers has had equal weight in determination of the mean. If the mean of all the observations is subtracted from each of the observations, the sum of the differences or deviations is equal to zero, which is the center of the distribution. An example of the deviation from the mean of 20 years is shown in Fig. 10-7. The

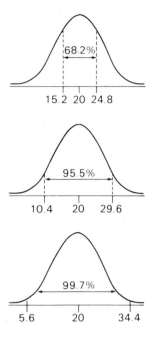

68.2%

15.2 20 24.8

95.5%

10.4   20   29.6

99.7%

5.6   20   34.4

Figure 10-7 Distribution of normal curve with standard deviation of 4.8 years.

distribution in this situation is fairly symmetric, as the frequencies on each side of the mean are similar.

The *median* is the middle observation of a series of observations when the observations are arranged in order of magnitude. If there is an even number of observations, the average of the two middle numbers is the median. For example the median number for the age at onset of the waterborne disease is 19.5 years.

The *mode* is the observation occurring with the greatest frequency in a set of observations. Thus in the example of age at onset of this waterborne disease, the mode is equal to 20 years. A summary of these three measurements is shown in Table 10-5.

The mean is the central measure of choice except when the distribution is asymmetric or skewed. The median is used when the distribution is asymmetric or when observations include occasional extreme values. For a more detailed discussion of the use and the calculation of the measures of central tendency, the reader is referred to the work of Hill, listed at the end of this chapter.

It is beyond the scope of this chapter to present the numerous statistical methods appropriate for analysis of different types of samples. It is suggested that the reader consult a statistician within the agency or a statistical consultant from the state health department for planning and analyzing data.

Mention will be made of one measure of variation, the *standard deviation,* which is commonly used. The standard deviation is most useful with reference to the normal frequency distribution. The measures of central tendency will vary from sample to sample, giving a distribution of the sample mean. These will vary around the true mean of the population from which the samples were drawn. The standard deviation of the distribution of means gives the measure of the degree of chance variation or sampling

Table 10-5 Cases of Waterborne Disease

Age at onset, years	
12	
15	
16	
16	
17	
18	
Range = 18 years 18	
19	*Median* = 19.5 years
20	
20	
20	*Mode* = 20 years
22	
24	
25	
28	
30	

320 ÷ 16 = 20.0 years, *arithmetic mean*

Arithmetic mean: The sum of the observations in a series divided by the total number of observations.

Median: The middle observation when observations are arranged in order of magnitude. In an even number of observations, the average of the two middle observations is taken.

Mode: The observation occurring with the greatest frequency.

Range: The difference between the largest and smallest observations.

within the population. The standard deviation is found by taking the square root of the sum of the squared deviations about the mean and dividing by the number in the sample or by the number of measurements. The formula, then, is:

$$SD = \sqrt{\frac{\text{sum of squared deviations}}{\text{no. of measurements}}}$$

or

$$Sx = \sqrt{\frac{\Sigma(x - \bar{x})^2}{n}}$$

When the standard deviation is calculated for a sample rather than for a population, the standard deviation is computed in the same way except that 1 is subtracted from the number of measurements, as a better estimate of the population is provided if the numbers are small. This would be the situation in the sample of age at onset of the waterborne disease. The formula would be:

$$SD = \sqrt{\frac{\text{sum of squared deviations}}{(\text{no. of measurements} - 1)}}$$

Even though the measures in the sample are discrete, the pattern is characteristic of the normal frequency distribution and is approximated by it. Substituting numbers from the same example, the formula is:

$$SD = \sqrt{\frac{\text{sum of squared deviations}}{(\text{no. of measurements} - 1)}} = \sqrt{\frac{348}{16 - 1}} = \sqrt{\frac{348}{15}} = 4.82$$

or 4.8 years

A summary of the distribution from the example is presented in Table 10-6. Since the sample is small and only approximates the frequency distribution, one is unable to generalize from the findings to large populations. The larger the sample, the closer is the approximation to normal frequency distribution.

If measurements are normally distributed, 68.26 percent of them will fall within

Table 10-6   Distribution of 16 Cases of Waterborne Disease According to Age in Years

Age at onset, years	Deviation from mean of 20 years	Squared deviation
12	-8	64
15	-5	25
16	-4	16
16	-4	16
17	-3	9
18	-2	4
18	-2	4
19	-1	1
20	0	0
20	0	0
20	0	0
22	+2	4
24	+4	16
25	+5	25
28	+8	64
30	+10	100
	0	348

Range: The difference between the largest and smallest measurements, e.g., 30 - 12 = 18 years.

Standard deviation: The square root of the average of the squared deviations of the measurements from the mean.

$$\sqrt{\frac{348}{16}} = \sqrt{21.75} = 4.66 = 4.7 \text{ years}$$

When the standard deviation is being computed for a sample, rather than for a population, it is computed as follows:

$$\sqrt{\frac{348}{16 - 1}} = \sqrt{\frac{348}{15}} = \sqrt{23.2} = 4.82 = 4.8 \text{ years}$$

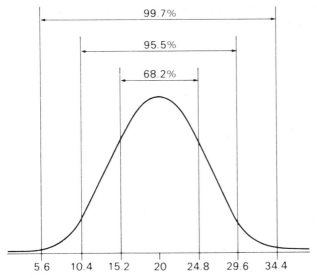

Figure 10-8   Distribution of normal curve with standard deviation of 4.8 years.

1 SD on either side of the mean, or approximately two-thirds of the measurements will not deviate from the mean by more than 1 SD. In other words, in the same example, within 1 SD, two-thirds of the observations will occur 4.8 years on either side of the mean of 20 years (Fig. 10-7).

Also, 95.5 percent of the measurements will fall within 2 SD on either side of the mean, or approximately 95 percent of the measurements will not deviate from the mean by more than 2 SD. Therefore, continuing with the sample example, 9.6 years on either side of the mean equals 2 SD.

Last, 99.7 percent of the measurements will fall within 3 SD on either side of the mean. Applying this principle to the example, almost all the measurements will be within 14.4 years of the mean. Figure 10-8 summarizes the measurements of normal distribution.

SUMMARY

A brief discussion with illustrations of some epidemiologic principles and statistical concepts useful to the nurse in conducting studies is presented. Variation in people, behavior and environment influences health and disease and makes it necessary to study the influence of special characteristics within the population. The purpose of the study, or the hypothesis, determines the study design, observational or experimental, and the type of data, quantitative or qualitative, to be collected. When planning the study, attention is given to the population and sample. After collecting the data, the findings must be systematically organized to show the interrelationships among the variables studied. Analysis of the data is the process of drawing conclusions so that intelligent judgments may be made. Rates and ratios allow for comparison of data with qualitative characteristics. Measurement data of all types, especially quantitative data, are summarized in terms of their distribution, e.g., measures of central tendency. Use of the data collected on a sample, as a basis for generalization to the entire population, requires statistical methods appropriate to different data. The standard deviation is the most useful in normal frequency distribution.

It is suggested that the nurse interested in conducting a study consult with an epidemiologist and a statistician. This chapter provides an elementary discussion of both disciplines.

SUGGESTED READINGS

Biles, Robert W., Patricia A. Buffler, and Alice A. O'Donell: "Epidemiology of Otitis Media: A Community Study," *American Journal of Public Health,* **70**(6):593–598, June 1980.

Branch, Laurence G., and Alan M. Jette: "The Framingham Disability Study: Social Disability among the Aging," *American Journal of Public Health,* **71**(11):1202–1210, November 1981.

Byron, William Brown, Jr., and Myles Hollander: *Statistics: A Biomedical Introduction,* John Wiley and Sons, New York, 1977.

Colvez, Alain, and Madeline Blanchet: "Disability Trends in the United States Population 1966–76: Analysis of Reported Causes," *American Journal of Public Health,* **71**(5):464–471, May 1981.

Fox, John P., Carrie E. Hall, and Lila R. Elveback: *Epidemiology: Man and Disease,* The Macmillan Company, New York, 1970.

Friedman, Gary D.: *Primer of Epidemiology,* McGraw-Hill Book Company, New York, 1974.

Hill, Sir Austin Bradley: *Principles of Medical Statistics,* 9th ed., Oxford University Press, New York, 1971.

Hodgman, Eileen Callahan: "Student Research in Service Agencies," *Nursing Outlook,* **26**(9):558–565, September 1978.

Hogue, Carol C.: "Epidemiology for Distributive Nursing Practice" in *A Systems Approach to Community Health* by Joanne E. Hall and Barbara R. Weaver, J. B. Lippincott Company, Philadelphia, 1977, pp. 193–208.

Jacox, Ada: "Nursing Research and the Clinician," *Nursing Outlook* **22**(6):382–385, June 1974.

Jette, Alan M., and Laurence G. Branch: "The Framingham Disability Study: Physical Disability Among the Aging," *American Journal of Public Health,* **71**(11):1211–1215, November 1981.

Kleinman, Joel C.: "Age-Adjusted Mortality Indexes for Small Areas: Applications to Health Planning," *American Journal of Public Health,* **67**(9):834–840, September 1977.

Kviz, Frederick J.: *Statistics for Nurses: An Introductory Text,* Little, Brown and Company, Boston, 1980.

McHugh, Norma G., and Jean E. Johnson: "Clinical Nursing Research: Beyond the Methods Books, *"Nursing Outlook,* **28**(6):352–356, June 1980.

Ostfeld, A. M., R. B. Shekelle, H. Klawans, and H. M. Tufo: "Epidemiology of Stroke in an Elderly Welfare Population," *American Journal of Public Health* **64**(5):450–458, May 1974.

Polich, J. Michael: "Epidemiology of Alcohol Abuse in Military and Civilian Populations," *American Journal of Public Health,* **71**(10):1125–1131, October 1981.

Standfast, Susan J., Susan Jereb, and Dwight T. Janerich: "The Epidemiology of Sudden Infant Death in Upstate New York: II: Birth Characteristics," *American Journal of Public Health,* **70**(10):1061–1067, October 1980.

Terris, Milton: "Approaches to an Epidemiology of Health," *American Journal of Public Health,* **65**(10):1037–1045, October 1975.

Chapter 11

Looking into the Past and into the Future

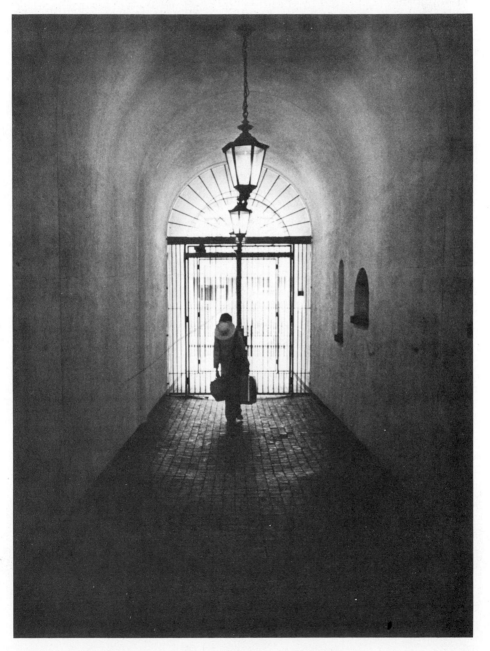

HISTORY OF COMMUNITY HEALTH NURSING

Early History

"Concern with matters of personal and community health appears to have been widely reflected in the records of every major civilization and the majority of cultures known to man."[1]

Similar references are to be found in the general literature and in the Bible. The Old Testament cites the efforts of Moses to prevent the spread of disease among his people by curbing their use of shellfish and pork as food. He did not know specifically why the ingestion of certain shellfish caused dysentery (probably typhoid) and death, or why the ingestion of pork caused illness and disability (probably trichinosis), but he did observe that when he prohibited the use of these foods, the incidence of these diseases declined among his people.

Community health nursing is also an outgrowth and a development of an ancient practice, that of visiting the sick. About 60 A.D. St. Paul mentions in his writings Phebe, a deaconess in the early Christian church, whose duties included a combination of parish work, friendly visiting, and district nursing. She has often been called the first visiting nurse; "from her day the work of visiting nursing has never been unknown."[2]

Nursing in Europe

For more than a thousand years after the time of Phebe, most of the nursing was done by men and women motivated by their religious faith. During the Crusades, illness and death were the fate of many pilgrims on their way to the Holy Land. Monasteries were established on some routes to provide care for these sick and travel-worn pilgrims. Here was the beginning of hospitals and nursing.

Following the Crusades, a spirit of great unrest dominated Western Europe. Many who had visited eastern Mediterranean countries, while on their pilgrimages, returned with a knowledge of new and easier modes of living, with stories of the luxuries of the East, its spices, jewels, and unfamiliar ideas about art and architecture. Important aftermaths of the Crusades were the improvement of economic conditions in many Western European countries; for example, the rise of the great maritime powers, Britain, France, Spain, and Italy, with their wealthy merchant class, and an eagerness for knowledge, especially in the sciences, in the universities.

Marked social reform came with the end of the sixteenth century and the beginning of the seventeenth. This was also a period of creativity, resulting in an increased production in literature and the other arts, a broadening of the horizons of science, and even more important to community health, a notable increase in social understanding, with a growing recognition of social responsibilities by those on different levels of power. The concept of the brotherhood of humanity and other such revolutionary ideas, for those times, as that people are born free and equal and entitled to equal chances, were gaining acceptance. Improvement in living conditions continued,

[1] Edward S. Rogers, *Human Ecology and Health,* The Macmillan Company, New York, 1960, p. 155.
[2] M. Adelaide Nutting and Lavinia L. Dock, *History of Nursing,* G. P. Putnam's Sons, New York, 1907, vol. 1, p. 102.

resulting in better housing, improved sanitation, and more nutritious food. In some instances these gains were the results of the English Poor laws of 1601 during the reign of Elizabeth I.

The sense of social responsibility for the welfare of others was demonstrated also by the sporadic attempts to provide nursing care for the sick, both in their homes and in hospitals. In 1610, in the little town of Annecy in eastern France, St. Francis de Sales (1567-1622) with the aid of Madame de Chantal, organized a nursing service for the care of the sick in their homes, the care to be given by a recently founded order of nuns drawn from women of the upper classes in the surrounding countryside. Unfortunately after 5 years, this order of nuns became cloistered and their home care of the sick was discontinued. Even though their project failed in such a short time, the work of St. Francis de Sales and Madame de Chantal created an interest in the venture, for in 1617 St. Vincent de Paul (1567-1660) founded a religious order of French women near Chatillon, France, to care for the sick on a home visiting nurse basis. St. Vincent de Paul had given much thought and study to the founding of this new organization while a university student in Paris. He introduced modern principles of social work and placed visiting nursing on a plane not reached in previous experiments of this nature. His order of nuns served local communities for many years, but after his death, it, too, became cloistered and could carry out its original purpose no longer.

Much of St. Vincent de Paul's philosophy of service to others is to be found in his writings, among which is the following, quoted from Nutting and Dock, which has significance and meaning for community health nurses today. "Lay off your jewels and fine clothing to visit the poor," said Vincent, "and treat them openly, respectfully and as persons of quality, avoiding all familiarity or stiffness. To send money is good, but we have not really begun to serve the poor until we visit them."[3]

In the centuries that followed, three movements or forces that stimulated interest in community health nursing were developing, slowly and unevenly, throughout Western Europe and were being carried to the New World. These were (1) a sense of humanity, a deepening consciousness of the social problems affecting the lives of many people, such as poverty, inadequate housing, evils of the industrial revolution, child labor, deplorable prison conditions, and lack of opportunities for education; (2) the growth of medical science, which was developing from the curing of disease to the prevention of disease and the promotion of health; and (3) the development of nursing as a profession and a discipline.

Social conditions in England showed definite improvement in the late eighteenth and early nineteenth centuries because of the work of both John Howard and Octavia Hill. John Howard (1726-1790), a sheriff of Bedfordshire, brought about, through his observations and writings, outstanding prison reforms, not only in his native England but in many countries in Europe as well. He has been called an "inspiration to the whole Humanitarian Movement." Octavia Hill (1838-1912), a social worker and contemporary of Florence Nightingale, instigated practical housing reforms in the Liverpool and London slums, bringing comfort, safety, and health to thousands of poor families.

[3] Ibid., p. 414.

Another evidence of a growing sense of social justice was the founding of the International Red Cross in Switzerland in 1863, through the efforts of Henri Dunant, a young man interested in promoting the welfare of others. As the Red Cross societies developed in each country, their emphasis on humanity and their efforts to prevent and to alleviate human suffering wherever it existed widened opportunities for providing nursing care in hospitals and in the community, particularly in many European countries.

The concept of present-day nonreligious community health nursing service was introduced in 1859 under the aegis of William Rathbone of Liverpool, England, who saw visiting nursing as a service that encompassed the new perception of humanity, the knowledge of modern medical science, and the "renewed art of nursing." He was actively supported in his work by Miss Nightingale.

Brainard has summarized the development of the three movements as follows:

> ... the "new community" had taught that universal brotherhood is but a name, unless it seeks to remove the causes of one's brother's degradation; and the new science had taught that disease and suffering are not a visitation from an angered God, but are the direct results of our own carelessness in not following the right principles of hygiene, sanitation and healthful living; and finally, the care of the sick had been raised from the despised occupation of unskilled, untrustworthy women, and placed in the hands of women of refinement and character, who looked upon it as a vocation, and were trained, not only to the gentle ways of the early nuns and deaconesses, but to the scientific care and treatment of the patient as well.[4]

Community Health Nursing in the United States

Nursing care of the sick in their own homes by a graduate nurse was commenced in New York City in 1877, sponsored by the Women's Board of the New York City Mission. The nurse was Frances Root, a graduate of the newly established Bellevue Training School for Nurses. The visiting nurse program, though modest, was a success, and similar ones were initiated on a sporadic basis in a few other American cities. Even in those early years, while providing bedside nursing care in city slums, these pioneer nurses recognized that many illnesses were caused by faulty economic and social conditions under which their patients and families lived, such as inadequate housing, lack of sanitation, insufficient food, and unfair, often vicious, labor conditions, and that measures for the prevention of these abuses were a necessity.

Nine years later the first district nursing associations were started, one in Boston and one in Philadelphia. They reflected a knowledge and understanding of the experience of the visiting nurse programs commenced previously in England. This was the period of prosperity in the reconstruction era following the Civil War. Standards of living were rising, and opportunities for education and travel, both in the United States and abroad, were becoming available to many people. Communication of ideas by post, telegraph, newspapers, and magazines were becoming a part of daily living. The idea of

[4] Annie M. Brainard, *The Evolution of Public Health Nursing,* W. B. Saunders Company, Philadelphia, 1922, pp. 102–103.

an organized district or visiting nurse service for the city poor spread rapidly west and south, and by 1900, twenty such agencies had been established in major cities.

Robert Koch, director of the Imperial Health Bureau in Berlin, in 1882 reported on his studies and those of his confreres, which demonstrated that tuberculosis was a transmissible disease, caused by a specific organism. This new concept of the cause of tuberculosis, with its bearing on the care and control of the disease, was quickly accepted by a large part of the medical profession, both in Europe and in the United States. Koch's discovery brought a new approach to the control of tuberculosis, that of public health measures, e.g., epidemiology and health education. The contribution that community health nurses could make to the control of this disease was recognized soon by the medical profession and the community. Community health nurses became responsible for much of the casefinding and case holding, for teaching patients and their families, and for providing both pre- and postsanatorium home nursing care. Nurses soon discovered that the families of their tuberculous patients, many of them in the upper socioeconomic brackets in the community, had other health problems, too. This widened the scope of the community health nursing program at the beginning of the twentieth century. This new aspect in the care and control of a specific disease by community health measures was important in the early development of community health nursing.

The leadership of Lillian Wald (1867-1940), both a nurse and social worker, at the beginning of this century was responsible for many developments in community health nursing. Miss Wald brought to her work a basic love of and faith in humankind, a brilliant mind trained in the sciences, a sense of the practical, and a vision of what community health nursing and social work could do for communities and their people. In 1893, she and Mary Brewster established a visiting nurse service as a part of their Henry Street Settlement in New York City. This became a model for similar organizations and a training center to which community health nurses were sent for many years, both on an apprenticeship basis and for advanced work in supervision and administration.

Miss Wald, in 1909, persuaded the Metropolitan Life Insurance Company to begin, at first on an experimental basis, a home nursing service for its policy holders through a working arrangement with the Henry Street Settlement. Twelve years later, a study and review of the project showed that the program had been highly successful and had been adopted by community health nursing agencies in many communities. When the number of policy holders warranted it and no community health nursing agency existed in the area, the company set up its own visiting nurse service to care for its policy holders. This program, with some variations, was adopted by other insurance companies in succeeding years.

With the assured income from the provision of nursing services to policy holders for which the insurance companies paid full cost, community health nursing agencies had a firm basis on which to build their overall budget. The remainder of the budget could then be raised in the community by charging full or part fees for visits to non-policy holders who could affort to pay, by gifts, and by allotments from community funds. This contributed to a healthy and steady growth of privately supported visiting nurse agencies throughout the country. With a group of persons (the insurance company policy holders) who were fairly secure economically and who were receiving home nursing service in times of illness from the visiting nurse, the feeling that nursing services were only for the sick poor began to change in many communities. Community health nursing organizations began to note an increase in requests for nursing services from families able and willing to pay for them.

The programs of caring for insurance companies' policy holders continued on a nationwide basis until several years after World War II, when changing social, economic and health conditions made them no longer feasible. Many communities, however, had learned the value of community nursing services and had come to realize responsibilities for supporting, by both public and private means, this health service to the community.

Lillian Wald, while on a visit to London, had an opportunity to observe a school nursing program that had been functioning in the London schools for nearly 10 years. She was impressed to see that the nurses' work showed an improvement in school attendance and a reduction in the spread of communicable diseases among the children, especially skin diseases such as scabies and impetigo.

Through the efforts of Miss Wald, school nursing as a full-time program for a community health nurse was demonstrated and adopted in the New York City schools in 1902. This had followed by a few years the beginning of an industrial or occupational health nursing program in 1895 and was succeeded later by the development, on a specialty basis, of tuberculosis nursing in 1904, following the founding of the National Tuberculosis Association, and of venereal disease nursing as a specialty in 1909, when improved laboratory methods of diagnosis and treatment for syphilis and gonorrhea were developed through the work of Ehrlich.

Maternal and child health had its beginning as a specialty following the first White House Conference on Children called in 1909 through the interest and support of President Theodore Roosevelt. The program received an impetus in its development with the founding of the Children's Bureau by the federal government in 1912 and 1913. Outstanding landmarks in the development of maternal and child health followed rapidly. The New York City Health Department had established a Division of Child Hygiene in 1908, and the New York State Health Department followed in 1914. In 1922, Congress passed the Sheppard-Towner Act for federal aid for local infant welfare work. This money was distributed nationwide, generally through the state departments of health. The Social Security Act of 1935 and its amendments in succeeding years included, among other measures, provisions for public assistance, social services, and means of strengthening family life. These all had an important bearing on maternal and child health work in all parts of the country, rural and urban.

During the 1960s, additional health and welfare programs were initiated by Congress and state legislatures, such as the provisions for medicare, medicaid, and similar programs sponsored by individual states. All this social legislation has increased the opportunities for the community health nurse to provide nursing care and health teaching to patients and families in all age groups.

In the years immediately preceding World War I, certain social, economic, and humanitarian forces, implemented by such leaders as Annie W. Goodrich, Lillian Wald, and Edith Abbott of the Children's Bureau, brought about several events that were important in the development of community health nursing. In 1910, Mrs. Helen

Hartley Jenkins, a friend of Miss Wald's, gave funds to Teacher's College, Columbia University, to establish an academic program of study in community health nursing. Thus a little more than thirty years after Frances Root began her work in district nursing, college preparation in that field became available to nurses. Prior to this, whatever preparation nurses had been able to secure had been provided on an apprenticeship basis by some of the big city nursing agencies, such as the Henry Street Settlement and the Instructive District Nursing Association of Boston.

Following World War I, many colleges and universities initiated study programs in community health nursing for graduate nurses. These were discontinued as community health nursing preparation became recognized as an integral part of the preparation for *all* nurses in the collegiate programs for nursing.

The National Organization for Public Health Nursing was founded in Chicago in 1912. Miss Wald was its first president. The new organization had three types of membership: nurse members, lay members, and corporate members. The key word in the name of the organization was "for." Lay members were active participants and were considered important to the new organization. They worked closely with community health nurses for forty years to improve the standards of nursing service and education. In 1952, the organization became a part of the National League for Nursing at the reorganization of the nursing organizations.

At the time of its founding, the National Organization for Public Health Nursing received a small but successful quarterly publication from the Cleveland, Ohio, Visiting Nurse Association. This became the official national magazine of the young organization, and was best known as *Public Health Nursing.* It devoted its contents to the interests of those in the public health field. In 1953 it was absorbed by a new publication, *Nursing Outlook,* founded to meet, on a broader basis, the needs of an expanding profession.

The American Red Cross pioneered in rural community health nursing when, in 1912, it provided demonstrations of community health nursing care to people in the villages and on the farms. Much of the work was done by "itinerant nurses," who were sent to an area for a period of several months to demonstrate home care of the sick, school nursing, and well-baby conferences. These nurses also conducted mothers' classes and home nursing classes. It was hoped that the communities would recognize the need to employ full-time community health nurses to carry on the program.

Following the introduction of the Red Cross program, rural nursing developed rapidly. County health departments, particularly in the Southern and Western states, were established. Nearly every county health department had a full-time nurse on its staff, though often she was the only full-time professional member of the department. Rural nursing was facilitated further by the production and marketing of the first inexpensive automobile, which made it possible for many nurses to reach patients and families on distant farms and ranches. Putting nurses "on wheels" opened up many new opportunities for nursing services in both rural and urban areas.

The organization of the Children's Bureau by the federal government was completed in 1913. The Bureau stimulated programs of mother and child care by preparing and distributing health literature, e.g., *Prenatal Care,* by investigating unsatisfactory conditions relating to mothers and children, and by assisting with community health studies. The Children's Bureau programs expanded rapidly following the Social Security Act of 1935. The Bureau is now a division of the U.S. Department of Health and Human Services.

Following World War I, a trend from specialization toward generalization occurred, with the staff nurse being responsible for all types of community health nursing services in her district, and the agency providing her with consultant service. This shift from specialization to generalization, and an increasing demand for community health nursing services, contributed to the rapid expansion of community health nursing programs of study for graduate nurses, as previously mentioned, in colleges and universities. The National Organization for Public Health Nursing offered consultant service in the development of such programs and helped to promote standards by an accreditation service and by studies and surveys.

For many years Annie W. Goodrich had pointed out that although nursing had a place in the institutions of the sick, it could not render its full service to the community until it had found a place also in colleges and universities. In 1923 Miss Goodrich founded the Yale School of Nursing as a collegiate school, and for the first time adequate preparation for community health nursing was included in the basic curriculum. This was an innovation closely watched by other collegiate schools of nursing. Slowly they adopted the program, but it was not until after World War II that community health nursing preparation became an integral part of the basic collegiate curriculum and a requirement for national accreditation for a collegiate school of nursing.

During and after World War II, the increased demand for nursing services by the military and by the civilian population made mandatory many improvements in the utilization of nursing services, both in hospitals and in community health agencies, including a discriminating use of the professional nurse's knowledge, abilities, and time. Wider use of the team concept and more carefully planned services by auxiliary personnel were instituted in many hospitals and community health agencies.

Across the country, there was a growing effort to prevent duplication of services offered by the official and nonofficial agencies, wherever possible, thereby conserving the nurses' time and efforts and reducing such overhead costs as those of rent, administration, and travel. Knowledge regarding health practices acquired by the laity during and since World War II and the new public health and community health nursing practices that developed from the nation's war experiences facilitated the movement for the combining of community health nursing agencies.

Some nursing studies had been made in the period between World War I and World War II, such as *Nursing and Nursing Education in the United States, Nurses, Patients and Pocketbooks,* and the *Survey of Public Health Nursing.* In order to determine how to meet adequately the country's needs for nursing in the period following World War II and how to provide the kind of professional education and preparation required by nurses, it was recognized that more studies and research regarding nursing and nursing education was needed. Such additional studies, e.g., *Nursing for the Future, Collegiate Education for Nurses, Twenty Thousand Nurses Tell Their Story,* and *Toward Quality in Nursing,* have been published. Many other studies relating to curriculum needs and development have been made; these have pointed out the need for deepening the content of the preparation for nursing, for supporting nursing knowledge with contributions from other disciplines in the natural and social sciences and the humanities, for developing skills and abilities in the problem-solving approach, and for preparing students in collegiate programs in basic nursing for beginning positions in both hospitals and community health agencies. Current developments in nursing education attempt to meet these needs on both basic and graduate levels of study.

The nursing profession recognized the need also for continued research in other aspects of nursing, nursing practice, and research methodology as well as education, thus the founding in 1952 of the periodical *Nursing Research Report,* sponsored by the National League for Nursing and later by the American Nurses' Association also. Through its pages, *Nursing Research* has made the results of many studies in the various fields of nursing available to the profession as a whole and to allied disciplines. In 1955, the American Nurses' Association created the American Nurses' Foundation to meet the needs for a permanent nonprofit organization devoted to research in nursing.[5] Research programs to determine community needs for nursing in all its aspects and ways for meeting these needs will continue for years to come.

ISSUES OF IMPORTANCE TO NURSES
TODAY AND TOMORROW

"The most frustrating fact of life is this: the more progress we make, the more we must make. The more needs we satisfy, the more needs we develop."[6] Changes in health care delivery along with the position of nursing in the health care system are occurring rapidly. As pointed out by Jones, nursing is struggling continuously for recognition as a true profession. For too long, other disciplines have been allowed to have too much influence in determining the nurse's role. Florence Nightingale and Lillian Wald were both nurse pioneers who successfully pushed forward into frontiers and broke down barriers that had limited nursing. It can be done again. For nursing to realize its full potential, nursing's identity must rest upon "what nurses are *together* as much as what nurses are *separately*."[7]

Nurses together as much as separately must (1) move toward professionalism and (2) develop a power base. In so doing, many issues must be addressed, some of which are identified in the following pages. The list of issues is by no means a complete one, but as new and/or controversial issues arise, nursing students must be prepared to study the facts, examine the pros and cons of each issue, and make a decision regarding the stand they will support.

Professionalism of Nursing

Pavalko, a sociologist, has specified eight criteria with which to measure the extent to which a work group or occupation has achieved the status of a profession. The eight

[5]Susan D. Taylor, "American Nurses' Foundation, 1955–1970," *Nursing Research Report,* 5(4): 1–6, December 1970.

[6]Richard E. Farson, "Bill of Rights for 1984," in Maryjane Dunstan and Patricia W. Garlan (eds.), *Worlds in the Making,* Prentice-Hall Inc., Englewood Cliffs, N.J., 1970, p. 367.

[7]Judith Nutt Jones, "The Not-So-Obvious Limits of Nursing," *Nursing and Health Care,* 2 (2):64–72, February 1981.

criteria are listed as follows in terms of their relevance to nursing: theory, relevance to basic social values, educational period, motivation, autonomy, sense of commitment, sense of community, and code of ethics.[8]

Theory Theories are intellectual tools used to develop a systematic body of knowledge for a given profession. Research is the means for defining the unique body of knowledge belonging to the stated profession. In nursing, theory development and research are revealing increasingly the domain of knowledge that belongs to nursing exclusively, the methodology with which to communicate, and the outcomes to be evaluated.[9]

The goal of theory development and research is professional practice which addresses consumer needs and concerns in health services and provides quality care with quality outcomes.

For research to be viable and respected as an indispensable reference source, it must be studied and utilized by all nurses practicing in educational and clinical settings. In many instances, research findings will provide support for current practices or will imply a change of established practices or ways of thinking about practice. For change to occur, legitimization of a proposed innovation must be provided by those persons in leadership positions who can manage organizational conditions as feasible to ensure that implementation is carried out as suggested by the research finding, and rewards given for reinforcing the desired new behavior.

When a research finding is utilized, it must be evaluated in terms of its quality of process and quality of outcome. The purpose of quality of process evaluation is to identify points to maximize the quality of professional practice. Criteria must be used or developed as a basis for making judgments about quality. The quality of outcome evaluation asks the difference which the use of the innovation makes on the outcome of practice. Evaluation on an ongoing basis is imperative when improvement of quality of care is the goal. Concurrent with ongoing evaluation of research, nurses must be alert to and protective of the consumer's human rights. Securing the consumer's understanding and consent, and assuring confidentiality and/or anonymity regarding an individual's participation in a study must never be forgotten or overlooked.

For research to have an impact on services provided by nurses in the health care delivery system, reports and findings must be studied and utilized by all nurses. There must be active sharing of ideas, viewpoints, knowledge, and findings between nurses in education and clinical practice on a mutually cooperative basis.[10]

Using theory as the criterion, nursing is moving rapidly toward professionalism.

Relevance to Basic Social Values Values are abstract ideals, positive or negative, representing a person's beliefs about ideal modes of conduct and ideal terminal goals. A value when internalized becomes a standard for guiding action, for maintaining

[8] R. M. Pavalko, *Sociology of Occupations and Professions*, F. E. Peacock Publishers, Inc., Itasca, Ill., 1971, p. 18.

[9] Ada K. Jacox and Catherine M. Norris, *Organizing for Independent Nursing Practice*, Appleton-Century-Crofts, New York, 1977, p. 27.

[10] Marjorie V. Batey, "Research: Its Dissemination and Utilization in Nursing Practice," *Washington State Journal of Nursing*, 47(1):6-9, Winter 1975.

attitudes toward relevant situations, and for justifying one's own and others' actions and attitudes.

Nursing has traditionally been concerned with providing care to people—all ages, races, creeds, colors. Society accepts and values nursing as a helping profession. Using relevance to basic social values as the criterion, nursing rates high on the professionalism scale.

One issue in nursing which may prove to be controversial for some nurses is that of client advocacy. The concept, advocacy, rates high intellectually when nurses perceive their role to be one of informing and supporting clients to make the best decisions possible for themselves. However, the actual performance of the role of client advocate can be potentially risky, precarious, and unpopular depending upon factors unique to each situation. Nurses who value the role of client advocate can approach each client situation requiring advocate behavior by thinking carefully through the following seven steps of the valuing process.

1　They can choose freely to perform the role of advocate. This entails looking at each situation critically, logically, creatively, and morally.

2　They can examine all options available in a given situation and choose an alternative action which they judge to be most appropriate.

3　They can consider the consequences of the selected alternative for action and commit themselves to their choice. This means looking at their choice in terms of the effect it will have on others, including clients, friends, nursing colleagues, etc.

4　They must be proud of and happy with their choice.

5　They must be willing to affirm their choice publicly.

6　They must demonstrate their choice by their behavior and action.

7　They must be able to repeat this behavior and action consistently.[11]

The issue of client advocacy is one example of a potentially difficult value with which nurses must contend. There are innumerable other values about which each nurse has to decide. The seven step valuing process is helpful for determining the degree of commitment each nurse is willing to assume.

Educational Period　This criterion is inclusive of the following dimensions; the amount and length of education, the degree of specialization, the use of symbolic and ideational processes, and the actual content.[12]

The length of education for the registered nurse varies from 2 years for an associate degree to 4 or 5 years for a baccalaureate degree. Graduate education in nursing provides a master's degree upon completion of 1 or 2 years, and a doctoral degree upon completion of 3 or more years. The specification of "professional nurse," based upon educational requirements, is a controversial issue currently. At the present time, nursing education ranges from 2 years to 8 years or more.

Nursing is rapidly becoming more and more specialized as evidenced by the

[11] Diane B. Uustal, "Values Clarification in Nursing: Application to Practice," *American Journal of Nursing,* 78(12):2058–2063, December 1978.
[12] Linda Anne Bernhard and Michelle Walsh, *Leadership, The Key to the Professionalization of Nursing,* McGraw-Hill Book Company, New York, 1981, p. 3.

increasing numbers of clinical specialists, nurse practitioners, nurse midwives, and nurses practicing in specialized fields of health care. Symbolic and ideational processes are characterized in nursing by the widespread use of the nursing process, problem-solving process, community organization process, theories, and conceptual frameworks. The actual content of nursing is based increasingly on findings gained through research which specify the unique domain of knowledge for which nursing is uniquely prepared.

Using educational period as the criterion, the nursing population in the United States has not reached a universal agreement in terms of its placement on the professionalism scale.

Motivation This criteron refers to the extent to which the work group emphasizes the ideal of service to the public.[13] All definitions of nursing refer, in one way or another, to the goal for "assisting the individual, sick or well," or "helping the individual and family to manage activities which contribute toward increased comfort and/or wellness." Safeguarding the life and health of individuals and promoting public welfare are indisputable goals which underlie the practice of nursing. For this reason, the criterion of motivation rates high on the scale of professionalism for nursing.

Autonomy The criterion, autonomy, means the freedom of the work group to regulate and control its own work behavior.[14] Autonomous means self-governing, independent, subject to its own laws only.

Because the majority of nurses are employed by bureaucratic institutions such as hospitals, agencies, industries, etc., they are subject to the control of their employer, and cannot claim to be totally autonomous. Nursing has been labeled a semiprofession based on its diluted authority for providing access to and market for valued nursing skills and knowledge. For a semiprofession to achieve professionalism, it must attain a monopoly over its service functions and a high social status for its members and leaders.[15] These goals can be accomplished through a consistent and sustained use of propaganda, public relations activities and political activism. As described by Larson, "Professionalization is an attempt to translate one order of scarce resources—special knowledge and skills—into another—social and economic rewards."[16]

Nursing is currently aspiring toward the goal of professionalism, but attainment of the goal has not yet been reached. Autonomy is a significant criterion in determining the achievement of professionalism.

"The core of autonomous practice is being able to offer a unique therapy. Not as central, but just as necessary, is the freedom to provide that service without interference or permission." As stated by Mundinger, nurses are autonomous but do not work in isolation. They function as unique professionals who give their richest

---

[13] Ibid., p. 5.
[14] Ibid., p. 5.
[15] Margaret Levi, "Functional Redundance and the Process of Professionalization: The Case of Registered Nurses in the United States," Unpublished paper presented to the 1978 International Sociological Association Meetings in Uppsala, Sweden, July 1978.
[16] Margali Sarfatti Larson, *The Rise of Professionalism: A Sociological Analysis,* University of California Press, Berkeley, 1977.

service in collaboration with others—physicians, clients, and other non-health-related professionals.[17]

To transform the public's image of nursing from one of serving the physician to one of providing unique services beneficial for clients and in collaboration with physicians, nurses must focus on health problems and nursing therapies with which they are most successful. They must make a conscious effort to publicize the efficacy of their services. They must maintain high standards of quality nursing practice, always mindful of the public trust.

Accountability and quality assurance are concepts associated with the idea of self-regulation. Self-regulation implies that each profession must establish standards and criteria for the outcomes, process, and structure of the services it provides.[18] Nursing as a service profession practices primarily for consumers—to improve their health, increase their comfort, or contribute toward a higher level of wellness. Consumers are the reason that nursing exists. Quality assurance activities involve assuring consumers of the specified degree of excellence in nursing practices through continuous measurement and evaluation of structural components, goal-directed nursing process, and/or consumer outcomes, using pre-established criteria and standards and available norms, and followed by appropriate alterations with the purpose of improvement.[19] Effective quality assurance programs provide valuable justification for nursing excellence as practiced in the competitive health care marketplace.

Peer review is a method of evaluation which is receiving increasing recognition among nurses and is a means of self-regulation. Peer review is a refined form of planned observation for review of nursing process, nurse performance, client outcomes, or other activities which may directly or indirectly relate to client care. Zimmer stated that peer review is nurse peers' review of the health/wellness outcomes of a population of clients—of nursing activities that assist clients to attain these benefits, and observable evidence of clients' progress toward these results.[20] Instituting peer review methods reflects the seriousness for which nurses wish to be accountable to consumers for provision of quality health care. From the perspective of the criterion, autonomy, nursing is making progress toward professionalism.

Sense of Commitment This criterion reflects the feelings of commitment that members have toward their work. If one were to interview a cross section of nurses working full time regarding their sense of commitment toward their work, a wide diversity of answers would probably be forthcoming. Many nurses view nursing as a job only, while others are career-oriented and have a deep interest in the growth of nursing as a profession. For nurses who feel proud of their career selection and their sense of accountability to consumers for excellence in nursing practice, opportunities

[17]Mary O'Neil Mundinger, *Autonomy in Nursing,* Aspen Systems Corporation, Germantown, Md., 1980, pp. 20, 196.

[18]Norma M. Lang, "Quality Assurance Review in Nursing," *Maternal Child Nursing,* March–April 1976, p. 75.

[19]John Charles Schmadl, "Quality Assurance: Examination of the Concept," *Nursing Outlook,* 27(7):462–465, July, 1979.

[20]Marie J. Zimmer, "Quality Assurance for Outcomes of Patient Care," *The Nursing Clinics of North America,* 9(2):305–315, June 1974.

for additional learning are seized to update their current knowledge and skills. Continuing education programs are the means provided for assuring excellence of nursing practice. The concept of lifelong learning is recognized as essential by practicing professional committed nurses.

Continuing education is formalized learning experiences or sequences designed to enlarge the knowledge or skills of nurses. Its purpose is to ensure the public that there will be a basic standard for the quality of nursing practice.[21]

Through the American Nurses' Association, a continuing education recognition program (CERP) was established to design and implement a system whereby nurses' accountability and quality continuing education activities would be recorded, recognized and documented in the event that mandatory continuing education becomes a reality. Guidelines were developed for continuing education contact hours in each state so that uniformity and reciprocity of recognition would be consistent throughout the nation. CE committees review proposed educational offerings in terms of specific criteria and factors assessed to be essential and determine a particular number of contact hours to be granted for each continuing education offering. For individual nurses seeking contact hours and proof of maintenance of professional competency, enrolling in a CE program is advantageous. Records of continuing education activities for which contact hours have been awarded can be maintained and retrieved through a computerized databank. Contact hours can be earned by attending CE approved offerings or pursuing an approved plan of independent study. In determining criteria for quality continuing education, nurses are demonstrating their commitment for seeking new knowledge and providing quality health care to consumers.[22]

The sense of commitment felt by the majority of nurses in the United States may change when and if professionalism comes closer to reality.

Sense of Community This criterion deals with the degree to which members of the work group share a common identity and destiny and possess a distinctive subculture. The subculture influences both the work and nonwork behaviors of group members.[23] Nurses possess a strong sense of identity and have definite perceptions of skilled nursing services. They enjoy interacting and mingling with nurse colleagues but do not necessarily demonstrate a sense of community regarding nursing's destiny.

The American Nurses' Association (ANA) is the national professional organization which lobbies for health legislation representing the special interests of nurses in the United States. However, only a small percentage of nurses currently belongs to the professional organization. To develop a greater sense of community and "nurse-power," nurses need to coalesce in a single body like the ANA or be supportive of a coalition of specialty nurse groups such as the Federation of Specialty Nursing Organizations. Nursing specialty organizations are composed mainly of registered nurses,

---

[21] Judith G. Whitaker, "The Issue of Mandatory Continuing Education," *The Nursing Clinics of North America,* "Current Legal and Professional Issues," Helen Creighton (ed.), 9(3): 475–478, September 1974.

[22] Cecilia Smith, "CERP: Where We Have Been, Where We Are, and Where We Are Going," *Washington State Journal of Nursing,* 47(1):17–18, Winter 1975.

[23] Bernhard and Walsh, op. cit. pp. 7–8.

have elected officers and bylaws which define their purpose and functions for the improvement of health care, and represent a body of knowledge and expertise in a defined area of clinical nursing practice. Examples of specialty nursing organizations include the Association of Operating Room Nurses, Association of Occupational Health Nurses, School Nurse Organization, Association of Critical Care Nurses, Association of Nephrology Nurses and Technicians, Association of Rehabilitation Nurses, Emergency Department Nurses Association, Association of Neurosurgical Nurses, Orthopedic Nurses Association, Recovery Room Nurses, Association of Nurse Anesthetists, and State Nurses Association.

By joining together regularly to discuss issues of concern which face nursing and nurses and provide a united front for influencing constructive changes in health care for consumers, nurses as a strong body of concerned health professionals can contribute significantly to the quality of health care in the United States. A sense of community currently exists in nursing specialty organizations and in the membership of state nurses' associations. This sense of community can be enlarged and professionalism furthered if nurses will join together as a unified body. To become recognized by society as a strong contingent of health professionals, nurses must present a united front in terms of their membership and articulate their unique concerns for improving the quality of health care through political activities. They must demonstrate their political strength by pooling communication resources which keep them informed of the emergence, dormancy, or necessity for action of significant health care legislation. Until nurses demonstrate a stronger coalition within their ranks, they will not be recognized by a society as a professional group with a strong sense of community.

Code of Ethics Codes of ethics delineate behaviors and relationships acceptable and recommended for members of a profession. ANA has a code of ethics for nurses which define the ethical duties of nurses to clients, to the profession, and to society. However, with the changing nature and values of the current society, ethical dilemmas often arise for nurses. Ethical dilemmas occur with a difficult problem that has no satisfactory solution, or with a situation involving choice between equally unsatisfactory alternatives.[24] Ethical dilemmas are represented by sometimes difficult decisions nurses must make about how they relate to and care for clients. Nurses are better prepared to deal with difficult problems when they are able to distinguish between legal and ethical rights, duties, and obligations.

Legal rights are claims recognized as valid by the legal system. *Ethical rights* are claims based on ethical principles or an enlightened conscience. Ethical rights may or may not be upheld in a court.

Legal duties and *obligations* are those called for by law. For nurses, the duties and obligations are for clients, health care institutions or agencies, and other health professionals. The legal duty relating to role, status, or position of nurses is defined in nurse practice acts and state board regulations. Ethical duties and obligations are based on ethical principles and define role, status, or position as delineated by professional codes of behavior. The ethical duties are often not specified by law.

[24] Anne J. Davis and Mila A. Aroskar, *Ethical Dilemmas and Nursing Practice,* Appleton-Century-Crofts, New York, 1978, p. 6.

Legal and ethical rights, duties, and obligations can and do conflict. Nurses as health care providers have a primary ethical obligation to clients. They also have legal obligations, however, to both the employing institution or agency and to the client.[25] Because of the complex nature of the nurse's position in relation to clients, employing institutions or agencies, or other health care professionals (physicians), nurses are faced daily with ethical dilemmas. To deal with these dilemmas intelligently, nurses need special education regarding legal and ethical issues which will assist them to examine their own ethical values and develop strategies for resolving the dilemmas satisfactorily. Nurse ethicists or interdisciplinary ethics committees should be available in every community for consultation whenever issues requiring clarification arise.

An example of an ethical dilemma which could confront a nursing student is the assignment and expectation that the student will request a client to sign an informed consent form preliminary to the performance of a medical or surgical procedure. The present principle of *informed consent* states that it is a contract between two people, without one dominating the other, and that the client makes the final decision to take a risk based on adequate information of risks and benefits, complete comprehension of that information, available alternatives to the proposed procedure, and time for client questions before signing the consent form.[26] Obviously, to fulfill the requirements of informed consent legally, the procedure for obtaining consent should be the responsibility of the physician doing the procedure. The dilemma of the nurse whether or not to proceed with acquiring a client's signature on an informed consent form will be based on knowledge of legal and ethical rights, willingness to take the risk, and courage to stand by the decision.

Code of ethics is a criterion of professionalism which sets standards of professional behavior, but in practice these standards are sometimes not easily attained. As nurses are faced with dilemmas requiring careful deliberation before making final decisions, the professional association may ultimately provide for nurse ethicists and/or nursing ethics committees to be available in institutions and/or communities.

An examination of nursing activities, issues, and concerns in terms of the eight criteria for professionalism as espoused by Pavalko show a definite progression toward professionalism. Nurses individually, collectively, and organizationally can become unified, can settle basic differences, and can achieve the distinction of becoming a profession. It will take concerted and persistent effort.

A Power Base for Nurses

Nurse power is an idea whose time has come. Changes in nursing education and health care delivery systems have contributed to the fact that large numbers of nurses have specialized expertise in practice. Through their commitment to improved practice, these nurses are realizing their own potential influence on the machinery of health care delivery and are asserting themselves in the formulation and implementation of

[25] Sharon Jeanne Smith and Anne J. Davis, "Ethical Dilemmas: Conflicts among Rights, Duties, and Obligations," *American Journal of Nursing,* 80(8):1463–1466, August 1980.
[26] Linda Briggs Besch, "Informed Consent: A Patient's Right," *Nursing Outlook,* 27(1): 32–35, January 1979.

policy in primary health care centers, critical care facilities, and independent and joint practice settings. Individually and in groups, they are exercising their power as practitioners.

Power in nursing means knowledge, strength, the courage to risk, and the ability as a collective body to influence improved health care for clients. Shared power or collective collaborative power has potential for far-reaching consequences. An early strategy to tap as a beginning resource toward an improved power base for nurses is networking. It is not the only resource, but is an effective one for beginners who want to move up the career ladder, and eventually play an influential role in articulating needed health care changes for clients in future years.

Networking is a process with which men are familiar and utilize traditionally. Women are beginning to network consciously as a means for developing and using contacts, providing support for each other, and organizing together to work toward an issue or a cause that needs publicity and/or legislation. It is proposed that nursing students start networking groups in their places of employment for the purpose of gaining information about the system in which they work, receiving advice when needed, and accepting moral support during periods of stress. Through network groups, informal connections are made with other nurses, topics are discussed openly and feelings shared, support for the reality shock that new graduates experience is given, and strength and self-confidence as nurses is gained personally and collectively.

As described by Welch, networking is easy and can be fun. One of the biggest benefits of effective networking is the development of a "sense of community." In the place of employment, information is power, and sharing those bits of information that network members accumulate as a group can prepare them to deal with anticipated activities and assignments efficaciously. When one individual of the group needs to know about informal and formal resources for some special purpose, network members often can refer that person to call Mr. X or Ms. Y. Knowing who to call is extremely useful. Network members can also give each other feedback about behavior, strategies for success, and encouragement when stressful activities are anticipated or have already occurred. Networking boosts self-confidence and expectations of great things to come.[27]

Starting a Network Group[28]   The following suggestions are offered for starting a network group.

1   Start with a core of two or three nurses who agree with you about the general need for a network group. An initial need may be the opportunity to discuss work activities and provide support for each other as nurses. As the group becomes committed to the purpose of the meetings, consider requesting additional nurses to join the group. Additional nurses can be peers, nurses at a higher level in the place of employment, or nurses from other institutions or agencies. Adding members to the group can be accomplished when regular network members are ready to add new dimensions to

[27]Mary-Scott Welch, *Networking: The Great New Way for Women to Get Ahead,* Warner Books, Inc., New York, 1980, p. 45.
[28]Ibid., pp. 285–292.

the group meetings. For example, when the group wants to expand, nurses who may act as potential mentors can be invited to join the network group. *Mentors* are nurses who are older, wiser, and already established in the nursing world. These persons can assist network members in their career advancement, can provide counseling and encouragement during times of need.[29] Mentors can be very helpful in providing new directions and/or purposes for the group when the members are ready to broaden their "power base."

2 Set a date, time, and place for three meetings in the beginning. It usually takes three meetings to get started and to smooth out uncertainties and questions.

3 For the first meeting, draw up an agenda and a tentative statement of purpose for the group. Provide the agenda to all group members preceding the first meeting. An example of an agenda appears as follows: (a) Self-introductions and reasons for attending the meeting; (b) Discussion and agreement regarding the purpose for the group; (c) Listing of questions that members want answered; (d) Suggestions or ideas for future meetings. The agenda will keep the members focused on the purpose for meeting.

4 During the first meeting, have someone take notes, or use a flip chart for key ideas and suggestions. Provide each member with a list of each person's name, address, and telephone number. Perform as the group leader during the first meeting to get the group started. The implementation of leadership functions in future meetings can be determined by the group. Be sure all persons attending have the agenda. Self-help refreshments always seem to facilitate discussion and sharing of ideas.

Before the end of the meeting, announce the date and time for the next meeting. A secret for success in keeping groups going is involving everyone as a participant. For this reason, tasks should be delegated such as sending out a summary of the meeting along with a reminder of the next meeting, assigning members to read about or request information that will be beneficial for the group, generating questions that the group would like answered, etc.

Once the group is organized and operating smoothly, remember to evaluate the functioning and purpose of the group at regular intervals. Purposes can change or be modified; membership of the group can be enlarged; issues of concern can take new directions. The point to be remembered is that networking is a process which helps nurses to progress in their careers. It is an effective means for nurses to utilize in the development of a power base individually, collectively, and organizationally.

As stated by Kalisch, "By 2003, the typical nurse will be described as confident, independent, autonomous, and even assertive. Nurses will be regarded as health professionals in their own right, who are as valuable to society for their unique contributions as physicians are for theirs. Nurses will be much more willing to accept responsibility and accountability for their performance than they are today and will engage in independent practice as well as in cooperative decision making with physicians and other health care providers."[30]

As stated by a nursing student,

Every nurse whether he or she is a student or a new graduate, a middle-aged nurse or an "old" one must see that the profession of nursing is changing. All

[29] Ruth Halcomb, *Women Making It,* Ballantine Books, New York, 1979, p. 107.
[30] Beatrice J. Kalisch, "The Promise of Power," *Nursing Outlook,* **26**:46, January 1978.

should be learning from others, growing, and working to improve oneself. And our best source of learning what we need to know is simply on the job from each other in the most cooperative and uplifting manner as possible. If we can feel value in ourselves as nurses then we will see much more power in our profession as a whole.

SUGGESTED READING

Besch, Linda Briggs: "Informed Consent: A Patient's Right," *Nursing Outlook,* **27**(1): 32–35, January 1979.

Bloch, Doris: "Criteria, Standards, Norms—Crucial Terms in Quality Assurance," *Journal of Nursing Administration,* **7**(7):22–30, September 1977.

Christy, Teresa E.: "Portrait of a Leader: M. Adelaide Nutting," *Nursing Outlook,* **17**:20–24, January 1969.

Christy, Teresa E.: "Portrait of a Leader: Annie Warburton Goodrich," *Nursing Outlook,* **18**:46–50, August 1970.

Christy, Teresa E.: "Portrait of a Leader: Lillian D. Wald," *Nursing Outlook,* **18**: 50–54, March 1970.

Ciske, Karen L.: "Accountability—The Essence of Primary Nursing," *American Journal of Nursing,* **79**(5):890–894, May 1979.

Collart, Marie E.: "An Overview in Planning, Implementing and Evaluating Continuing Nursing Education," *Journal of Continuing Education in Nursing,* **7**(6):9–22, 1976.

Cooper, Signe, and May Hornback: *Continuing Nursing Education,* McGraw-Hill Book Company, New York, 1973.

Craig, James H., and Marge Craig: *Synergic Power Beyond Domination and Permissiveness,* Proactive Press, Berkeley, Calif., 1974.

Davis, Anne J., and Mila A. Aroskar: *Ethical Dilemmas and Nursing Practice,* Appleton-Century-Crofts, New York, 1978.

del Bueno, Dorothy J.: "Continuing Education, Spinach and other Good Things," *Journal of Nursing Administration,* **7**(4):32–34, April 1977.

del Bueno, Dorothy J.: "How to Get Your Money's Worth Out of Continuing Education," *RN,* **41**(4):37–42, April 1978.

del Bueno, Dorothy J.: "Performance Evaluation: When All Is Said and Done, More Is Said than Done," *Journal of Nursing Administration,* **7**(10):21–23, December 1977.

Fromer, Margot Joan: "Teaching Ethics by Case Analysis," *Nursing Outlook,* **28**(10): 604–609, October 1980.

Goeppinger, Jean: "Community Health Nursing, Primary Nursing Care in Society," in Beverly Flynn and Michael H. Miller (eds.), *Current Perspectives in Nursing: Social Issues and Trends,* vol 2, The C. V. Mosby Company, St. Louis, 1980.

Gortner, Susan R.: "Scientific Accountability in Nursing," *Nursing Outlook,* **22**(12): 764:768, December 1974.

Halcomb, Ruth: *Women Making It,* Ballantine Books, New York, 1979.

Jacox, Ada K., and Catherine M. Norris: *Organizing for Independent Nursing Practice,* Appleton-Century-Crofts, New York, 1977.

Jacox, Ada: "Theory Construction in Nursing: An Overview," *Nursing Research,* **23**(1): 4–12, January–February 1974.

Jones, Judith Nutt: "The Not-So-Obvious Limits of Nursing," *Nursing and Health Care,* 2(2):64–72, February 1981.

Lang, Norma M.: "Quality Assurance Review in Nursing," *Maternal Child Nursing,* 1(2):75–79, March–April 1976.

Lieb, Renee: "Power, Powerlessness and Potential—Nurse's Role Within the Health Care Delivery System," *Image,* 10(3):75–83, October 1978.

Mundinger, Mary O'Neil: *Autonomy in Nursing,* Aspen Systems Corporation, Germantown, Md., 1980.

Popiel, Elda S.: *Nursing and the Process of Continuing Education,* 2d ed., The C. V. Mosby Company, St. Louis, 1977.

Roberts, Mary M.: *American Nursing: History and Interpretation,* The Macmillan Company, New York, 1954.

Schmadl, John Charles: "Quality Assurance: Examination of the Concept," *Nursing Outlook,* 27(7):462–465, July 1979.

Thompson, John D.: "The Passionate Humanist: From Nightingale to the New Nurse," *Nursing Outlook,* 28(5):290–295, May 1980.

Welch, Mary-Scott: *Networking: The Great New Way for Women to Get Ahead,* Warner Books, New York, 1980.

Part Two

INTRODUCTION

Case situations, experiential exercises, and case studies are provided in the following section to be used as examples for discussion and learning. It is hoped that these descriptions of community health situations will provide insight about aspects of community health nursing, will arouse thought regarding the effective use of self as a nurse with families in communities, and will demonstrate the utilization of selected theories with consumers.

The case studies are based on papers written by nursing students and are descriptive of actual situations encountered with families in the local community. Grateful acknowledgment is expressed for the direct and indirect contributions of the following students: Janet Arusell, Diana Ciganik, Lynda Gentz, Nancy Hoover, Sandra Kennedy, Michelle Kroll, Sonia Mounsey, Sandra Withers, Deborah Strong, and Thomas Visaya.

Community Situations

USING ROSS'S COMMUNITY ORGANIZATION PROCESS

In searching for an idea which would be acceptable in fulfilling the requirements of a community project, a small group of senior nursing students enthusiastically decided to start working toward the establishment of a drop-in center for teenagers in the local community. They felt a deep concern and empathy for the youth in the community because recreational and social facilities were limited. They thought that if a drop-in center for teenagers were available where they could "come and rap," perhaps some would be prevented from choosing self-destructive alternative lifestyles (drugs and alcohol).

Their first steps in proceeding to identify the needs of the community in regard to youth were to investigate the existence of resources currently in operation. They found that the youth in the community had no "constructive" recreational or social facilities. There were no resources dealing with drug and alcohol problems. There were facilities for youth in nearby communities; however, because of the rivalry of community competition, the youth did not feel welcome in nearby community facilities. The next activities of the nursing students were to interview a cross section of local community citizens. They interviewed school teachers and administrators, psychologists, police, clergy, representatives of the local coordinating and planning agencies, and a member of the YWCA. The nursing students returned from these interviews either depressed or enthusiastic, depending upon to whom they talked. As they discussed their goal and experiences among themselves, regardless of the up-and-down swings of emotion, they became increasingly convinced that a drop-in center was desperately needed in that community. An empathy for the plight of the local teenagers was particularly poignant at that stage of the community organization process. An opportunity arose to attend an evening community meeting sponsored by the local YWCA in relation to the need for a drop-in center in the community. The director and two high school students from a nearby community facility were on the agenda to explain their organization, purpose, and functions. During the meeting the local citizens were informed that all that was necessary to start a drop-in center was a group of interested young people and a house, and other details could be worked out thereafter. The discussion during the meeting accepted the assumption that a drop-in center was needed; however, the securing of a house and the financial and legal implications involved a risk with which no one wanted to deal. As the meeting terminated on an indecisive note, a young woman counselor of the local community recreational center volunteered her services to work toward the goal of a drop-in center. At a subsequent meeting with the counselor, the nursing students were advised to contact a clergyman who had expressed an interest in the project. It was at this point that the nursing students were searching for potentially productive local resources to deal with their objectives. They were also vacillating in emotions about the behavior of local citizens at meetings. With uncertainty, but with hope, they met with the local clergyman who had with him a public school counselor and physical educational coordinator. In their report of this meeting they described the discussion as follows:

> We discussed the drop-in center in abstract terms. Father R. and Mr. J. mentioned influential people in the community who might be of some aid to our project. Father R. stated that if he was going to help us financially, he wanted to know more about how we were going to be organized. He mentioned lawyers, incorporating the center, and made what we thought to be a relatively simple organization a very complex endeavor. However, his assistance was vital in making us aware of the problems that would arise.

A series of meetings were held with the clergyman and school counselor at regular intervals thereafter, and an increasing number of local citizens were drawn into the project, including a lawyer, a judge, a policeman, a Catholic clergyman, a local businessman, a physician, representatives from the local school district, local service clubs, and the local coordinating agency, as well as local high school students. All aspects of planning and implementing the project were discussed thoroughly. The nursing students learned many things, including the following: (1) The importance of planning which envisions all obstacles, possibilities, and events that may aid or infringe upon the project. (2) How citizens behave and talk when dealing with a controversial project during community meetings—the desire of some citizens to become involved in changes when they are asked to assume some responsibility. (3) Action seems slow when a large number of citizens are involved. (4) When asking for support, words must be carefully chosen; for instance, if comparison is made with facilities of nearby communities, citizen response is inclined to be negative. (5) Influential persons are essential because of their emotional support, financial backing, and knowledge about existing local politics. (6) Risk taking is involved in any project and some citizens assume more responsibility and risk than others. (7) Organization is a must; all procedures are best anticipated in advance and planned for before implementation of action takes place. (8) There is an orderly procedure involved in establishing a center, which takes into consideration the need for rules and regulations, criteria for eligibility of staff workers, an advisory board, a board of directors, and other considerations.

(9) With a firm foundation, a newly established center is less vulnerable to negative legal procedures or negative public opinion.

A center was opened in the local community eight months after the first nursing students became actively involved in initiating the establishment of such a facility. The nursing students participated actively in the community organization process. In their evaluation of their activities they stated:

> The students' efforts in organizing this project have had a tremendous influence on our ideas about how to organize a community, how to contact key people in the establishment, and how to become involved. As nurses, we find that our training and our individual personalities can lead us far from the emergency room or the operating room of a large hospital, and very much into the community to work with the people with whom we live. We can work at any level of community organization, in that we have the ability to recognize problems, to make people aware of them, and then to do something about them.

DISCUSSION

1 Identify the steps of the community organization process as outlined by Ross in this community study.
2 In reading this community study, what factor or factors were most important in accomplishing the desired end-result?
3 If you were to critique this community study, what points or steps would you emphasize as needing further investigation?

A Weight Control Group for Senior Women

In planning for the initiation and implementation of a weight control support group for senior women living in a low-income high-rise apartment building for elderly citizens, a nursing student wrote the following objectives: By the end of a series of group meetings, participants will

1 Support each other toward the mutual goal of weight loss
2 Use resources to aid them in meal planning and other aspects of weight control
3 Be committed to weight loss by identifying a goal, pinpointing areas that need change and planning for the change, and evaluating progress toward their goal
4 Enjoy their times together

The nursing student described her activities with the group as follows:

In preparing for the first group meeting, I focused my attention on recruiting group members. Each woman that I knew who wanted to lose weight I contacted personally to see if they would be interested in getting together with other women who wanted to do the same. Each one I talked with expressed interest in the idea, and I consulted with them about the best time to meet. We set up a meeting time at 11 o'clock on Tuesday mornings.

Four out of five women I had invited came to the first meeting. I did not post a sign advertising the first meeting because I had procrastinated so long in my preparation that I felt a sign would not be up long enough to attract anyone else. Although unintentional on my part, I eventually was glad that my first meeting was "by invitation only." I felt that this gave the group members a sense that the group was special, and that it was "their" group. They suggested at the meeting that I post a sign in the lobby to invite more people to come, so I posted a sign as a result of their encouragement. The sign was an invitation from the group to other would-be reducers to stop wishing and come join us. Eight women came to the second meeting, five of them there for the first time. I am not sure that all came in response to the sign, as I believe that a considerable amount of inviting went out by word-of-mouth.

This early expression of interest really encouraged me. The women came to the meetings very talkative, sharing their ideas, and introducing themselves to one another with little prompting from me. The development of a warm, informal atmosphere was a goal I hoped for.

I had very specific plans for what I would say and do in the first meeting as I had read that the leader must be very directive in early stages of group development. I asked group members to write down what they weighed at age 17, at 40, and now, in order to get a picture of when they had gained weight. None of them had always been as heavy as they were now, and could see that they did have the potential to weigh less. We also discussed previous attempts to lose weight—everyone had tried, and most had been successful at some time. For a group of five people, we managed to keep the conversation flowing. Everyone was willing to share. They shared their failures, their successes, the reasons they thought that they had gained weight, and their successful techniques. This became a sort of group norm through the next two meetings, and showed fulfillment of one of the objectives I had set for the group.

The group did not need me to fill up the silent spots, but I did try to wrap up that first meeting by directing everyone in a similar path. I asked everyone to set a weight goal with a date and write it down. Although some women had already set some long-term goals for weight loss, I encouraged them to set a goal that could be met in a short amount of time. I also talked a few minutes about how calories can add up inadvertently by using an example of drinking several cups of coffee a day with varying amounts of cream and sugar.

I began the second meeting with a brief recap of the week before, since we had five new members. I asked them to do the exercise of remembering their weights at different ages and comparing them to now. We had a lively discussion about *when* it was that we gained so much weight. One woman said it was when she retired from her job. Two others felt that it was when they began to live alone. I passed out some recipes for low-calorie dips and dressings which had been requested the week before, along with a handout that compared how many minutes of various activities were required to burn off an apple, a baked potato, a strawberry shortcake. We spent a little time talking about increasing our activity level and how we could do it. A few residents were interested in swimming, and decided to look into the free senior swims at the city pools.

Six women came to the third group meeting; all of them had come before. Several weighed themselves before the group meeting that day, and I asked how many had lost weight. Nearly all of them had. I questioned them about what specifically they thought it was that made them lose this week and received these answers: "Not snacking after watching TV at night." "Cutting down portion sizes." "Cutting out desserts." and "Keeping so busy that I didn't nibble." Everyone shared their experiences of the week and there was a lot of laughter. One group member brought pamphlets on a low-calorie, low-sodium seasoning she was recommending. Another gave a recipe for a buttermilk and strawberry drink. Conversation came easily.

DISCUSSION

1 Were the objectives written behaviorally? Is there evidence that a taxonomy categorizing levels of knowledge was considered? Are the objectives measurable?
2 What community organization model, if any, was used to get this group started? Would a needs assessment prior to the initiation of the group, have been helpful?
3 List the activities of the leader that contributed to the attainment of objectives. How would you critique the activities of the leader? What additional activities would you suggest?

Screening for
Cardiovascular Risk Factors

In preparing for a project screening employees of a governmental agency for cardio-vascular risk factors, a nursing student wrote the following eloquent introduction:

In the dawn of time humans stood in darkness, stone axes in hand, pupils dilated, ears cocked, hearts racing, muscles tense, awaiting the light of day, when they would pit themselves against the environment that was contrary to their survival. Since then, we have scientifically and technologically come to an era of light and wheels and gadgets and push buttons. We have progressed from requiring superior arm and leg muscles for sheer survival to now requiring but a superior mind for the same purpose. We have traded the physical tensions of threat of life and limb for the emotional tensions which commonly require months, even years, for resolution. All too often they are never resolved at all.

Humans have moved from the jungle of trees, where they fought against many odds for survival, to the jungles of civilization—the technological computer age comprised of steel and concrete—where they wrestle with frustration, anxiety, and tension in a never-ending stream. First we ran, then we walked, for a short time we rode upon two wheels, but now we passively ride on four. Our once physically keen arms and legs which were utilized for fight or flight have become for the majority a means for lifting a fork or reaching the nearest auto for transportation.

In a society that has come to place a premium on brains and to frown on hand labor, humans have left their feet in favor of their seat. We have become fat, lazy, and indolent. We would rather be spectators than participants. In short, we have become overripe tomatos—soft, physically inept, desk-bound, cigarette-bound, and blissfully ignorant of the effects of lifestyle on cardiovascular health status.

It is never too late to learn, and prevention begins with education. Living is learning, and learning could mean living longer.

DISCUSSION

1 What needs assessment approach would be most useful for an employee population, based on the nature of this introduction?
2 How can potential clients be alerted to the need to change lifestyles?
3 What strategies would you employ to get a health promotion program started
   with a selected target population?

Using Social Learning Theory and Festinger's Theory of Cognitive Dissonance

Mrs. F., a 69-year-old widow who had been living alone for 12 years, was referred for a visit by the community health nurse to assess her ability to continue living independently. Mrs. F. was in desperate need of help financially and physically. She was having blackout spells almost daily. She had a 2-inch pile of medical bills from recent hospitalizations for a cerebrovascular accident and later hospitalizations for smoke inhalation, from a fire she caused by dropping a lighted cigarette on her mattress.

When I first went into her home, Mrs. F. and I were aware that I was evaluating her ability to be independent. On a series of visits, from interviews and personal observations, I found that Mrs. F. was existing on a diet of Chinese noodles and canned milk. She was not taking medication for her hypertension, ulcers, anxiety, or osteoporosis in the proper dosages or time intervals.

She was highly motivated to change her behavior because of the high value she placed on independent living. She stated, "I'd rather die right here in this house, than have to leave right now." I believe one reason she wanted to stay so badly was because of her dog, whom she had raised for 9 years in this same home. She loved him as a mother loves a child, and would rather feed him than herself. She therefore was receptive to the idea of setting mutual goals for demonstration of capability of independent living, and together, we established a contract.

I decided to use the social learning theory because social reinforcement is an important source of motivation for human behavior. Social learning also considers environmental factors and their effect on behavior. Verbal and nonverbal attention and recognition can serve as social reinforcers.

APPLICATION OF THEORY

Mrs. F. and I decided to attempt to change two basic behaviors—eating habits and taking medications—both being essential to her health maintenance and ability to care for herself competently and safely. I suggested that we employ the use of flow charts, in the hope that this would enable Mrs. F. to actively participate and assume maximum responsibility for her own daily activities. In addition, the charts would serve as a reminder to take her medications at the proper times. Modification of dietary patterns is difficult. Therefore, we felt it was most realistic to include one new food each week, and gradually build until a varied, well-balanced diet including all food groups was achieved.

I had two basic hypotheses. The first was that my verbal recognition of her efforts to achieve independence and the attention she received weekly from me during my visits were social reinforcers which could motivate Mrs. F. to change her behavior. I held this to be true because Mrs. F. was a lonely woman, unable to get out of the house and actively seek companionship, and was blessed "with the gift of gab" and loved to converse. I fulfilled her desire and need for companionship so she would act in a manner pleasing to me in order to achieve the reward of my continued visits and pleasure in her successes.

My second hypothesis was based on Festinger's theory of cognitive dissonance which states that a person's related beliefs are mostly consistent with each other, and if they are not, the person feels discomfort which often motivates him or her to change. Festinger sees the inconsistency as a motivating drive. When the nurse introduces dissonance as a motivating factor, she states her view of the situation, as opposed to the view of the client, and examines the differences in viewpoints. If rapport has been established, these differences are likely to cause unpleasant psychological tension (cognitive dissonance). The inconsistencies felt should prompt action in such a way that the unpleasant tension will be reduced.

In Mrs. F.'s case, her lack of responsibility in self-care, specifically in preparing nutritious meals and taking her medications as prescribed, is inconsistent with the concept of independence. It was my hypothesis that this inconsistency would produce cognitive dissonance, and serve as a further motive for Mrs. F. to change her behavior, in order to decrease psychological tension and behave within the context of independence.

Social reinforcement was very effective in Mrs. F.'s case. We initially discussed the basic elements of good nutrition, inexpensive yet high-protein dishes, likes and dislikes, planning for shopping, and her accessibility to stores. She asked many questions and showed a great deal of enjoyment in planning menus and shopping lists. I felt that she appreciated my acknowledgement that it was difficult to stretch a limited budget, but together we agreed on some economical, yet delicious, dishes.

We also spent time reviewing Mrs. F.'s medications, their purposes, proper dosages, and frequency. I was glad I took the time to explain these thoroughly and carefully because Mrs. F. had several misconceptions about both purposes and frequency of her prescriptions. At each visit, I would also take Mrs. F.'s blood pressure which on my initial visit was 180/110.

Twice a week I visited Mrs. F. to review her charts, take her blood pressure, and listen to her questions, concerns, and family problems. The biggest problem, I soon discovered, was her very limited vision, due to one glass eye and a severe cataract on the other. This posed a problem in reading medication labels, food cans, writing grocery lists, reading hospital bills that came in the mail, as well as reading the flow sheets. I had made the print very large on the sheets, so she was able to fill them in with little trouble, but this was not the case with bills or labels. I discussed this with Mrs F., and she felt that a magnifying glass would be a great aid to reading. She had already discussed the visual problem with her physician, who said the cataract "was not ripe yet."

Only a week after my initial visit with Mrs. F., she blacked out and was taken to the hospital. The cause was probably a transient ischemic attack secondary to chronic hypertension, but it was an incentive for her physician to change her anti-hypertensive medication. Mrs. F. subsequently had no more blackout spells and her blood pressure remained at about 140/85 on all my later visits.

I found that as Mrs. F. kept the charts, she would recognize if she ate poorly, that she had indeed done so. "I was depressed after my son called because he was so drunk," she would state. I neither agreed with the excuses nor reprimanded her, but merely acknowledged the fact that she had eaten poorly, and allowed her to accept the responsibility. Mrs. F. also cut down tremendously on her ingestion of pain medications, stating that she only occasionally suffered severe pain. She could recall that no one ever explained what the pills were for but had said to take them four times a day. This is indeed what the label stated. They had made her groggy, so she decided to take them only at bedtime. Her other medications were now taken regularly in the proper dosage, and she could now explain the purpose of each.

I felt that Mrs. F. was making great progress in moving toward independence. An added benefit which evolved was that Mrs. F.'s granddaughter, who was pregnant, had assumed the job of cleaning Mrs. F.'s home twice weekly and was paid by the Department of Social and Health Services. She was there during my visits and became very interested in the nutritional guidelines I discussed with Mrs. F. at each visit— menu planning, budgeting, and buying a variety of economical, yet nutritious, foods. She asked questions, and when Mrs. F. and I reviewed the weekly flow sheet for food intake, she would reinforce my suggestions and augment my encouragement of Mrs. F., offer her own suggestions, and offer to shop for whatever Mrs. F. needed to follow through with her menu plans. She began to eat lunch with Mrs. F. 2 to 3 times a week.

This support by a family member was an essential step in Mrs. F.'s gain of independence. The focus of reward was gradually being turned away from social reinforcement by my presence and praise, to reinforcement by her granddaughter and an actual sharing by her in the learning experience.

DISCUSSION

1 Was social learning theory used appropriately with this client? Cognitive dissonance?
2 Specify other ways that the theories may have been used more effectively.
3 Were any principles of learning evident in this case study?
4 Identify the steps of the nursing process used in this case study.
5 If you were to critique this case, what points would you emphasize as needing further investigation?

Using Rogers's Law of Interpersonal Relationships

Carl Rogers states, "It is the quality of the interpersonal encounter with the client which is the most significant element in determining effectiveness." He talks of several components which the counselor must have and utilize to facilitate such a relationship and to promote true growth of the client. The counselor must have genuineness or congruence, empathy, and positive regard. In addition, an important element in the interpersonal encounter is the client's perception of the counselor. How has the client perceived the attitudes that have been communicated to her or him?

APPLICATION OF THEORY

I used this theory with a client and her two sons with whom I had previously been ineffective. I initially began the relationship with this family by feeling that I was the "helper," and they were to be "helped." They would tell me what their problems were, and I would deal with those problems for them, and we would live happily ever after. Therefore, I entered the home with a preconceived idea of how I wanted them to talk and react, and I was actually fearful that they would not cooperate with my plans. I was surprised to find on our first two visits, the mother was very compliant to all my wishes, mechanically answered all my questions with all the "right" answers, and then promptly admitted herself in the local hospital, as she felt very depressed and suicidal. Although I realized that in such a short time, I as a counselor probably could never have prevented such feelings, it bothered me that I had not had an inkling during my visits of what was going on inside her.

I began thinking through step-by-step what our relationship had been and came to the conclusion that we had been sharing facades. I also sought help from people who had had dealings with my client. Her psychiatrist replied, "Talk to R."; her mother said, "Be her friend"; her psychiatric nurse answered, "Everyone makes plans for R. without consulting her." These answers reminded me of Carl Rogers's theory. They were saying, "R. is a person and she must be dealt with as a person."

In my next visit I tried putting Rogers's theory to practice. This required much inner thinking and searching as to my true feelings in regard to our relationship. This was the beginning of genuineness and congruence. I felt the best way to begin communicating this feeling of genuineness would be to tell R. these feelings, which include "I have been trying to be a helper to you without knowing your feelings. I have been acting as the Saviour to the sinner, and I have been wrong. I realize that you are capable of seeking help for yourself, and I have stepped where I was not invited." It was somewhat uncomfortable at first but R. replied with genuineness. She replied that she felt most of the problem was that she could not be open because she did not want to be hurt; that she knew she could not help herself, but she hated people. With that, she burst into tears. It was at this moment that I truly saw R. as a person.

I found that this first act of true genuineness-congruence and openness led easily to the other elements. I did not have to consciously think about these next elements, but I could see them happening as our communication progressed. I found several ways of communicating empathy—through reiteration, such as "I feel that you are meaning this . . ." and clarification statements. For example, R. said, "I hate people." I replied, "Do you mean you hate all people?" She replied by saying that she did hate all people because they tell her what to do all the time without giving her a chance, but it was all right for me to tell her what to do because she needed help. I reiterated her statement, then said, "I feel that you mean you hate people who butt into your life and try to take command but as long as you are the one who first asks for help, you are still the one governing your life and therefore, have a feeling of worth." R. seemed to pick up the fact that I was really trying to understand her feelings and went on to describe some examples of real people she hated. It was difficult to be truly empathic at first as I could not know R.'s true feelings, but the fact that I let her know that I was trying to grasp an understanding told R. that I cared.

True positive regard was one of the most important elements of the "growing" relationship between R. and me. I looked at all the things which made R. a person—an individual—the fact that she cried, became nervous, smiled, had her own thoughts and feelings, loved her sons, had a special way of dealing with her sons, had her own unique facial features, walk, air of being. Something I said placed an absolute flow of pleasure on R.'s face—something I had not observed before. It was, "R, I am so glad that you do not want to live with your mother because you feel she dominates the children. I think that you are the most loving, caring, concerned mother. You know your children better than anyone else—they are a part of you—and you are the most able to care for them. I would hate to see that ability taken away from you." On paper, this sounds like a "buttering-up" routine. However, it was exactly how I felt about her as a person in the role of a mother. This kind of positive feedback truly seemed to bolster her morale and it seemed easier for R. to communicate her true feelings. Also, I felt she began to see herself as a worthwhile person with some positive strengths.

DISCUSSION

1 Was Rogers's interpersonal approach the appropriate one to use in this case study?
2 Are there other communication theories that may have been used more effectively?
3 Describe examples in the case study demonstrating the nurse's use of therapeutic interactions.
4 Identify the steps of the nursing process used in this case study.
5 If you were to critique this case study, what points would you emphasize as needing further investigation?

Using Maslow's Hierarchy
of Human Needs

L. was referred to the community health nurse for the purpose of offering antepartum care and counseling. On the initial home visit it was obvious that there were explicit overwhelming needs which were not being met for the maintenance of a safe, comfortable, and healthy daily life. The observations and nursing history which I gained are itemized as follows:

1 Water was coming through the bedroom ceiling—the room was uninhabitable. The water was from an overflow of the toilet in the upstairs apartment.
2 Nothing could be stored in bottom cupboards of the kitchen because shelves were covered with "rat" droppings. The family had seen "rats" and had heard them at night.
3 Windows were broken and taped.
4 The porch and steps were collapsing—the porch had a 35° slant.
5 L. had fears about her fetus. She was 8 months pregnant, had had x-rays during the first trimester, and was worried about her baby's normality.
6 One of the children had a skin rash.
7 L.'s husband had deserted the family 3 months previously.
8 The family was financially supported by welfare and owned no car.

I selected Maslow's theory because of its realistic approach and assistance in knowing how to proceed. I hypothesized that L. would not be able to experience and/or fulfill higher needs such as love and belonging, esteem, and self-actualization, until the lower, basic physiological and safety needs were met. By systematically going over each problem and determining the level of human need, I planned my activities with the family.

APPLICATION OF THEORY

1 *The environmental and living conditions.* L. stated that her brother had been bitten by a rat as a baby and she did not want that to happen to her children. She had

a choice of motivating the landlord to improve the environment or changing residences. This problem fell into the physiological and safety levels, and I gave it top priority by helping L. to find a new home.

2 *L.'s pregnancy.* When L. found out that she was pregnant, she had been advised to have an abortion, and all arrangements had been made. On the day it was scheduled, after completing some of the preliminary procedures, she could not go through with it because of moral and religious convictions. She subsequently had a fear that radiation had affected her baby. This problem represented a physiological need. I listened to L.'s feelings, gave explanations as appropriate, and encouraged her to visit the doctor for examination and reassurance.

3 *L.'s feelings about her husband.* "I still love him but can't live with him as we argue too much." This problem was of the higher level, that of love and belonging, so I deferred any action on this problem until a later time when the physical comfort and safety needs were met.

By using Maslow's theory I was impressed that some clients just accept and tolerate life on a day-by-day basis and are not motivated to act until they receive help, encouragement, and support from persons who can offer hope and direction. I was also amazed that clients do not realize that they themselves can change their predicament; they have the capabilities, but wait for stimulation or encouragement from an outside source.

DISCUSSION

1 Was the application of Maslow's theory appropriate in this case study?
2 At what phase of the nursing process was Maslow's theory most facilitative?
3 Are there other theories that may have been used effectively with this family?
4 Were any principles of learning evident in this case study?
5 If you were to critique this case study, what points would you emphasize as needing further investigations?

Using Otto's Strengthening Theory

This case study was written by a senior nursing student.

Cindy is 11 years old with a diagnosis of meningomyelocele and has had a problem with stool incontinence at home and school. She had not taken the initiative on her own to clean herself up until I started working with her. This had led to increasing problems of social isolation at school and much frustration and embarrassment for the family. Since her family thinks Cindy is very apathetic and could care less when it comes to being clean, I decided to try Otto's strengthening theory.

I hypothesized that if Cindy had a good self-concept, she would be more motivated to carry out her own self-care and hygiene. In saying this, I am proposing that she has a poor concept of herself and needs motivational tools which will assist her to improve her hygiene.

Since Cindy is a child, I wracked my brain to think of a way to present this theory to an 11-year-old. Cindy loves to play games, so a game it became. She would name ten things she liked about herself or was good at, and I would name ten things I liked about her. We would share them together and then tie them in a bright pink ribbon. This would be her nice list. Then on mutual agreement we would draw up a work list, and this would be things she needs to work on or would like to change.

On my next home visit, the minute I got in the door, she could not wait to tell me that her bowel program was working. She had not been incontinent since the day it was started, and she was pleased. Cindy lives on a farm, so I asked her to show me the animals. We chased the cows, petted the pigs, and held and petted the chickens, with her dog, Smokey, accompanying us. Then we sat down on a huge rock which she explained to me was her favorite, because she spends a lot of time sitting there.

We talked about the animals, and when she started talking about games that she liked to play, I told her that I had brought a game for us to play. She was all ears. After explaining my game to her, she said, "but I do not like anything about myself." She stated that she could write a list of things she did not like about herself. She felt that people are always finding things wrong with her now. However, she

381

Table CS4-1

Mine	Cindy's
Fun to be with	Nose
Pretty smile	Nails
Likes to play games	Feet
Tries hard at things she wants to do	Toes
Cheerful	Fingers
Likes to be with people	Ears
Likes to eat	Arms
Has a family	Legs
Pretty eyes	Eyes
Pretty, thick hair	Hair

said, after a time, that she might be able to name some good things about herself but not her personality, because she did not like it at all. We went for a short walk, then went into the house to play the game.

It took her quite some time to think of five items, but after she had done those, she wanted five more to complete. I filled out my cards at the same time. Then we shared them with one another, alternating as if playing a card game. Table CS4-1 gives each of our lists.

I found it surprising that she mentioned only parts of her body. She was amazed at the things I said about her, and said, "You know I do like those things! I love to eat and be with people." We took the nice list and tied a hot pink ribbon around it.

We then composed a short list of things which she would like to change. These were that her bowels would be regular, that she would wash herself to decrease her odor, and that people would spend more time with her. It was agreed that we would share this list with her mother. Cindy wanted to call this her bad list, but I explained that these things were not bad because they were part of her. They only needed to be worked on, if she wanted them to change. At this time, she expressed the fact that she did wish that people would tell her good things about herself once in a while.

I have not worked with children for quite some time. I had forgotten how intense their own feelings can be. It really hurt when Cindy came right out and said, "I really do not like anything about myself, and especially my personality." I was sort of taken aback at that moment. I realize how very important it is to take the time to really listen to a child, for so much can be learned from them. I never considered it before, but self-esteem is really important to develop as one grows. If we do not feel good about ourselves, what will motivate us to achievement?

DISCUSSION

1 How was application of the strengthening theory modified in this case study?
2 Were any principles of learning evident in this case study?
3 Identify the steps of the nursing process used.
4 Are there other theories that could have been used just as effectively?
5 If you were to critique this case study, what points would you emphasize as needing further investigation?

Using a Client-Centered Approach

In the clinical experiences I have had during the past year, I have become increasingly reluctant to use certain "techniques" in my approach to clients. I have felt particularly uncomfortable using those methods in which I formed a judgment about what was "good" or "acceptable" behavior in a client and then proceeded to mechanically reinforce and reward that "desired" behavior, so that the client would see it as desirable behavior also.

In my relationships with clients, with my son, and with mentally retarded persons, I have preferred to use a less manipulative, less mechanical approach—one that does not see the other as an object for control. I have frequently observed with my son that positive reinforcement is a very heavy burden for him to carry, and he frequently rejects my positive evaluation for one of his own that is less demanding and less threatening. He has taught me that the appropriate place for evaluation and judgment is within ourselves and that a truly helping, growth facilitating relationship must allow the individual space and freedom for this to occur.

In visiting a multiproblem family for the first time, I ran into problems with my own feelings at the very start. Mrs. O. is very obese, and I place a very high value on physical fitness. Mrs. O.'s house is in a state of total chaos—it appears that nothing is in place or even has a place. The entire house is very dirty and the smells are most unpleasant to me. I was repulsed by the conditions of the house and even by Mrs. O. herself. When I thought of trying to see the world through the client's eyes, I felt a little afraid and very reluctant. If I *really* saw her world through her eyes, how could I justify my own world: and if I felt this need for justification, how helpful could I be to her? If I saw her world through her eyes, would my feelings of compassion be touched, and would I not then perhaps be vulnerable to demands I could not meet?

As I made more visits to her home, I still had not come face to face with these feelings, and I could tell that my goal of forming a relationship with her that would increase her self-esteem was far from being met.

However, I found my regard for her was increasing as I observed her interacting

with her children, and by their responses to her. She showed obvious pleasure in being
with them, in playing with the baby, and in talking with each of them about their
activities. The youngest, who is 18 months, was born 6 weeks prematurely, and she
was concerned about his developmental progress. I suggested a Denver Developmental
Screening Test and she agreed. It was during the administration of this test that our
relationship became closer. Our mutual focusing on this child and the shared pleasure
of seeing him perform each of the activities brought a dimension to our relationship
that helped me to overcome some of my earlier negative feelings.

DISCUSSION

1 Was the client-centered approach an appropriate one in this case study?
2 Are there other theories or approaches that might have been used successfully?
3 Explain how the relationship with a client affects each step of the nursing process.
4 Were principles of learning evident in this case study?

A Family with a Newborn Baby

A description of a young family with a new baby who had been visited by a beginning student in community health nursing was written as follows:

Mrs. H. is an 18-year-old pale young girl with bangs hanging to her eyes, who was startled to have a nurse visit but accepted it compliantly. She stated that she had never had a nurse visit her before. She lives in a housing project and has two kittens. She states she feels OK. Her breasts have been engorged, but she has been wearing tight bras, and the discomfort is lessened. Her flow has been intermittent, varying from light to heavy. She admits to tensions, varying at times, because she wants to be a good mother. She says she gets enough rest. She does not want to be the same kind of mother as her own mother. She has done a lot of baby-sitting and likes having her own baby. Mrs. H. likes to read, but not books about mother-child care. She seems lonely. She was encouraged to give the baby a lot of love and not worry about spoiling the infant.

D. is a normal-appearing contented newborn who sleeps 3 to 4 hours and drinks 3 to 3½ ounces of formula every 3 to 4 hours. Birthweight: 6 lb ¾ oz. Mother is concerned about dry, peeling skin and has been applying lotion. Skin appeared soft and nonpeeling to nurse. Baby was dressed warmly. Cord dropped off today. Mother plans to see physician this weekend. Would like to have cereal added to diet. Mrs. H. agreed to another visit next week.

DISCUSSION

1 How might this visit be converted to the problem-oriented style of recording?
2 What would be your plan for the next visit with this family?
3 Did the nurse give satisfactory service on this first visit to a "new" family?

Clarifying Nursing Visits

In meeting a family for the first time who had had nursing visits for the purpose of assisting with disciplinary measures with the children, I had this experience.

K. greeted me at the door and asked me into the dining area. She offered some tea, and while she was fixing it, she quite candidly asked me what the community health nurse is supposed to do. I was a little surprised by the question and in answering it, I simply told her that it was primarily up to the person or members of the family to decide or determine what kind of help was needed or what they wanted the community health nurse to help them with. She explained how the nurse happened to visit in the first place. When she had B. (1 year old) at the pediatrician's for his immunizations, she mentioned to the doctor that some days she felt like she could discard the kids, especially S. (2½ years old). The pediatrician asked her if she would like a nurse to visit her and give some suggestions on how to manage the kids. She consented to have this done. Then she went on to explain what the nurse had done thus far. On her visits, the nurse had asked a few questions, commented about the sweet kids, given advice on how to handle S., marked things down on a clipboard, and left.

DISCUSSION

1 How would you clarify the purpose of nursing visits with clients?
2 Explain the bearing that perception has on relationships and interpretation of behavior.

A Family with Communication Problems

Mrs. A. is a 19-year-old mother of two children. She acts immature for her age and has had great difficulty just getting through the ninth grade (most of her school work was at a failure level). Mr. A. is presently unemployed. The family lives with Mrs. A.'s parents and are on welfare for support. The oldest child is a little boy of 3 years and was born before the couple were married. He is not Mr. A.'s son. The second child is a little girl of 8 months who is Mr. A.'s daughter. This child was diagnosed as having hydrocephalus. At the birth of the little girl, Mr. A.'s mother began blaming Mrs. A. for all the baby's problems.

On my first visit with Mrs. A., I sat on the front steps with her and devoted my attention to her. I listened to what she had to say and how she was feeling about her situation. She seemed depressed (did not smile much, kept her head down, and frowned whenever she spoke of her mother-in-law). In talking with her I could tell she had some very angry feelings toward her mother-in-law, as was indicated by gritting her teeth and by her glare. She said she could not talk to her mother-in-law about the baby's defect because her mother-in-law kept blaming her and making her feel guilty. I asked her if she did feel guilty. She replied, "No, not really." The reason she gave was because the doctors had told her it was a birth defect and that she was not to blame. I asked her if she was sure she felt this way, as she had been a little hesitant in her answer. She then said, "Yes," but that she felt bad because it was hard to take the blame which came from her mother-in-law. I agreed with her that it indeed would be hard to take. She said that the doctor had written Mr. A.'s mother a letter explaining about the baby's defect, and that she and her husband had tried talking with the mother-in-law; however, nothing seemed to change the mother-in-law's opinion that Mrs. A. was to blame. Mrs. A. said she was unable to communicate any longer because it always ended up with a lot of yelling and name-calling which emphasized the bad feelings between them.

In later visits, as I got better acquainted with Mr. and Mrs. A., I observed their supportive relationship with each other and Mrs. A.'s increasing acceptance of the baby, which was demonstrated by the spontaneity with which she played and talked with the baby. Imagine my surprise when, about this time, Mr. and Mrs. A. asked if I would please talk with the mother-in-law and see if somehow I could help her understand about the baby's condition. My first thought was, "You have got to be kidding, me?—When already doctors have tried talking with her?" I told them I would see what I could do.

DISCUSSION

1 Describe examples of behavior description evident in this case situation.
2 Describe examples demonstrating the nurse's use of therapeutic interactions.
3 How would you plan a contact with the mother-in-law?

A Potentially "Abusing" Family

The L. family had initially been referred for a community health nursing visit by Dr. T., who wanted the nurse to assess the home situation for child-abuse potential. The baby boy in 10-months' time had been cared for by Dr. T. in regard to a skull fracture, frequent bruising, allergy, and two episodes with pneumonia requiring hospitalization. The first community health nurse made a contract with Mrs. L. to visit the home to see how R. (baby boy) was recovering from his latest problem. Mrs. L. agreed to this, and the nurse made several visits to the home. At this point in time, the case was assigned to a student nurse.

After several home visits, my assessment of the family and observations of behavioral dynamics are described as follows:

N., the mother, has attractive hair and facial features. She has a flawless complexion but is obese, having a weight of 167 lb and a height of 5 ft. 2 in. She is open to talking about herself and the family. N. was raised with a lot of responsibility and feels this is how children learn to cope with life. In the home many fragile and dangerous items are left out. N. will say "No, No!" to R. repeatedly as a warning not to touch something. If he touches it and the object breaks, she spanks him. If he hurts himself, she says to him, "I told you that you were going to hurt yourself." The baby is walking and bumping into things quite frequently. When he falls and hurts himself, he does not get picked up. If N. does anything at all. she will get him a bottle of juice and put it by him on the floor.

R. is a 10-month-old, pale, tense-looking baby. He is advanced for his age level developmentally. When he walks and falls, he really whacks his head frequently but rarely cries. If his mother screams at him, he just throws himself on the floor and bangs his head a few times. He has a phony kind of smile. He rarely smiles spontaneously. He will reach for his mother when he hurts himself. He is allowed to play with the coasters on the living room floor. The house is full of hazards. As an example, on my first visit, he fell off the rocker once, teetered and hit his head on the corner of the coffee table, hit his head on the stone corner of the fireplace ledge, and fell down, hitting his head again. After this episode, N. did nothing—as if the baby did not exist. R almost never verbalizes anything, unless it is with the cat.

C. (the 5-year-old sister) is tan, attractive, slim, average height, and cannot pronounce some of her consonants because of a hearing loss due to colds. N. related C.'s daily tasks to me—feeding R. and getting him up, changing diapers, vacuuming his and her bedrooms, dusting the house, and feeding the animals. C. starts school this fall, and N. related she will really miss all the help around the house. C. picks out her clothes for each day and has always had matched clothing. C. seems devoted to her brother, giving him the physical affection he does not get from his mother. She will pick him up and carry him, although he is half her size. She looks out for him. When R. cracked his head on the corner of the coffee table again, C. put her hands on her hips, walked up to her mother pointing at the table, and told her mother that it was a "bad coffee table." N. relates there is only one thing with which she has trouble with C., and that is when C. just will not stop going up to R. and hugging him after she (N.) has disciplined him. C. minds well, seems to love her mother, and is happy.

B., the father, is 5 ft. 5 in., good-looking, medium build, and very quiet. He is very attentive to N., carrying in the groceries for her and performing similar activities. There is no physical greeting such as a kiss or hug when he returns from work. He is unassuming, affectionate with the children, plays with the children, and substitutes other toys for R. if R. is not to play with a particular toy.

DISCUSSION

1 Is this family a potentially abusing one?
2 What other information do you need to complete your assessment of the family?
3 What communication theory might be useful in working with this family?
4 What would be your approach as a helping person in working with this family?

A Family with an Alcoholic Member

During a teacher-nurse conference one afternoon, the teacher mentioned Jean N.'s periodic absences from school for no apparent reason and said that she was falling behind in her schoolwork.

"I used to have her brother, Jimmie, in my class last year," the teacher commented, "and he was absent this way, too. Usually the mother telephones that the children will not be in school that day, but gives no reason. They come on the school bus, and I've asked the driver if he knows anything about them. He said the mother told him if the children were not at the bus stop in the morning not to wait for them. I'm sure it's not a matter of money, they are always nicely dressed. Do you think a home call would be in order?"

The nurse agreed that it would be; she, too, had wondered about the children lately, as neither of them looked well and both seemed unhappy. She planned for a home call that afternoon.

The nurse found the home, a large well-kept farmhouse, about 15 miles from the school. Mrs. N., a neat-looking somewhat tense woman answered the nurse's knock. The two children were with her. The nurse introduced herself and was invited into a pleasant living room. The mother was courteous but unresponsive. She gave some vague excuses for the children's absences. After about 10 minutes, the nurse, realizing that nothing was being accomplished, took her leave, baffled by the situation. She made another home call en route to her office. It was nearly 5 o'clock when she reached her desk, to find a note to call Mrs. N. as soon as she came in. Somewhat puzzled, the nurse returned the call. Mrs. N. was almost sobbing as she said, "I didn't know what to say to you this afternoon. My children and I are in great trouble. My husband is really a very good man, but often he drinks too much, and I have to keep the children home on those days to help me with the chores. Could you come back in the morning to see me?" The nurse promised to do so, and made an appointment for about 10:30 the next day.

DISCUSSION

1 What should the nurse include in her preparation for the next day's visit?
2 How should the nurse approach the situation?
3 In reporting back to the teacher, what information should be shared with her regarding the family?
4 What can a nurse contribute to a family faced with problems due to alcoholism?
5 List the official and nonofficial resource agencies available in your community for helping a family with this sort of problem.

Nursing Management of an Elderly Client

The granddaughter of an 84-year-old patient called me (a nursing student) frantically about 3 P.M. one day. She told me that her grandmother was "in withdrawal": shaking, crying, and unable to talk clearly. I knew of Mrs. J. as a tiny 84-year-old woman who had been taking about 2800 milligrams of meprobamate daily until a month earlier when the strength of her tablets had been cut in half. Through consultation with her physician and her granddaughter, we had initiated this change at the pharmacy in order to decrease her falls. She had not gone into noticeable withdrawal from the cutback in dosage, and had been functioning normally, looking more cheerful and steadier on her feet. I had just visited with her earlier in the day.

The M. pharmacy refused to refill the prescription, because it had been refilled so recently. The granddaughter wanted me to do something! I tried calling my instructor, then the doctor, then the supervisor of the agency. I could not get anyone. I was all alone and had a sinking sensation that this was an emergency. My last resort was to call the M. pharmacy again. I explained the situation to the pharmacist on the phone. "Well," I asked him, "what do you think I should do? Take her to the emergency room?" He informed me that the physician had put pressure on him not to refill as often because the nursing agency had been putting pressure on him. I told him that I was on the staff of the nursing agency, that I realized her dosage had already been cut in half, and that neither our intention nor the physician's was for Mrs. J. to go into withdrawal. He agreed to refill.

The granddaughter ran right up to the pharmacy for the prescription, and then I met her at Mrs. J.'s apartment. Mrs. J. was noticeably shaky and her pulse was 100 when we arrived. She counted her pills immediately and took one, thanking her granddaughter, and later me, for getting them for her. Since then I have made several home visits to Mrs. J., who continues to insist that she takes only 6 tablets a day while my pill counts show that she takes about 12. She does not know where all the pills go, but she refuses to let me set them up for each day. Last week she began to look unsteady on her feet again and it is difficult to say whether it is from withdrawal or from overdose.

DISCUSSION

1 In your opinion, was this situation an emergency? Could it have been handled differently?
2 In considering long-term management of this client, how would you prevent a recurrence of this situation?
3 Assume the role of the nurse. Discuss your strategy for improved maintenance of this client's health status.

A Family's Reaction to Death

In May, Mrs. B. brought Mark to a preschool registration conference. While talking to the community health nurse, Mrs. B. said she expected a new baby early in October. When the nurse offered to call to help her plan for the baby, Mrs. B. eagerly accepted.

The nurse found the family living in an attractive duplex in a pleasant area, one block from the school. They had lived in this home about a year. Mr. B., age 30, had been a federal government employee for the past 9 years. He had been attending night school classes at a nearby college. The nurse did not meet him, but from his wife's comments, he appeared to be conscientious, stable, and intelligent. He helped at home when he could, took the children to the park to play, and seemed to understand the importance of physical and emotional health.

Mrs. B., 28, was a bright, energetic woman with a variety of interests, her main ones being her family and their welfare. The children, Eileen, 7, and Mark, 5, appeared to be normal, healthy, and active.

Although Mrs. B. had seen her physician several times, she had questions relating to her pregnancy and was interested in having help. Her other pregnancies had been normal, and she had breast-fed her babies. With this pregnancy, she experienced great fatigue and was completely exhausted by evening. This concerned her. As she was talking, she suddenly interrupted herself and said, "I should tell you why we are having this baby, and why it is so important to us."

She explained that 5 months previously, their 14-month-old daughter had died of sudden infant death syndrome. She said that she and her husband did not talk about the tragedy, but that both of them got up at repeated intervals during the night to check and recheck that Eileen and Mark were all right. Since the accident, Eileen had refused to mention her baby sister, had frequent nightmares and unexplained severe crying spells, once at school. The doctor had ordered sedatives for her. The neighbors were supportive and included the family in their social activities.

The physician had advised the parents, shortly after the death, to consider having another baby as soon as possible.

DISCUSSION

1 How can Mr. and Mrs. B. be helped to accept the loss of their little daughter and to accept the new baby?

2 Is the frequent checking on the children during the night by the parents a normal reaction 5 months after the death?

3 What could be done to help Eileen overcome her sense of grief and loss?

4 Assume the role of the nurse. What is your reaction to this family's problems?

Cuban Refugee Family

Mr. F., age 40, laborer
Mrs. F., age 35, mother
Manuel, age 15
Tito, age 14
Rosita, age 12
Carlos, age 7, client (cerebral palsy)
Maria, age 5
Juan, age 3
Panchita, new baby

The F. family, Cuban refugees, was referred by their social worker to the nursing service of the city-county health department. She reported that Mrs. F., about 7-months pregnant, had been in the county hospital for a week because of high blood pressure, and was being discharged that day. The social worker said the parents spoke little English. They were living in a three-bedroom apartment in a large public housing complex. The family was Protestant.

Visit 1 The nurse made a home visit the next day. Talking in broken Spanish and English with Mr. and Mrs. F., the nurse learned that the family had been in the United States less than a year. In Cuba, Mr. F. had made a fairly comfortable living as a fisherman and had had additional employment in a factory. The family escaped from Cuba in Mr. F.'s small fishing boat, which was wrecked off the Florida coast. Two of their children were lost in the accident. After a short stay in Miami, the family moved to the West Coast. At the time of the nurse's visit, Mr. F. did not have steady employment and the family had been on welfare for 3 months. The three elder children attended a nearby grade school but were not doing well because of language difficulties.

During the visit, the nurse became aware of strange gutteral sounds and an unusual crying. Mrs. F. finally left the room and returned with Carlos in her arms. The child was undersized, emaciated, unable to walk, and had uncontrolled head movements. The nurse thought he had a cerebal palsy condition. Throughout the visit, Maria and Juan clung, whimpering, to their mother and watched the nurse fearfully.

The nurse reviewed the doctor's orders for Mrs. F. regarding diet and rest with Mr. and Mrs. F. and felt there was little more she could do at the time because of language difficulties. She promised to return in a week. As she was leaving, the Protestant minister arrived. The nurse explained to him that her knowledge of Spanish was insufficient for her to help the family as she wished to do, and asked if there were someone who might act as interpreter. He suggested Mrs. L., a neighbor who spoke English and Spanish fluently and would be acceptable to the family.

Later The nurse called on Mrs. L., a friendly young woman of Spanish-American descent. She said she and her husband felt sorry for the F. family. Her husband had tried to help Mr. F. find work, but his lack of knowledge of English made it difficult. Mrs. L. worked part-time in a neighborhood grocery store. She said if the nurse could arrange her visits to the family when she was free, she would do all she could to help. She gave the nurse her telephone number.

Later The nurse reported to the social worker, who had not known of Carlos' condition. She offered to work with the nurse in getting him to the children's clinic for a diagnosis.

Later The nurse telephoned the school nurse, who reported the children were absent a great deal and were seriously handicapped in their school work by their lack of English. The teachers were concerned and wished the children could have extra help in learning English.

Visit 2 With Mrs. L.'s help, the nurse had arranged for another visit to the family a week later. With an interpreter, the nurse found it easier to build interpersonal relationships. She discovered Mrs. F. had been eating some foods not on her prescribed diet, but thought this resulted from a misunderstanding. With Mrs. L.'s help, she was able to explain the importance of following the doctor's orders. The nurse told the parents that the social worker had made a tentative appointment for Carlos at the children's clinic the latter part of the week if they could take him at that time. The parents quickly agreed, and Mrs. L. said she would either take them herself or find someone who could provide transportation.

Later The nurse confirmed the appointment with the social worker and notified Mrs. L.

Because of unusual pressure of work in the agency, the nurse was unable to visit the family for 2 weeks. However, she telephoned Mrs. L., who said the family had taken Carlos to the clinic and that institutional care had been recommended for him. The family was given an application to River Falls, a state school for handicapped children about 20 miles away. A neighbor had taken them to visit the school and they were satisfied that Carlos would have good care there, and they were eager to file an application and wanted the nurse's help in filling it out. Several days later, Mrs. L. phoned to say that Mrs. F. had been taken to the hospital by ambulance, and had had a baby girl by caesarean section. Mrs. F.'s condition was good and she was expected home in a few days.

Later The school nurse telephoned that the F. children had been absent for several days and wanted to know if they were ill. The nurse explained that Mrs. F. was in the hospital for delivery and thought it was possible Mr. F. had kept them at home. She planned a visit soon and would let the school nurse know if the children were ill.

The nurse learned that a summer Head Start program would begin soon at the school and that Maria would be eligible and also that there were plans to offer English classes for the foreign-born at the school building in the evenings during the summer.

Visit 3 When the nurse and Mrs. L. called they found the children had returned to school. Mr. F. had kept them at home during Mrs. F.'s hospitalization because he was lonely and afraid. With the help of their minister, they filled out Carlos' application for River Falls, and mailed it, and were waiting to hear from the institution. The nurse explained the Head Start program for Maria and the English classes for the parents and older children. Mrs. F.'s condition appeared good. She was obviously trying hard to follow the doctor's orders and the prescribed diet. Panchita appeared to be a normal, healthy baby.

Visit 4 A few days later, as the nurse was in the neighborhood, she stopped to see Mrs. F. and check on her clinic appointments. When Maria saw the nurse, she ran out the door and soon returned with Mrs. L. Mrs. F. showed the nurse a letter from River Falls to the effect that Carlos was on the waiting list, and that there would be a place for him in about a month. Mrs. L. and Mrs. F. had a conversation in rapid Spanish. Then Mrs. L. explained that Mr. and Mrs. F. felt that they should not have any more children, and could the nurse tell them of a clinic where they could go for help. The nurse explained about the planned parenthood clinic and gave Mrs. F. a card to the clinic. The nurse arranged for a call about a month later.

Visit 5 Mr. and Mrs. F. were home when the nurse called. Mr. F. had found work as a fisherman and thought it would be permanent. He had arranged for time off so that he could be home when the nurse called. Manuel and Tito had summer jobs, thanks to Mrs. L.'s help and that of the minister. Carlos had been admitted to River Falls. A neighbor had taken them to visit him, and they were happy with the care he was receiving. They and the older children were attending the evening classes and Maria was enrolled in the Head Start program. The parents had attended the planned parenthood clinic. Mr. F. hoped they would be able to go off welfare the following month. The nurse urged Mrs. F. to take the preschool children to the children's clinic for immunizations. It appeared to the nurse that this family had achieved a certain amount of independence and could probably handle future health problems. She left her card and asked the family to call the nursing service if a need arose.

Later The nurse reported to the social worker and the school nurse that she had closed the case, as Mr. and Mrs. F. now seemed able to manage their own situation. Case closed.

DISCUSSION

1 What resources did this family appear to have within itself?
2 What emotional problems might you expect this family to have as a result of their experiences since leaving Cuba?
3 Should the nurse have closed the case when she did? Why?

Infant Health Supervision

Mr. H., age 26, laundry driver
Mrs. H., age 23, housewife.
Tommie, age 4 months.

A student nurse made the visit described here. She wished to do a self-evaluation of her call, and wrote it up on a process recording basis.

Purpose of Visit On my previous visit I had suggested that Mrs. H. attend the well-baby clinic with Tommie, which she did. On this visit I planned to discuss the clinic experience and any problems that Mrs. H. might have in caring for her baby.

Introduction Mr. and Mrs. H. are high school graduates and have been married for 2 years. They are buying their home, which is in an old part of the city, in a middle-class neighborhood and close to a college where Mr. H. attends night school. He hopes to be a certified public accountant some day. Prior to her marriage, Mrs. H. worked for the telephone company. She is an intelligent young woman, eager to learn to care for her first child.

The Visit Mrs. H. greeted me warmly at the door, but then her facial expression became one of grave concern. After we were seated, Mrs. H. opened the conversation.

Mother-Nurse Verbal and Nonverbal Exchange and Interaction	Nurse Comments and Analysis
Mrs. H.: Last week at the well-child clinic, the doctor took my baby's diaper and handed it to the nurse. He told her to do a PKU test. At the time I didn't	Mrs. H. was obviously quite anxious about this test and the baby's health. I wondered if the test were the real cause of her anxiety or if she had some other

think to ask him what that meant, but I have been wondering: does this mean he thinks something is wrong with my baby?

Nurse: You're concerned about your baby's health?

Mrs. H.: Yes, I am [Silence, but she seemed to want to say more.]

Mrs. H.: You see I've been leaving the window open in the bedroom at night because the baby's been perspiring so much. My husband keeps telling me the baby is going to get sick sleeping in that draft, and I knew deep down he was right. When I went to the clinic I was afraid the doctor would find something wrong with him.

Nurse: I see.

Nurse: What did the doctor say about Tommie's health?

Mrs. H.: Oh, he said the baby was in absolutely perfect health and gaining weight.

Nurse: That's fine, Mrs. H.

Mrs. H. (her face clouded): I was so happy until I came home and remembered that PKU test. What does it mean?

Nurse: Do you remember, Mrs H., when you had your chest x-ray at the health department?

Mrs. H. (puzzled): Yes, but that was a routine check for TB. My baby doesn't have TB, does he?

reason for inquiring. I needed more information before answering her question.

This interpretation would allow Mrs. H. to expand upon the problem further, and allow me to evaluate it.

I nodded, telling her nonverbally to go on.

It seems Mrs. H. may feel guilty that she might have caused an illness in her baby. Before clarifying her first question I wanted information about the general condition of her baby in order to relieve her fears.

This was said in an understanding tone to let her know that I understood her explanation.

I wanted to ascertain if the baby had a cold or other symptoms that could be related to the draft.

The mother smiled for the first time—she seemed very pleased.

I shared her delight and showed my approval.

She still may have connected the test with the draft in the bedroom, and now was the time to clarify this misunderstanding of her initial question.

I knew she had an x-ray for tuberculosis.

I was going to use this to correlate it with her baby's test, and I accepted her momentary puzzlement.

Nurse: No, but you see, just as you had a routine x-ray to check for tuberculosis, so the PKU test is a routine check for a disease in children called phenylketonuria.

I was going from the known (her own x-ray) to the unknown, the PKU test, so that she could understand better.

Mrs. H.: What does that mean?

Mother wants more explanation.

Nurse: Well, remember when we talked about the importance of protein, fats, and sugar foods in the diet?

Again, I attempted to enable the mother to recall what she knew in order to help her understand this condition.

Mrs. H: Yes, I understand that.

She was eager for me to go on and I now knew she was following and understanding my explanation so far.

Nurse: This disease is concerned with proteins. Before they can be used to build strong bodies they have to be broken down to smaller parts, and to do this there is a substance called an enzyme. Do you understand so far?

Mrs. H.: Yes, I think I do. What you're saying is that a substance breaks proteins down in order to give my baby a strong body.

This feedback from Mrs. H. was evidence that she understood and was able to relate her learning to incident concerning the baby.

Nurse (smiling): That's right. In the disease phenylketonuria this substance, or enzyme, that breaks down a particular part of the protein isn't there and can't be used by the body. Therefore this part of the protein keeps building up in the body and can cause brain damage. Some of it comes out in the baby's urine, too, and that's one way to know if the baby has the disease. Do you understand so far?

I wanted to show my approval.

I was explaining it in lay terms, but before proceeding I asked for indication of her understanding.

Mrs. H.: I see, then this is what the nurse was testing for?

Again, feedback from Mrs. H. showed she understood.

Nurse: That's right.

I smiled to show my approval.

Mrs. H.: Can the nurse do the test there, or did she take something off the diaper and send it somewhere?

It seemed she was worried that she might be informed later about the test, and was concerned about whether her baby had the condition.

Nurse: No, they do the test right away at the clinic. Do you remember when your mother stayed with you after she had diabetes and you did her urinalysis for her—and how the urine changed color after you dropped the tablet into the tube?

Mrs. H. (with interest): Yes.

Nurse: They tested the baby's urine like that. They drop a testing solution on a small spot on a wet diaper, and if the spot turns green, they know the baby has the disease. That is, they are pretty sure of it.

Mrs. H.: Then my baby doesn't have it, because the nurse brought the diaper back, smiled at me, and didn't say anything. Come to think of it, it was after the nurse talked to the doctor that he came back and said Tommie was in perfect health. Oh! I feel so much better now that I understand it wasn't the draft that had anything to do with this.

Again going from the known to the unknown and using my knowledge of family history.

Using correlation in explanation.

Evidence she understood the test; she seemed happy—perhaps in knowing that the draft had caused no harm.

There was marked relief in her voice. I nodded.

My suspicions were confirmed, and this was the opportunity to deal with the draft problem, which I did.

Summary Although Mrs. H. was concerned about the test for PKU, her concern stemmed from her guilt feelings about the draft. By allowing the mother to talk further about her feelings and not answering the question directly at the beginning of the visit, I found a problem that could be dealt with. After answering Mrs. H.'s questions about the test, I focused on the draft problem. It was discovered that Mrs. H. had kept the four wool blankets she had used during the winter months on Tommie's bed. She had not removed any of the blankets with the approaching spring weather, and this was the reason for the baby's perspiration. Hence the open window, which was creating a draft, would not be necessary if some of the blankets were removed. This action served two purposes: first, alleviating the draft on the baby, and second, alleviating the guilt feeling of Mrs. H. that she might cause the baby illness. Mrs. H. was pleased and happy at the end of the visit and appeared relieved. From the course of the discussion, Mrs. H. now understood something about PKU. I planned to discuss it further with her next time so that she would be a well-informed mother regarding this current problem.

DISCUSSION

1 What purpose did this visit serve?
2 What principles of learning did this nurse utilize?

3 What concomitant learning is it reasonable to hope took place?
4 How does the process recording method help in self-evaluation?
5 Should or should not the nurse have completed the discussion of PKU (e.g., incidence, symptoms, treatment, and problems) on this visit? Why?

A Home Health Agency Client with a Terminal Diagnosis

A nursing student was assigned the following client from a home health agency. A review of the record disclosed the following information:

Patient: Female. Birthdate: 5-13-08

Diagnosis: Terminal Cancer—possible liver metastasis. Hysterectomy—Cancer of the uterus several years ago. Diabetes.

Current home situation: Lives alone in apartment. Son and daughter from an adjacent state visit occasionally. Has choreperson 3 times a week. Neighbor helps. Has few friends.

Orders: Referred by local hospital. Nurse to visit 2 times weekly to supervise home care, diet, and medication management. Assess ambulation status and instruct in home safety. Monitor vital signs, bowel and bladder status, respiratory status, nutritional status. Home health aide to visit once weekly to assist with personal care.

Assessment of admitting nurse on first visit: BP 110/60; pulse 88; respirations 18; weight 174 lb.; medications: Compazine 5 mg prn for nausea. Demerol 50 mg prn for pain. Darvon 1 capsule prn for pain. Belap 1 tablet ac and hs. Complains of weakness, fatigue, short of breath, severe mid/epigastric pain with occasional pain in right chest area. Epigastric pain controlled with pain medication for approximately 3 hours. Appetite poor. No nausea, vomiting. Occasional productive cough—yellowish phlegm. Lungs clear.

Plan: Refuses nursing home care. Is aware of impending death. Will transfer client to nursing student for case management.

DISCUSSION

1 Assume the role of nurse. Write a nursing care plan for your first visit. Is the assessment of the admitting nurse adequate or do you want additional information?
2 How will you introduce yourself to this client?
3 Will you do a complete physical assessment? Will you encourage any self-care activities?
4 What theory might be used effectively with this client?
5 Are there other resources, providing the client consents, that can be utilized appropriately?

Getting Acquainted
with a New Community

You are a 70-year-old widow who is hardy, curious (nosy), and full of energy. You want to volunteer your services wherever there seems to be a need. You can do just about anything that a nonprofessional person does (cook meals, serve coffee, visit lonely people, baby-sit with handicapped persons, etc.).

You want to visit community facilities that may be interested in your volunteer services, i.e., senior service centers, handicapped children's facilities, nursing homes, free clinics, etc. Or perhaps you want to get an idea about what elderly people do in this community for health, recreation, social outlets, or constructive activities?

Activity assignment Find a variety of community facilities that may be responsive to receiving volunteer services from an able geriatric citizen. Visit these places and get a "feel" of the environment. Be prepared to report about these places in writing and verbally.

DISCUSSION

1 Describe briefly the community facilities that were visited.
2 Is the local community responsive to the needs of the elderly?
3 In general, how were your inquiries received in the local community?

Getting Acquainted
with a New Community

You are a 17-year-old girl who has lived all aspects of the alternative lifestyle—meaning drugs, alcohol, sex, poverty, etc. You have a vaginal discharge that is getting worse, and you do not know where to go for medical help (or health care.) You are considering going off drugs since you are fed up with the life you have been living. The guy you have been living with does not want you around anymore—he has a new girlfriend. If you go straight, who will help you?

Activity Assignment Visit a variety of community facilities that may be of assistance to you, i.e., free women's clinics, drug and alcohol information centers, health department, etc. Find out if these places are actually helpful for young women in distress. Be prepared to write a written report and/or describe your findings verbally.

DISCUSSION

1 Describe briefly the community facilities that were visited.
2 Is the local community responsive to the needs of youth?
3 In general, how were your inquiries received in the local community?

Getting Acquainted
with a New Community

You are a young wife and mother who recently arrived in this community. Your husband is out of work but is making the rounds regarding job possibilities. Your child is 16 months old, is developing normally, but tends to have too many bouts of upper respiratory infections. You wonder if you are feeding the child on an adequate diet. You are in the second trimester of pregnancy and beginning to think about supplies needed for the new baby. You have just visited the office of social and health services (welfare) and received a check of x dollars, which is the monthly allotment for a husband, wife, and one child. You wish to rent an apartment or home and want to find one today. According to the welfare worker, you can pay up to y dollars a month for a place. The remaining z dollars should be enough for food since you can buy food stamps.

Activity Assignment Look for a place to live today that will not cost over y dollars. Look for a place that you think will satisfy your needs. Is there a grocery store nearby? How about a physician's office? Since your husband uses the car daily, are you able to walk to your destinations? Is there a play area outside that is satisfactory for your child? Do you like the looks of the neighborhood? Be prepared to report your findings in writing or verbally.

DISCUSSION

1 Describe briefly the activities undertaken in finding a place to live.
2 Was a suitable place found? If so, what criteria were used in making the selection?
3 Is the local community concerned about the needs of low-income families?

Index